Pocket

INJECTABLE
DRUGS

Companion to the

Handbook on
INJECTABLE
DRUGS

14TH EDITION

Lawrence A. Trissel

American Society of Health-System Pharmacists®
Bethesda, MD

Lawrence A. Trissel, FASHP, is the author of the *Pocket Guide to Injectable Drugs*.

Mr. Trissel gratefully acknowledges the contribution of **N. Pauline Thomas Parks**, M.S., Consultant Pharmacist, Houston, Texas, who served as a reviewer for the *Pocket Guide*.

Any correspondence regarding this publication should be sent to the publisher, American Society of Health-System Pharmacists®, 7272 Wisconsin Avenue, Bethesda, MD 20814, attn: Special Publishing.

Director, eHealth Solutions Division: Jeffery A. Shick

eHealth Data Manager and Clinical Informaticist: Edward D. Millikan

Production: Johnna Hershey

Cover and Page Design: David A. Wade

The information presented herein reflects the opinions of the author and reviewer. It should not be interpreted as an official policy of ASHP or as an endorsement of any product.

Drug information and its applications are constantly evolving because of ongoing research and clinical experience and are often subject to professional judgment and interpretation by the practitioner due to the uniqueness of a clinical situation. The author, reviewer, and ASHP have made every effort to ensure the accuracy and completeness of the information presented in this book. However, the reader is advised that the publisher, author, editor, and reviewer cannot be responsible for the continued currency of the information, for any errors or omissions, and/or for any consequences arising from the use of the information in the clinical setting.

The reader is cautioned that ASHP makes no representation, guarantee, or warranty, express or implied, that the use of the information contained in this book will prevent problems with insurers and will bear no responsibility or liability for the results or consequences of its use.

ISBN 978-1-58528-146-6

Contents

How to Use the *Pocket Guide*

The *Pocket Guide to Injectable Drugs* is an easy-to-use and highly portable reference source for reliable information about many frequently used injectable drug products. The book should be valuable to busy nurses, pharmacists, and physicians in the hospital setting. The information has been distilled from over 2620 primary published research reports on the stability and compatibility of injectables. The results in these reports have been simplified into brief and graphic representations in the *Pocket Guide*.

The *Pocket Guide to Injectable Drugs*, 2007 edition, is the most recent contribution in this continuing series. With its publication, all previous editions are considered out of date.

Organization of the *Pocket Guide*

The information in the *Pocket Guide to Injectable Drugs* is organized in monographs for 137 drug products, including 7 drugs new to this edition. The monographs are arranged alphabetically by nonproprietary names. (Nonproprietary names and many corresponding trade names are cross-referenced at the end of the book.)

The information is an abbreviated version of the parent publication, the *Handbook on Injectable Drugs*, 14th edition. The first item for each drug refers to the related *Handbook* monograph. This citation allows easy reference back to the *Handbook* for a more complete summary of the literature. Also, a listing of the primary published sources can be found in the *Handbook*.

The monographs in the *Pocket Guide* are divided into the following subheadings:

Description

A brief statement describing the agent.

Products

Some trade names and many of the sizes, strengths, and volumes in which the drug is supplied. (This list is not necessarily comprehensive and should not be considered an endorsement of any product.) Sizes of products cited may not be available in all packaging types. The pH range of the products is cited under this subheading.

Preparation

Instructions for reconstitution and dilution for administration, where appropriate.

Administration

Recommended routes of administration, primarily from the official labeling and the *American Hospital Formulary Service*.

Stability

Important stability considerations for the drug, including sorption characteristics when available.

Compatibility Table

Results of published reports regarding compatibility, incompatibility, and conditional or variable findings with other drugs or solutions.

Organization of Compatibility Tables

The Compatibility Tables are composed of two parts: IV infusion solutions and drugs. The listings of IV infusion solutions are, of necessity, brief; only the most common solutions are noted. Therefore, the absence of a solution does not imply either compatibility or incompatibility. The listings of the drugs are more comprehensive, reflecting most drug combinations that have been studied.

The various entries, whether IV infusion solutions or drugs, are designated "Compatible," "Incompatible," or "Variable" in the *Pocket Guide* based on how the drug is tabulated in the *Handbook on Injectable Drugs*. The drug or solution is listed as Compatible if one or more of the following were indicated:

- Physical compatibility (no visible sign of incompatibility).
- Stability of components for at least 24 hours in an IV solution (decomposition of 10% or less) under the test conditions.
- Stability of components for the entire test period, although this period was less than 24 hours in some cases.

The items are noted as Incompatible if one or both of the following were indicated:

- Physical incompatibility (haze, precipitate, color change, etc.).
- Greater than 10% decomposition of one or more components in an IV solution within 24 hours under the test conditions.

The items are noted as Variable if either of the following was indicated:

- Compatibility characteristics are dependent on certain specific conditions.

- Contradictory information is present regarding the compatibility or incompatibility of the combination.

Therapeutic incompatibilities or other drug interactions are not included in the *Pocket Guide*.

Limitations

The *Pocket Guide to Injectable Drugs* is convenient to use. It is also quite obviously (and intentionally) brief. Some important information, such as drug concentrations, storage conditions, and the exact nature of the results, is not included. Therefore, it is suggested that the *Pocket Guide* be used as a portable companion to the *Handbook on Injectable Drugs*. The *Handbook* can then be used for a more thorough evaluation of compatibility and stability considerations.

Monographs

Acyclovir Sodium

Handbook on Injectable Drugs pp. 6–12.

Description: A nucleoside analog of guanine that acts as an antiviral.

Products: Zovirax; 500-mg and 1-g vials. *pH:* From 10.5 to 11.6.

Preparation: Reconstitute the 500-mg vials with 10 mL and the 1-g vials with 20 mL of sterile water for injection and shake to obtain a 50-mg/mL solution. Further dilute the dose in 50 to 125 mL of compatible diluent to a concentration of 7 mg/mL or less.

Administration: Administer by IV infusion over one hour or more; ensure adequate hydration.

Stability: Vials should be stored at room temperature. Use the reconstituted solution within 12 hours. Refrigeration of this solution may cause a precipitate, which will dissolve at room temperature. Diluted in infusion solutions, the drug may be stored at room temperature and should be used within 24 hours. In dextrose solutions of 10% or more, a yellow discoloration may appear but does not affect potency. No sorption to plastic or glass containers or elastomeric reservoirs has been found.

Compatibility Table

Solutions	Compatible	Incompatible	Variable
Dextrose 5%	●	…	…
Dextrose 5% in sodium chloride 0.2, 0.45, & 0.9%	●	…	…
Ringer's injection, lactated	●	…	…
Sodium chloride 0.9%	●	…	…

Drugs	Compatible	Incompatible	Variable
Amifostine	…	●	…
Amikacin sulfate	●	…	…
Amphotericin B cholesteryl sulfate complex	●	…	…
Ampicillin sodium	●	…	…

Drugs	Compatible	Incompatible	Variable
Anidulafungin	●	...	...
Aztreonam	...	●	...
Caffeine citrate	...	●	...
Cefamandole nafate	●	...	...
Cefazolin sodium	●	...	...
Cefepime HCl	...	●	...
Cefotaxime sodium	●	...	...
Cefoxitin sodium	●	...	...
Ceftazidime	●	...	...
Ceftizoxime sodium	●	...	...
Ceftriaxone sodium	●	...	...
Cefuroxime sodium	●	...	...
Chloramphenicol sodium succinate	●	...	...
Cimetidine HCl	●	...	...
Cisatracurium besylate	...	...	●
Clindamycin phosphate	●	...	...
Dexamethasone sodium phosphate	●	...	...
Diltiazem HCl	...	...	●
Dimenhydrinate	●	...	...
Diphenhydramine HCl	●	...	...
Dobutamine HCl	...	●	...
Docetaxel	●	...	...
Dopamine HCl	...	●	...
Doxorubicin HCl liposome injection	●	...	...
Doxycycline hyclate	●	...	...
Erythromycin lactobionate	●	...	...
Etoposide phosphate	●	...	...
Famotidine	●	...	...
Filgrastim	●	...	...
Fluconazole	●	...	...
Fludarabine phosphate	...	●	...
Foscarnet sodium	...	●	...
Gallium nitrate	●	...	...
Gemcitabine HCl	...	●	...
Gentamicin sulfate	●	...	...
Granisetron HCl	●	...	...
Heparin sodium	●	...	...
Hydrocortisone sodium succinate	●	...	...
Hydromorphone HCl	●	...	...

Drugs	Compatible	Incompatible	Variable
Idarubicin HCl	...	●	...
Imipenem–cilastatin sodium	●	...	...
Lansoprazole	●	...	...
Levofloxacin	●	...	...
Lorazepam	●	...	...
Magnesium sulfate	●	...	...
Meperidine HCl	...	...	●
Meropenem	...	...	●
Methylprednisolone sod. succ.	●	...	...
Metoclopramide HCl	●	...	...
Metronidazole	●	...	...
Milrinone lactate	●	...	...
Morphine sulfate	...	...	●
Multivitamins	●	...	...
Nafcillin sodium	●	...	...
Ondansetron HCl	...	●	...
Oxacillin sodium	●	...	...
Paclitaxel	●	...	...
Pantoprazole sodium	...	●	...
Pemetrexed disodium	●	...	...
Penicillin G potassium	●	...	...
Pentobarbital sodium	●	...	...
Piperacillin sodium	●	...	...
Piperacillin sod.–tazobactam sod.	...	●	...
Potassium chloride	●	...	...
Propofol	●	...	...
Ranitidine HCl	●	...	...
Remifentanil HCl	●	...	...
Sargramostim	...	●	...
Sodium bicarbonate	●	...	...
Tacrolimus	...	...	●
Teniposide	●	...	...
Theophylline	●	...	...
Thiotepa	●	...	...
Tobramycin sulfate	●	...	...
Trimethoprim–sulfamethoxazole	●	...	...
Vancomycin HCl	●	...	...
Vinorelbine tartrate	...	●	...
Zidovudine	●	...	...

Allopurinol Sodium

Handbook on Injectable Drugs pp. 22–27.

Description: A xanthine oxidase inhibitor used to treat gout and hyperuricemia.

Products: Aloprim; 500-mg vials. *pH:* From 11.1 to 11.8.

Preparation: Reconstitute the vial contents with 25 mL of sterile water for injection. The reconstituted solution is diluted in dextrose 5% or sodium chloride 0.9% to a concentration no greater than 6 mg/mL.

Administration: The drug diluted properly for administration is given as a single daily infusion or in equally divided infusions at 6-, 8-, or 12-hour intervals. The rate is determined by the volume to be infused.

Stability: The vials should be stored at room temperature. The reconstituted solution and diluted infusion admixture should not be refrigerated. Administration should begin within 10 hours of reconstitution.

Compatibility Table

Solutions	Compatible	Incompatible	Variable
Dextrose 5%	●	...	...
Sodium chloride 0.9%	●	...	...

Drugs	Compatible	Incompatible	Variable
Acyclovir sodium	●	...	...
Amikacin sulfate	...	●	...
Aminophylline	●	...	...
Amphotericin B	...	●	...
Aztreonam	●	...	...
Bleomycin sulfate	●	...	...
Bumetanide	●	...	...
Buprenorphine HCl	●	...	...
Butorphanol tartrate	●	...	...
Calcium gluconate	●	...	...

Drugs	Compatible	Incompatible	Variable
Carboplatin	●	...	...
Carmustine	...	●	...
Cefazolin sodium	●	...	...
Cefotaxime sodium	...	●	...
Cefotetan disodium	●	...	...
Ceftazidime	●	...	...
Ceftizoxime sodium	●	...	...
Ceftriaxone sodium	●	...	...
Cefuroxime sodium	●	...	...
Chlorpromazine HCl	...	●	...
Cimetidine HCl	...	●	...
Cisplatin	●	...	...
Clindamycin phosphate	...	●	...
Cyclophosphamide	●	...	...
Cytarabine	...	●	...
Dacarbazine	...	●	...
Dactinomycin	●	...	...
Daunorubicin HCl	...	●	...
Dexamethasone sodium phosphate	●	...	...
Diphenhydramine HCl	...	●	...
Doxorubicin HCl	...	●	...
Doxorubicin HCl liposome injection	●	...	...
Doxycycline hyclate	...	●	...
Droperidol	...	●	...
Enalaprilat	●	...	...
Etoposide	●	...	...
Famotidine	●	...	...
Filgrastim	●	...	...
Fluconazole	●	...	...
Fludarabine phosphate	●	...	...
Fluorouracil	●	...	...
Gallium nitrate	●	...	...
Ganciclovir sodium	●	...	...
Gentamicin sulfate	...	●	...
Granisetron HCl	●	...	...
Haloperidol lactate	...	●	...
Heparin sodium	●	...	...
Hydrocortisone sodium phosphate	●	...	...
Hydrocortisone sodium succinate	●	...	...

Drugs	Compatible	Incompatible	Variable
Hydromorphone HCl	●	...	...
Hydroxyzine HCl	...	●	...
Idarubicin HCl	...	●	...
Ifosfamide	●	...	...
Imipenem–cilastatin sodium	...	●	...
Lorazepam	●	...	...
Mannitol	●	...	...
Mechlorethamine HCl	...	●	...
Meperidine HCl	...	●	...
Mesna	●	...	...
Methotrexate sodium	●	...	...
Methylprednisolone sod. succ.	...	●	...
Metoclopramide HCl	...	●	...
Metronidazole	●	...	...
Mitoxantrone HCl	●	...	...
Morphine sulfate	●	...	...
Nalbuphine HCl	...	●	...
Ondansetron HCl	...	●	...
Piperacillin sodium	●	...	...
Potassium chloride	●	...	...
Prochlorperazine edisylate	...	●	...
Promethazine HCl	...	●	...
Ranitidine HCl	●	...	...
Sodium bicarbonate	...	●	...
Streptozocin	...	●	...
Teniposide	●	...	...
Thiotepa	●	...	...
Ticarcillin disod.–clavulanate pot.	●	...	...
Tobramycin sulfate	...	●	...
Trimethoprim–sulfamethoxazole	●	...	...
Vancomycin HCl	●	...	...
Vinblastine sulfate	●	...	...
Vincristine sulfate	●	...	...
Vinorelbine tartrate	...	●	...
Zidovudine	●	...	...

Amikacin Sulfate

Handbook on Injectable Drugs pp. 37–50.

Description: A semisynthetic aminoglycoside antibiotic.

Products: Amikin; Available in concentrations of 50 and 250 mg/mL. *pH:* From 3.5 to 5.5.

Preparation: For adults, prepare IV infusions by adding 500 mg to 100 to 200 mL of compatible diluent. For pediatric patients, the volume of diluent depends on the patient but should allow a one- to two-hour infusion in infants or a 30- to 60-minute infusion in older children.

Administration: Administer by IM injection or by IV infusion over 30 to 60 minutes for adults and older children. Infants should receive a one- to two-hour IV infusion.

Stability: Store intact vials at room temperature. Amikacin is a colorless to pale yellow or light straw-colored solution. The solution may darken in color because of air oxidation, but this change does not affect potency. Amikacin is stable for 30 days frozen or 60 days under refrigeration in most infusion solutions. No sorption to plastics has been found.

Compatibility Table

Solutions	Compatible	Incompatible	Variable
Dextrose 5 & 10%	●	...	...
Dextrose 5% in Ringer's injection	●	...	...
Dextrose 5% in Ringer's injection, lactated	●	...	...
Dextrose 5% in sodium chloride 0.2, 0.45, & 0.9%	●	...	...
Sodium chloride 0.45 & 0.9%	●	...	...

Drugs			
Acyclovir sodium	●	...	...
Aldesleukin	●	...	...
Allopurinol sodium	...	●	...
Amifostine	●	...	...
Aminophylline	...	...	●

8

Drugs	Compatible	Incompatible	Variable
Amiodarone HCl	●	...	...
Amobarbital sodium	●	...	...
Amphotericin B	...	●	...
Amphotericin B cholesteryl sulfate complex	...	●	...
Ampicillin sodium	...	●	...
Anidulafungin	●	...	...
Ascorbic acid injection	●	...	...
Azithromycin	...	●	...
Aztreonam	●	...	...
Bivalirudin	●	...	...
Bleomycin sulfate	●	...	...
Caffeine citrate	●	...	...
Calcium chloride	●	...	...
Calcium gluconate	●	...	...
Cefazolin sodium	...	●	...
Cefepime HCl	●	...	...
Cefotaxime sodium	...	...	●
Cefoxitin sodium	●	...	...
Ceftazidime	...	...	●
Ceftriaxone sodium	●	...	...
Chloramphenicol sodium succinate	●	...	...
Chlorothiazide sodium	...	●	...
Cimetidine HCl	●	...	...
Ciprofloxacin	●	...	...
Cisatracurium besylate	●	...	...
Clindamycin phosphate	●	...	...
Cloxacillin sodium	●	...	...
Colistimethate sodium	●	...	...
Cyclophosphamide	●	...	...
Dexamethasone sodium phosphate ...	...	...	●
Dexmedetomidine HCl	●	...	...
Diltiazem HCl	●	...	...
Dimenhydrinate	●	...	...
Diphenhydramine HCl	●	...	...
Docetaxel	●	...	...
Doxapram HCl	●	...	...
Enalaprilat	●	...	...
Epinephrine HCl	●	...	...

Drugs	Compatible	Incompatible	Variable
Esmolol HCl	●	...	...
Etoposide phosphate	●	...	...
Fenoldopam mesylate	●	...	...
Filgrastim	●	...	...
Fluconazole	●	...	...
Fludarabine phosphate	●	...	...
Foscarnet sodium	●	...	...
Furosemide	●	...	...
Gemcitabine HCl	●	...	...
Granisetron HCl	●	...	...
Heparin sodium	...	●	...
Hetastarch in sodium chloride 0.9%	...	●	...
Hextend	●	...	...
Hyaluronidase	●	...	...
Hydrocortisone sodium phosphate ...	●	...	...
Hydrocortisone sodium succinate	●	...	...
Hydromorphone HCl	●	...	...
Idarubicin HCl	●	...	...
IL-2	●	...	...
Labetalol HCl	●	...	...
Lansoprazole	●	...	...
Levofloxacin	●	...	...
Lincomycin HCl	●	...	...
Lorazepam	●	...	...
Magnesium sulfate	●	...	...
Melphalan HCl	●	...	...
Meperidine HCl	●	...	...
Metronidazole	●	...	...
Midazolam HCl	●	...	...
Milrinone lactate	●	...	...
Morphine sulfate	●	...	...
Nicardipine HCl	●	...	...
Norepinephrine bitartrate	●	...	...
Ondansetron HCl	●	...	...
Oxacillin sodium	...	...	●
Paclitaxel	●	...	...
Pantoprazole sodium	...	●	...
Pemetrexed disodium	●	...	...
Penicillin G potassium	...	...	●

Drugs	Compatible	Incompatible	Variable
Pentobarbital sodium	●	...	...
Phenobarbital sodium	●	...	...
Phenytoin sodium	...	●	...
Phytonadione	●	...	...
Polymyxin B sulfate	●	...	...
Potassium chloride	...	...	●
Prochlorperazine edisylate	●	...	...
Promethazine HCl	●	...	...
Propofol	...	●	...
Ranitidine HCl	●	...	...
Remifentanil HCl	●	...	...
Sargramostim	●	...	...
Sodium bicarbonate	●	...	...
Succinylcholine chloride	●	...	...
Teniposide	●	...	...
Thiopental sodium	...	●	...
Thiotepa	●	...	...
Vancomycin HCl	●	...	...
Verapamil HCl	●	...	...
Vinorelbine tartrate	●	...	...
Warfarin sodium	●	...	...
Zidovudine	●	...	...

Amikacin Sulfate

Aminophylline

Handbook on Injectable Drugs pp. 99–112.

Description: The ethylenediamine salt of theophylline.

Products: 10-mL (250 mg) and 20-mL (500 mg) containers for IV injection. *pH:* From 8.6 to 9.

Administration: Administer slowly IV (undiluted or diluted in a compatible solution).

Stability: Store at room temperature; do not refrigerate because of possible crystallization. No sorption to plastic syringes, bags, sets, or filters has been noted.

Compatibility Table

Solutions	Compatible	Incompatible	Variable
Dextrose 5%	●	...	...
Dextrose 5% in Ringer's injection	●	...	...
Dextrose 5% in Ringer's injection, lactated	●	...	...
Dextrose 5% in sodium chloride 0.2, 0.45, & 0.9%	●	...	...
Fat emulsion 10%, IV	...	...	●
Invert sugar 10% in sodium chloride 0.9% or water	...	●	...
Sodium chloride 0.45 & 0.9%	●	...	...

Drugs	Compatible	Incompatible	Variable
Allopurinol sodium	●	...	...
Amifostine	●	...	...
Amikacin sulfate	...	...	●
Amiodarone HCl	...	●	...
Amobarbital sodium	●	...	...
Amphotericin B cholesteryl sulfate complex	●	...	...
Anidulafungin	●	...	...
Ascorbic acid injection	...	...	●
Atracurium besylate	...	●	...

Drugs	Compatible	Incompatible	Variable
Aztreonam	●	...	...
Bivalirudin	●	...	...
Bleomycin sulfate	...	●	...
Caffeine citrate	●	...	...
Calcium gluconate	●	...	...
Cefepime HCl	...	●	...
Ceftazidime	...	...	●
Ceftriaxone sodium	...	●	...
Chloramphenicol sodium succinate	●	...	...
Chlorpromazine HCl	...	●	...
Cimetidine HCl	●	...	...
Ciprofloxacin	...	●	...
Cisatracurium besylate	...	...	●
Cladribine	●	...	...
Clindamycin phosphate	...	●	...
Corticotropin	...	...	●
Dexamethasone sodium phosphate ...	●	...	...
Dexmedetomidine HCl	●	...	...
Diltiazem HCl	...	...	●
Dimenhydrinate	...	...	●
Diphenhydramine HCl	●	...	...
Dobutamine HCl	...	●	...
Docetaxel	●	...	...
Dopamine HCl	●	...	...
Doxapram HCl	...	●	...
Doxorubicin HCl	...	●	...
Doxorubicin HCl liposome injection	●	...	...
Enalaprilat	●	...	...
Epinephrine HCl	...	●	...
Erythromycin lactobionate	●	...	...
Esmolol HCl	●	...	...
Etoposide phosphate	●	...	...
Famotidine	●	...	...
Fenoldopam mesylate	...	●	...
Filgrastim	●	...	...
Fluconazole	●	...	...
Fludarabine phosphate	●	...	...
Flumazenil	●	...	...

Drugs	Compatible	Incompatible	Variable
Foscarnet sodium	●	...	...
Furosemide	●	...	...
Gallium nitrate	●	...	...
Gemcitabine HCl	●	...	...
Granisetron HCl	●	...	...
Heparin sodium	●	...	...
Hextend	●	...	...
Hydralazine HCl	...	●	...
Hydrocortisone sodium succinate	●	...	...
Hydroxyzine HCl	...	●	...
Insulin, regular	...	●	...
Isoproterenol HCl	...	●	...
Labetalol HCl	●	...	...
Lansoprazole	...	●	...
Levofloxacin	●	...	...
Lidocaine HCl	●	...	...
Linezolid	●	...	...
Melphalan HCl.......................	●	...	...
Meperidine HCl	...	●	...
Mephentermine sulfate	●	...	...
Meropenem	●	...	...
Methyldopate HCl	●	...	...
Methylprednisolone sod. succ.	...	...	●
Metoclopramide HCl	●	...	...
Midazolam HCl	...	...	●
Morphine sulfate	...	...	●
Nafcillin sodium	...	...	●
Nitroglycerin	●	...	...
Norepinephrine bitartrate	...	●	...
Ondansetron HCl	...	●	...
Paclitaxel	●	...	...
Pancuronium bromide	●	...	...
Pantoprazole sodium	●	...	...
Pemetrexed disodium	●	...	...
Penicillin G potassium	...	●	...
Pentazocine lactate	...	●	...
Pentobarbital sodium	●	...	...
Phenobarbital sodium	●	...	...
Piperacillin sodium–tazobactam sodium	●	...	...

Drugs	Compatible	Incompatible	Variable
Potassium chloride	●	...	...
Procaine HCl	...	...	●
Prochlorperazine edisylate	...	●	...
Promethazine HCl	...	●	...
Propofol	●	...	...
Ranitidine HCl	●	...	...
Remifentanil HCl	●	...	...
Sargramostim	●	...	...
Sodium bicarbonate	●	...	...
Tacrolimus	●	...	...
Teniposide	●	...	...
Terbutaline sulfate	●	...	...
Thiopental sodium	●	...	...
Thiotepa	●	...	...
Vancomycin HCl	...	...	●
Vecuronium bromide	●	...	...
Verapamil HCl	...	...	●
Vinorelbine tartrate	...	●	...
Warfarin sodium	...	●	...

Amiodarone Hydrochloride

Handbook on Injectable Drugs pp. 112–118.

Description: A cardiac antiarrhythmic agent.

Products: **Cordarone Intravenous;** 50 mg/mL in 3-mL ampuls. *pH:* About 4.

Preparation: Dilute the concentrate in dextrose 5%. The loading dose at a concentration of 1.5 mg/mL is generally admixed in 100 mL. Maintenance infusions are usually at concentrations of 1 to 6 mg/mL. Concentrations greater than 2 mg/mL require a central venous catheter.

Administration: Administer by IV infusion using a volumetric infusion pump, a dedicated central catheter, if possible, and an inline filter. NOTE: Drop counter infusion devices may underdose significantly.

Stability: Store the pale yellow concentrate at room temperature with protection from light and excessive heat. Light protection is not necessary during administration. Amiodarone hydrochloride sorbs to PVC containers and sets; losses of 10% in two hours have been found. It also leaches plasticizer from PVC tubing. The use of non-PVC containers and administration sets is recommended.

Compatibility Table

Solutions	Compatible	Incompatible	Variable
Dextrose 5%[a]	●	...	...
Sodium chloride 0.9%	...	...	●

[a]Non-PVC containers only.

Drugs			
Amikacin sulfate	●	...	...
Aminophylline	...	●	...
Amphotericin B	●	...	...
Ampicillin sodium–sulbactam sodium	...	●	...

Drugs	Compatible	Incompatible	Variable
Atracurium besylate	●	...	...
Atropine sulfate	●	...	...
Bivalirudin	...	●	...
Calcium chloride	●	...	...
Calcium gluconate	●	...	...
Cefamandole nafate	...	●	...
Cefazolin sodium	...	...	●
Ceftazidime	...	●	...
Ceftizoxime sodium	●	...	...
Ceftriaxone sodium	●	...	...
Cefuroxime sodium	●	...	...
Ciprofloxacin	●	...	...
Clindamycin phosphate	●	...	...
Dexmedetomidine HCl	●	...	...
Digoxin	...	●	...
Dobutamine HCl	●	...	...
Dopamine HCl	●	...	...
Doxycycline hyclate	●	...	...
Drotrecogin alfa (activated)	...	●	...
Epinephrine HCl	●	...	...
Eptifibatide	●	...	...
Erythromycin lactobionate	●	...	...
Esmolol HCl	●	...	...
Famotidine	●	...	...
Fenoldopam mesylate	●	...	...
Fentanyl citrate	●	...	...
Fluconazole	●	...	...
Furosemide	...	...	●
Gentamicin sulfate	●	...	...
Heparin sodium	...	●	...
Hextend	●	...	...
Imipenem–cilastatin sodium	...	●	...
Insulin, regular	●	...	...
Isoproterenol HCl	●	...	...
Labetalol HCl	●	...	...
Lepirudin	●	...	...
Lidocaine HCl	●	...	...
Lorazepam	●	...	...
Magnesium sulfate	...	...	●
Methylprednisolone sodium succinate	●	...	...

Drugs	Compatible	Incompatible	Variable
Metronidazole HCl	●	...	...
Midazolam HCl	●	...	...
Milrinone lactate	●	...	...
Morphine sulfate	●	...	...
Nitroglycerin	●	...	...
Norepinephrine bitartrate	●	...	...
Pantoprazole sodium	...	●	...
Penicillin G potassium	●	...	...
Phenylephrine HCl	●	...	...
Piperacillin sodium	...	●	...
Piperacillin sodium–tazobactam sodium	...	●	...
Potassium chloride	●	...	...
Potassium phosphates	...	●	...
Procainamide HCl	●	...	...
Quinidine gluconate	...	...	●
Sodium bicarbonate	...	●	...
Sodium nitroprusside	...	...	●
Sodium phosphates	...	●	...
Tirofiban HCl	●	...	...
Tobramycin sulfate	●	...	...
Vancomycin HCl	●	...	...
Vasopressin	●	...	...
Vecuronium bromide	●	...	...
Verapamil HCl	●	...	...

Amphotericin B

Handbook on Injectable Drugs pp. 126–133.

Description: A fungistatic antibiotic.

Products: Amphocin, Fungizone; 50 mg/vial. *pH:* Amphotericin B 100 mg/L in dextrose 5% has a pH of 5.7.

Preparation: Reconstitute with 10 mL of sterile water for injection without preservatives and shake to yield a 5-mg/mL colloidal dispersion. NOTE: Other diluents such as sodium chloride 0.9% and those with preservatives may cause precipitation. Further dilute with dextrose 5% (with a pH above 4.2), usually to 0.1 mg/mL.

Administration: Administer by slow IV infusion over approximately two to six hours. A concentration of 0.1 mg/mL is recommended. CAUTION: Ensure that the correct drug, dose, and administration procedure are used; do not confuse with other products.

Stability: Store intact vials under refrigeration and protect from light. The reconstituted solution is stable for at least 24 hours at room temperature or one week under refrigeration.

Compatibility Table

Solutions	Compatible	Incompatible	Variable
Dextrose 5%	●	…	…
Dextrose 5% in Ringer's injection, lactated	…	●	…
Dextrose 5% in sodium chloride 0.9%	…	●	…
Fat emulsion 10 & 20%, IV	…	●	…
Ringer's injection, lactated	…	●	…
Sodium chloride 0.9%	…	●	…

Drugs			
Aldesleukin	●	…	…
Allopurinol sodium	…	●	…
Amifostine	…	●	…
Amikacin sulfate	…	●	…
Amiodarone HCl	●	…	…

Drugs	Compatible	Incompatible	Variable
Anidulafungin	...	●	...
Aztreonam	...	●	...
Bivalirudin	...	●	...
Calcium salts	...	●	...
Cefepime HCl	...	●	...
Chlorpromazine HCl	...	●	...
Cimetidine HCl	...	●	...
Ciprofloxacin	...	●	...
Cisatracurium besylate	...	...	●
Dexmedetomidine HCl	...	●	...
Diltiazem HCl	●	...	...
Diphenhydramine HCl	...	●	...
Docetaxel	...	●	...
Dopamine HCl	...	●	...
Doxorubicin HCl liposome injection	...	●	...
Edetate calcium disodium	...	●	...
Enalaprilat	...	●	...
Etoposide phosphate	...	●	...
Fenoldopam mesylate	...	●	...
Filgrastim	...	●	...
Fluconazole	...	...	●
Fludarabine phosphate	...	●	...
Foscarnet sodium	...	●	...
Gemcitabine HCl	...	●	...
Gentamicin sulfate	...	●	...
Granisetron HCl	...	●	...
Heparin sodium	●	...	...
Hextend	...	●	...
Hydrocortisone sodium phosphate	●	...	...
Hydrocortisone sodium succinate	●	...	...
Kanamycin sulfate	...	●	...
Lansoprazole	...	●	...
Lidocaine HCl	...	●	...
Linezolid	...	●	...
Magnesium sulfate	...	●	...
Melphalan HCl	...	●	...
Meropenem	...	●	...
Methyldopate HCl	...	●	...
Ondansetron HCl	...	●	...
Paclitaxel	...	●	...

Drugs	Compatible	Incompatible	Variable
Pantoprazole sodium	...	●	...
Pemetrexed disodium	...	●	...
Penicillin G potassium	...	●	...
Penicillin G sodium	...	●	...
Piperacillin sod.–tazobactam sod.	...	●	...
Polymyxin B sulfate	...	●	...
Potassium chloride	...	●	...
Procaine HCl	...	●	...
Prochlorperazine mesylate	...	●	...
Propofol	...	●	...
Ranitidine HCl	...	●	...
Remifentanil HCl	...	...	●
Sargramostim	...	...	●
Sodium bicarbonate	●	...	...
Streptomycin sulfate	...	●	...
Tacrolimus	●	...	...
Teniposide	●	...	...
Thiotepa	●	...	...
Verapamil HCl	...	●	...
Vinorelbine tartrate	...	●	...
Zidovudine	●	...	...

Amphotericin B Cholesteryl Sulfate Complex

Handbook on Injectable Drugs pp. 133–139.

Description: This product consists of the fungistatic antibiotic, amphotericin B, complexed in a 1:1 ratio to cholesteryl sulfate.

Products: Amphotec; 50- and 100-mg vials.

Preparation: Reconstitute with sterile water for injection using 10 mL for the 50-mg vials and 20 mL for the 100-mg vials. Shake the vials gently to yield an opalescent or clear colloidal dispersion containing amphotericin B 5 mg/mL. NOTE: Other diluents such as sodium chloride 0.9%, other electrolyte solutions, and solutions with preservatives may cause precipitation and should be avoided. For administration, dilute the reconstituted product in dextrose 5% to a concentration between 0.16 and 0.83 mg/mL.

Administration: Administer IV after appropriate dilution to approximately 0.6 mg/mL (range 0.16 to 0.83 mg/mL). A test dose of 10 mL (1.6 to 8.3 mg) should be given over 15 to 30 minutes preceding each new course of treatment. IV infusion is performed at a rate of 1 mg/kg/hour, but it may be shortened to two hours in patients with no evidence of intolerance or reactions. The infusion period may need to be extended for patients who experience reactions or cannot tolerate the fluid volume. CAUTION: Ensure that the correct drug, dose, and administration procedure are used; do not confuse with other products.

Stability: Store the vials at room temperature. The reconstituted dispersion should be stored under refrigeration, protected from freezing, and used within 24 hours. After the drug is diluted to a concentration of 0.16 to 0.83 mg/mL in dextrose 5% for administration, it should be stored under refrigeration and used within 24 hours. Filtration of this colloidal dispersion should not be performed.

Compatibility Table

Solutions	Compatible	Incompatible	Variable

NOTE: Other lipid complex and liposomal amphotericin B products are sufficiently different from amphotericin B cholesteryl sulfate complex that extrapolating compatibility data to these other forms is inappropriate.

	Compatible	Incompatible	Variable
Dextrose 5%	●	...	...
Sodium chloride 0.9%	...	●	...

Drugs	Compatible	Incompatible	Variable
Acyclovir sodium	●	...	...
Alfentanil HCl	...	●	...
Amikacin sulfate	...	●	...
Aminophylline	●	...	...
Ampicillin sodium	...	●	...
Ampicillin sod.–sulbactam sod.	...	●	...
Atenolol	...	●	...
Aztreonam	...	●	...
Buprenorphine HCl	...	●	...
Butorphanol tartrate	...	●	...
Calcium chloride	...	●	...
Calcium gluconate	...	●	...
Carboplatin	...	●	...
Cefazolin sodium	...	●	...
Cefepime HCl	...	●	...
Cefoxitin sodium	●	...	...
Ceftazidime	...	●	...
Ceftizoxime sodium	●	...	...
Ceftriaxone sodium	...	●	...
Chlorpromazine HCl	...	●	...
Cimetidine HCl	...	●	...
Cisatracurium besylate	...	●	...
Cisplatin	...	●	...
Clindamycin phosphate	●	...	...
Cyclophosphamide	...	●	...
Cyclosporine	...	●	...
Cytarabine	...	●	...
Dexamethasone sodium phosphate ...	●	...	...
Diazepam	...	●	...
Digoxin	...	●	...

Drugs	Compatible	Incompatible	Variable
Diphenhydramine HCl	...	●	...
Dobutamine HCl	...	●	...
Dopamine HCl	...	●	...
Doxorubicin HCl	...	●	...
Doxorubicin HCl liposome injection	...	●	...
Droperidol	...	●	...
Enalaprilat	...	●	...
Esmolol HCl	...	●	...
Famotidine	...	●	...
Fentanyl citrate	●	...	...
Fluconazole	...	●	...
Fluorouracil	...	●	...
Furosemide	●	...	...
Ganciclovir sodium	●	...	...
Gentamicin sulfate	...	●	...
Granisetron HCl	●	...	...
Haloperidol lactate	...	●	...
Heparin sodium	...	●	...
Hydrocortisone sodium succinate	●	...	...
Hydromorphone HCl	...	●	...
Hydroxyzine HCl	...	●	...
Ifosfamide	●	...	...
Imipenem–cilastatin sodium	...	●	...
Labetalol HCl	...	●	...
Leucovorin calcium	...	●	...
Lidocaine HCl	...	●	...
Lorazepam	●	...	...
Magnesium sulfate	...	●	...
Mannitol	●	...	...
Meperidine HCl	...	●	...
Mesna	...	●	...
Methotrexate sodium	●	...	...
Methylprednisolone sod. succ.	●	...	...
Metoclopramide HCl	...	●	...
Metoprolol tartrate	...	●	...
Metronidazole	...	●	...
Midazolam HCl	...	●	...
Mitoxantrone HCl	...	●	...
Morphine sulfate	...	●	...
Nalbuphine HCl	...	●	...

Drugs	Compatible	Incompatible	Variable
Naloxone HCl	...	●	...
Nitroglycerin	●	...	...
Ondansetron HCl	...	●	...
Paclitaxel	...	●	...
Pentobarbital sodium	...	●	...
Phenobarbital sodium	...	●	...
Phenytoin sodium	...	●	...
Piperacillin sodium	...	●	...
Piperacillin sod.–tazobactam sod.	...	●	...
Potassium chloride	...	●	...
Prochlorperazine edisylate	...	●	...
Promethazine HCl	...	●	...
Propranolol HCl	...	●	...
Ranitidine HCl	...	●	...
Remifentanil HCl	...	●	...
Sodium bicarbonate	...	●	...
Sufentanil citrate	●	...	...
Ticarcillin disod.–clavulanate pot.	...	●	...
Tobramycin sulfate	...	●	...
Trimethoprim–sulfamethoxazole	●	...	...
Vancomycin HCl	...	●	...
Vecuronium bromide	...	●	...
Verapamil HCl	...	●	...
Vinblastine sulfate	●	...	...
Vincristine sulfate	●	...	...
Vinorelbine tartrate	...	●	...
Zidovudine	●	...	...

Ampicillin Sodium

Handbook on Injectable Drugs pp. 141–158.

Description: A broad spectrum semisynthetic penicillin.

Products: 125 mg to 2 g/vial. *pH:* From 8 to 10 when reconstituted.

Preparation: For IM use, reconstitute with sterile or bacteriostatic water for injection. Reconstitution volumes vary slightly with the brand of drug, yielding concentrations of 125 or 250 mg/mL. For IV use, reconstitute 125-, 250-, and 500-mg vials with 5 mL of sterile water for injection. The 1- and 2-g vials require 7.4 mL or 14.8 mL, respectively.

Administration: Administer IM, by IV infusion, or by direct IV injection slowly over three to five minutes for doses up to 500 mg and over 10 to 15 minutes for larger doses.

Stability: The reconstituted solution is stable for at least one hour at room temperature or four hours under refrigeration. No sorption to plastic syringes, bags, sets, or filters has been noted.

Compatibility Table

Solutions	Compatible	Incompatible	Variable
Dextrose 5%*	...	●	...
Dextrose 5% in sodium chloride 0.45* & 0.9%	...	●	...
Dextrose 10%	...	●	...
Ringer's injection	...	...	●
Ringer's injection, lactated*	...	...	●
Sodium bicarbonate 1.4%	...	●	...
Sodium chloride 0.9%	...	...	●

*Although room temperature stability in these solutions is insufficient to be considered truly compatible, the drug is sufficiently stable to permit use within a few hours.

Drugs	Compatible	Incompatible	Variable
Acyclovir sodium	●	...	...
Amifostine	●	...	...
Amikacin sulfate	...	●	...
Amphotericin B cholesteryl sulfate complex	...	●	...

Drugs	Compatible	Incompatible	Variable
Anidulafungin	●	...	...
Aztreonam	...	...	●
Bivalirudin	●	...	...
Calcium gluconate	...	...	●
Cefepime HCl	...	...	●
Chloramphenicol sod. succ.	●	...	...
Chlorpromazine HCl	...	●	...
Cimetidine HCl	...	...	●
Cisatracurium besylate	...	...	●
Clindamycin phosphate	...	...	●
Colistimethate sodium	●	...	...
Cyclophosphamide	●	...	...
Dexmedetomidine HCl	●	...	...
Diltiazem HCl	...	...	●
Dimenhydrinate	●	...	...
Docetaxel	●	...	...
Dopamine HCl	...	●	...
Doxapram HCl	●	...	...
Doxorubicin HCl liposome injection	●	...	...
Enalaprilat	●	...	...
Epinephrine HCl	...	●	...
Erythromycin lactobionate	...	...	●
Esmolol HCl	●	...	...
Etoposide phosphate	●	...	...
Famotidine	●	...	...
Fenoldopam mesylate	...	●	...
Filgrastim	●	...	...
Fluconazole	...	●	...
Foscarnet sodium	●	...	...
Furosemide	●	...	...
Gemcitabine HCl	●	...	...
Gentamicin sulfate	...	●	...
Granisetron HCl	●	...	...
Heparin sodium	...	...	●
Hextend	●	...	...
Hydralazine HCl	...	●	...
Hydrocortisone sodium succinate	...	...	●
Hydromorphone HCl	...	...	●
Insulin, regular	●	...	...

Ampicillin Sodium

Drugs	Compatible	Incompatible	Variable
Kanamycin sulfate	...	●	...
Labetalol HCl	●	...	...
Lansoprazole	...	●	...
Levofloxacin	●	...	...
Lidocaine HCl	...	...	●
Lincomycin HCl	...	●	...
Linezolid	●	...	...
Magnesium sulfate	●	...	...
Melphalan HCl	●	...	...
Meperidine HCl	●	...	...
Metoclopramide HCl	...	●	...
Metronidazole	...	...	●
Midazolam HCl	...	●	...
Milrinone lactate	●	...	...
Morphine sulfate	●	...	...
Nicardipine HCl	...	●	...
Ondansetron HCl	...	●	...
Pantoprazole sodium	●	...	...
Pemetrexed disodium	●	...	...
Polymyxin B sulfate	...	...	●
Potassium chloride	●	...	...
Procaine HCl	●	...	...
Prochlorperazine edisylate	...	●	...
Propofol	●	...	...
Ranitidine HCl	...	...	●
Remifentanil HCl	●	...	...
Sargramostim	...	●	...
Streptomycin sulfate	...	...	●
Tacrolimus	●	...	...
Teniposide	●	...	...
Theophylline	●	...	...
Thiotepa	●	...	...
Vancomycin HCl	...	...	●
Verapamil HCl	...	...	●
Vinorelbine tartrate	...	●	...

Ampicillin Sodium– Sulbactam Sodium

Handbook on Injectable Drugs pp. 158–162.

Description: A combination of a semisynthetic penicillin with an inhibitor of penicillin inactivation.

Products: **Unasyn;** 1.5- and 3-g vials and piggyback bottles. *pH:* From 8 to 10.

Preparation: For IM injection, reconstitute the 1.5- or 3-g vial with 3.2 or 6.4 mL, respectively, of sterile water for injection or lidocaine hydrochloride 0.5% or 2% to yield a 375-mg/mL solution (ampicillin 250 mg/mL, sulbactam 125 mg/mL).

For IV use, reconstitute the 1.5- and 3-g piggyback bottles with a compatible diluent to yield a combined concentration of 3 to 45 mg/mL (ampicillin 2 to 30 mg/mL, sulbactam 1 to 15 mg/mL). Vials may be reconstituted as for IM injection and diluted to yield a combined concentration of 3 to 45 mg/mL.

Allow foaming to dissipate after reconstitution.

Administration: Administer by deep IM injection, IV injection over at least 10 to 15 minutes, or IV infusion over 15 to 30 minutes.

Stability: The reconstituted solution should be used within one hour. After dilution in a compatible diluent for IV infusion, administration should be completed within eight hours.

Compatibility Table

Solutions	Compatible	Incompatible	Variable
Dextrose 5%*	...	●	...
Dextrose 5% in sodium chloride 0.45%*	...	●	...
Ringer's injection, lactated	●	...	...
Sodium chloride 0.9%	●	...	...

*Although room temperature stability in these solutions is insufficient to be considered truly compatible, the drug is sufficiently stable to permit use within a few hours.

Drugs			
Amifostine	●	...	...
Amiodarone HCl	...	●	...
Amphotericin B cholesteryl sulfate complex	...	●	...
Anidulafungin	●	...	...

Drugs	Compatible	Incompatible	Variable
Aztreonam	●	...	...
Bivalirudin	●	...	...
Cefepime HCl	●	...	...
Ciprofloxacin	...	...	●
Cisatracurium besylate	...	...	●
Dexmedetomidine HCl	●	...	...
Diltiazem HCl	...	...	●
Docetaxel	●	...	...
Drotrecogin alfa (activated)	●	...	...
Enalaprilat	●	...	...
Etoposide phosphate	●	...	...
Famotidine	●	...	...
Fenoldopam mesylate	●	...	...
Filgrastim	●	...	...
Fluconazole	●	...	...
Fludarabine phosphate	●	...	...
Gallium nitrate	●	...	...
Gemcitabine HCl	●	...	...
Granisetron HCl	●	...	...
Heparin sodium	●	...	...
Hextend	●	...	...
Idarubicin HCl	...	●	...
Insulin, regular	●	...	...
Lansoprazole	...	●	...
Linezolid	●	...	...
Meperidine HCl	●	...	...
Morphine sulfate	●	...	...
Nicardipine HCl	...	●	...
Ondansetron HCl	...	●	...
Paclitaxel	●	...	...
Pemetrexed disodium	●	...	...
Remifentanil HCl	●	...	...
Sargramostim	...	●	...
Tacrolimus	●	...	...
Teniposide	●	...	...
Theophylline	●	...	...
Thiotepa	●	...	...
Vancomycin HCl	...	...	●

Argatroban

Handbook on Injectable Drugs pp. 169–170.

Description: A semisynthetic derivative of L-arginine used as an anticoagulant.

Products: 100-mg/mL concentrate in 2.5-mL (250-mg) vials. *pH:* After dilution for use, the pH is 3.2 to 7.5.

Preparation: For use, the concentrate must be diluted 100-fold in dextrose 5%, sodium chloride 0.9%, or Ringer's injection, lactated, resulting in a final concentration of 1 mg/mL. For a 2.5-mL vial, the contents are mixed with 250 mL of infusion solution. Mix thoroughly after dilution by repeated inversion of the solution container for one minute. Slight haziness may form due to transient microprecipitation, but the solution should clear with adequate mixing.

Administration: Administer by continuous IV infusion after 100-fold dilution.

Stability: The clear, colorless to pale yellow slightly viscous injection in intact vials should be stored at room temperature and retained in the original carton to protect from light. Freezing should be avoided. Argatroban diluted for administration in a suitable infusion solution is stable for 24 hours at room temperature exposed to normal room light and 48 hours under refrigeration in the dark. The solutions should not be exposed to direct sunlight.

Compatibility Table

Solutions	Compatible	Incompatible	Variable
Dextrose 5%	●	...	...
Ringer's injection, lactated	●	...	...
Sodium chloride 0.9%	●	...	...

Drugs	Compatible	Incompatible	Variable
Amiodarone HCl	...	●	...
Atropine sulfate	●	...	...
Diltiazem HCl	●	...	...
Diphenhydramine HCl	●	...	...
Dobutamine HCl	●	...	...

Drugs	Compatible	Incompatible	Variable
Dopamine HCl	●	...	...
Fenoldopam mesylate	●	...	...
Fentanyl citrate	●	...	...
Furosemide	●	...	...
Hydrocortisone sodium succinate	●	...	...
Lidocaine HCl	●	...	...
Metoprolol tartrate	●	...	...
Midazolam HCl	●	...	...
Milrinone lactate	●	...	...
Morphine sulfate	●	...	...
Nesiritide	●	...	...
Nitroglycerin	●	...	...
Norepinephrine bitartrate	●	...	...
Phenylephrine HCl	●	...	...
Sodium nitroprusside	●	...	...
Vasopressin	●	...	...
Verapamil HCl	●	...	...

Atracurium Besylate

Handbook on Injectable Drugs pp. 178–182.

Description: A synthetic, nondepolarizing, neuromuscular blocking agent.

Products: **Tracrium;** 10 mg/mL in 2.5- and 5-mL single-use vials and 10-mL multiple-dose vials. *pH:* From 3.25 to 3.65.

Administration: Administer by rapid IV injection or IV infusion in concentrations of 0.2 to 0.5 mg/mL in a compatible infusion solution. It must not be given by IM injection.

Stability: The clear, colorless solution should be refrigerated but protected from freezing. Intact vials are stable for up to three months at room temperature. At a concentration of 0.2 to 0.5 mg/mL in compatible infusion solutions, it is stable for up to 24 hours at 5 and 25 °C. The drug should not be mixed with alkaline solutions.

Compatibility Table

Solutions	Compatible	Incompatible	Variable
Dextrose 5%	●	…	…
Dextrose 5% in sodium chloride 0.9%	●	…	…
Ringer's injection, lactated	…	●	…
Sodium chloride 0.9%	●	…	…

Drugs	Compatible	Incompatible	Variable
Alfentanil HCl	●	…	…
Aminophylline	…	●	…
Amiodarone HCl	●	…	…
Barbiturates	…	●	…
Cefazolin sodium	…	…	●
Cefuroxime sodium	●	…	…
Cimetidine HCl	●	…	…
Ciprofloxacin	●	…	…
Diazepam	…	●	…
Dobutamine HCl	●	…	…
Dopamine HCl	●	…	…
Epinephrine HCl	●	…	…
Esmolol HCl	●	…	…
Etomidate	●	…	…
Fenoldopam mesylate	●	…	…

Drugs	Compatible	Incompatible	Variable
Fentanyl citrate	●	...	...
Gentamicin sulfate	●	...	...
Heparin sodium	...	...	●
Hextend	●	...	...
Hydrocortisone sodium succinate	●	...	...
Isoproterenol HCl	●	...	...
Lidocaine HCl	●	...	...
Lorazepam	●	...	...
Midazolam HCl	●	...	...
Milrinone lactate	●	...	...
Morphine sulfate	●	...	...
Nitroglycerin	●	...	...
Potassium chloride	●	...	...
Procainamide HCl	●	...	...
Propofol	...	●	...
Quinidine gluconate	...	●	...
Ranitidine HCl	...	...	●
Sodium nitroprusside	...	...	●
Sufentanil citrate	●	...	...
Thiopental sodium	...	●	...
Trimethoprim–sulfamethoxazole	●	...	...
Vancomycin HCl	●	...	...

Atropine Sulfate

Handbook on Injectable Drugs pp. 182–188.

Description: An anticholinergic drug with spasmolytic and central effects.

Products: Available from various manufacturers in a variety of concentrations from 0.4 mg/0.5 mL to 1 mg/mL in single-dose and multiple-dose containers. *pH:* From 3 to 6.5.

Administration: Atropine sulfate injection may be administered SC, IM, or by direct IV injection.

Stability: Atropine sulfate injection is stable when stored at room temperature and protected from temperatures above 40 °C and freezing.

Compatibility Table

Solutions	Compatible	Incompatible	Variable
Sodium chloride 0.9%	●	...	...

Drugs			
Abciximab	●	...	...
Amiodarone HCl	●	...	...
Argatroban	●	...	...
Buprenorphine HCl	●	...	...
Butorphanol tartrate	●	...	...
Chlorpromazine HCl	●	...	...
Cimetidine HCl	●	...	...
Dimenhydrinate	●	...	...
Diphenhydramine HCl	●	...	...
Dobutamine HCl	●	...	...
Droperidol	●	...	...
Etomidate	●	...	...
Famotidine	●	...	...
Fenoldopam mesylate	●	...	...
Fentanyl citrate	●	...	...
Furosemide	●	...	...
Glycopyrrolate	●	...	...
Heparin sodium	●	...	...
Hydrocortisone sodium succinate	●	...	...
Hydromorphone HCl	●	...	...

Drugs	Compatible	Incompatible	Variable
Hydroxyzine HCl	●	. . .	. . .
Meperidine HCl	●	. . .	. . .
Meropenem	●	. . .	. . .
Methadone HCl	●	. . .	. . .
Methohexital sodium	. . .	●	. . .
Metoclopramide HCl	●	. . .	. . .
Midazolam HCl	●	. . .	. . .
Milrinone lactate	●	. . .	. . .
Morphine sulfate	●	. . .	. . .
Nafcillin sodium	●	. . .	. . .
Nalbuphine HCl	●	. . .	. . .
Norepinephrine bitartrate	. . .	●	. . .
Ondansetron HCl	●	. . .	. . .
Pantoprazole sodium	. . .	●	. . .
Pentazocine lactate	●	. . .	. . .
Pentobarbital sodium	. . .	. . .	●
Potassium chloride	●	. . .	. . .
Prochlorperazine edisylate	●	. . .	. . .
Promethazine HCl	●	. . .	. . .
Propofol	. . .	. . .	●
Ranitidine HCl	●	. . .	. . .
Scopolamine HBr	●	. . .	. . .
Sodium bicarbonate	. . .	. . .	●
Sufentanil citrate	●	. . .	. . .
Thiopental sodium	. . .	●	. . .
Tirofiban HCl	●	. . .	. . .
Verapamil HCl	●	. . .	. . .

Azithromycin

Handbook on Injectable Drugs pp. 189–191.

Description: A semisynthetic azalide antibiotic with a broader spectrum than erythromycins or clarithromycin.

Products: Zithromax; 500-mg vials. *pH:* From 6.4 to 6.6.

Preparation: Reconstitute the vacuum-packed 500-mg vials with 4.8 mL of sterile water for injection and shake to yield a 100-mg/mL solution.

Administration: Administer by IV infusion at a concentration of 1 to 2 mg/mL in a compatible infusion solution over not less than 60 minutes.

Stability: The lyophilized powder in intact vials should be stored at room temperature at or below 30 °C. The reconstituted solution is stable for 24 hours at room temperature. Diluted to a concentration of 1 or 2 mg/mL for use, the drug is stable for 24 hours at room temperature and for seven days under refrigeration.

Compatibility Table

Solutions	Compatible	Incompatible	Variable
Dextrose 5%	●	…	…
Dextrose 5% in Ringer's, lactated	●	…	…
Dextrose 5% in sodium chloride 0.45%	●	…	…
Ringer's injection, lactated	●	…	…
Sodium chloride 0.9%	●	…	…

Drugs	Compatible	Incompatible	Variable
Amikacin sulfate	…	●	…
Aztreonam	…	●	…
Bivalirudin	●	…	…
Cefotaxime sodium	…	●	…
Ceftazidime	…	●	…
Ceftriaxone sodium	…	●	…
Cefuroxime sodium	…	●	…
Ciprofloxacin	…	●	…
Clindamycin phosphate	…	●	…
Dexmedetomidine HCl	●	…	…

Drugs	Compatible	Incompatible	Variable
Diphenhydramine HCl	●	...	...
Dolasetron mesylate	●	...	...
Droperidol	●	...	...
Famotidine	...	●	...
Fentanyl citrate	...	●	...
Furosemide	...	●	...
Gentamicin sulfate	...	●	...
Hextend..........................	●	...	...
Imipenem–cilastatin sodium	...	●	...
Ketorolac tromethamine	...	●	...
Levofloxacin	...	●	...
Morphine sulfate	...	●	...
Piperacillin sod.–tazobactam sod.	...	●	...
Potassium chloride	...	●	...
Ticarcillin disod.–clavulanate pot.	...	●	...
Tobramycin sulfate	...	●	...

Aztreonam

Handbook on Injectable Drugs pp. 191–203.

Description: A monobactam antibiotic.

Products: **Azactam;** 500-mg, 1-g, and 2-g sizes in vials, infusion bottles, and frozen premixed solutions. *pH:* From 4.5 to 7.5 when reconstituted.

Preparation: For IM use, reconstitute each gram of drug in vials with 3 mL of bacteriostatic (benzyl alcohol) or sterile water for injection or sodium chloride 0.9%. For direct IV injection, reconstitute each gram of drug in vials with 6 to 10 mL of sterile water for injection. For IV infusion, reconstitute each gram of drug in infusion bottles with at least 50 mL of compatible infusion solution. Alternatively, the contents of reconstituted vials may be diluted further in a compatible infusion solution.

Administration: Administer IV or by deep IM injection. By direct IV injection, the dose is injected slowly over three to five minutes. Intermittent infusion should be completed within 20 to 60 minutes.

Stability: Store intact vials at room temperature. Solutions range from colorless to yellow. A slight pink color may develop without affecting potency. Aztreonam solutions of 2% or less should be used within 48 hours at room temperature or seven days under refrigeration. More concentrated solutions should be used immediately, except in sodium chloride 0.9% or sterile water for injection which may be used within 48 hours at room temperature or seven days under refrigeration.

Compatibility Table

Solutions	Compatible	Incompatible	Variable
Dextrose 5 & 10%	●	...	...
Dextrose 5% in Ringer's injection, lactated	●	...	...
Dextrose 5% in sodium chloride 0.2, 0.45, & 0.9%	●	...	...
Ringer's injection	●	...	...
Ringer's injection, lactated	●	...	...
Sodium chloride 0.9%	●	...	...

Drugs	Compatible	Incompatible	Variable
Acyclovir sodium	...	●	...
Allopurinol sodium	●	...	...
Amifostine	●	...	...
Amikacin sulfate	●	...	...
Aminophylline	●	...	...
Amphotericin B	...	●	...
Amphotericin B cholesteryl sulfate complex	...	●	...
Ampicillin sodium	...	...	●
Ampicillin sod.–sulbactam sod.	●	...	...
Anakinra	...	...	●
Azithromycin	...	●	...
Bivalirudin	●	...	...
Bleomycin sulfate	●	...	...
Bumetanide	●	...	...
Buprenorphine HCl	●	...	...
Butorphanol tartrate	●	...	...
Calcium gluconate	●	...	...
Carboplatin	●	...	...
Carmustine	●	...	...
Cefazolin sodium	●	...	...
Cefepime HCl	●	...	...
Cefotaxime sodium	●	...	...
Cefotetan disodium	●	...	...
Cefoxitin sodium	...	...	●
Ceftazidime	●	...	...
Ceftizoxime sodium	●	...	...
Ceftriaxone sodium	●	...	...
Cefuroxime sodium	●	...	...
Chlorpromazine HCl	...	●	...
Cimetidine HCl	●	...	...
Ciprofloxacin	●	...	...
Cisatracurium besylate	●	...	...
Cisplatin	●	...	...
Clindamycin phosphate	●	...	...
Cyclophosphamide	●	...	...
Cytarabine	●	...	...
Dacarbazine	●	...	...
Dactinomycin	●	...	...
Daptomycin	●	...	...

Drugs	Compatible	Incompatible	Variable
Daunorubicin HCl	...	●	...
Dexmethasone sodium phosphate	●	...	...
Dexmedetomidine HCl	●	...	...
Diltiazem HCl	●	...	...
Diphenhydramine HCl	●	...	...
Dobutamine HCl	●	...	...
Docetaxel	●	...	...
Dopamine HCl	●	...	...
Doxorubicin HCl	●	...	...
Doxorubicin HCl liposome injection	●	...	...
Doxycycline hyclate	●	...	...
Droperidol	●	...	...
Enalaprilat	●	...	...
Etoposide	●	...	...
Etoposide phosphate	●	...	...
Famotidine	●	...	...
Fenoldopam mesylate	●	...	...
Filgrastim	●	...	...
Fluconazole	●	...	...
Fludarabine phosphate	●	...	...
Fluorouracil	●	...	...
Foscarnet sodium	●	...	...
Furosemide	●	...	...
Gallium nitrate	●	...	...
Ganciclovir sodium	...	●	...
Gemcitabine HCl	●	...	...
Gentamicin sulfate	●	...	...
Granisetron HCl	●	...	...
Haloperidol lactate	●	...	...
Heparin sodium	●	...	...
Hextend	●	...	...
Hydrocortisone sodium phosphate ...	●	...	...
Hydrocortisone sodium succinate	●	...	...
Hydromorphone HCl	●	...	...
Hydroxyzine HCl	●	...	...
Idarubicin HCl	●	...	...
Ifosfamide	●	...	...
Imipenem–cilastatin sodium	●	...	...
Insulin, regular	●	...	...
Lansoprazole	...	●	...

Drugs	Compatible	Incompatible	Variable
Leucovorin calcium	●	...	...
Linezolid	●	...	...
Lorazepam	...	●	...
Magnesium sulfate	●	...	...
Mannitol	●	...	...
Mechlorethamine HCl	●	...	...
Melphalan HCl	●	...	...
Meperidine HCl	●	...	...
Mesna	●	...	...
Methotrexate sodium	●	...	...
Methylprednisolone sod. succ.	●	...	...
Metoclopramide HCl	●	...	...
Metronidazole	...	●	...
Mitomycin	...	●	...
Mitoxantrone HCl	...	●	...
Morphine sulfate	●	...	...
Nafcillin sodium	...	●	...
Nalbuphine HCl	●	...	...
Nicardipine HCl	●	...	...
Ondansetron HCl	●	...	...
Pemetrexed disodium	●	...	...
Piperacillin sodium	●	...	...
Piperacillin sod.–tazobactam sod.	●	...	...
Potassium chloride	●	...	...
Prochlorperazine edisylate	...	●	...
Promethazine HCl	●	...	...
Propofol	●	...	...
Quinupristin–dalfopristin	●	...	...
Ranitidine HCl	●	...	...
Remifentanil HCl	●	...	...
Sargramostim	●	...	...
Sodium bicarbonate	●	...	...
Streptozocin	...	●	...
Teniposide	●	...	...
Theophylline	●	...	...
Thiotepa	●	...	...
Ticarcillin disod.–clavulanate pot.	●	...	...
Tobramycin sulfate	●	...	...
Trimethoprim–sulfamethoxazole	●	...	...
Vancomycin HCl	...	...	●
Vinblastine sulfate	●	...	...
Vincristine sulfate	●	...	...
Vinorelbine tartrate	●	...	...
Zidovudine	●	...	...

Bivalirudin

Handbook on Injectable Drugs pp. 207–213.

Description: A synthetic analog of hirudin used as an anticoagulant.

Products: **Angiomax;** 250-mg vials. *pH:* From 5 to 6.

Preparation: Reconstitute the 250-mg vials with 5 mL of sterile water for injection and swirl to dissolve, yielding a 50-mg/mL solution. The reconstituted solution must be diluted for use to a concentration of 0.5 to 5 mg/mL in dextrose 5% or sodium chloride 0.9% for infusion.

Administration: Administer by IV injection and infusion. The drug should not be administered by other routes.

Stability: The white powder in intact vials should be stored at room temperature. The reconstituted solution is clear or opalescent and colorless to slightly yellow and is stable for 24 hours under refrigeration; freezing should be avoided. Diluted in a suitable infusion solution to a concentration of 0.5 to 5 mg/mL, bivalirudin is stable for 24 hours at room temperature.

Compatibility Table

Solutions	Compatible	Incompatible	Variable
Dextrose 5%	●	...	...
Sodium chloride 0.9%	●	...	...

Drugs	Compatible	Incompatible	Variable
Abciximab	●	...	...
Alfentanil HCl	●	...	...
Alteplase	...	●	...
Amikacin sulfate	●	...	...
Aminophylline	●	...	...
Amiodarone HCl	...	●	...
Amphotericin B	...	●	...
Ampicillin sodium	●	...	...
Ampicillin sodium–sulbactam sodium	●	...	...

Drugs	Compatible	Incompatible	Variable
Azithromycin	●	...	...
Aztreonam	●	...	...
Bumetanide	●	...	...
Butorphanol tartrate	●	...	...
Calcium gluconate	●	...	...
Cefazolin sodium	●	...	...
Cefepime HCl	●	...	...
Cefotaxime sodium	●	...	...
Cefotetan disodium	●	...	...
Cefoxitin sodium	●	...	...
Ceftazidime	●	...	...
Ceftizoxime sodium	●	...	...
Ceftriaxone sodium	●	...	...
Cefuroxime sodium	●	...	...
Chlorpromazine HCl	...	●	...
Cimetidine HCl	●	...	...
Ciprofloxacin	●	...	...
Clindamycin phosphate	●	...	...
Dexamethasone sodium phosphate	●	...	...
Diazepam	...	●	...
Digoxin	●	...	...
Diphenhydramine HCl	●	...	...
Dobutamine HCl	●	...	...
Dopamine HCl	●	...	...
Doxycycline hyclate	●	...	...
Droperidol	●	...	...
Enalaprilat	●	...	...
Ephedrine sulfate	●	...	...
Epinephrine HCl	●	...	...
Epoprostenol sodium	●	...	...
Eptifibatide	●	...	...
Erythromycin lactobionate	●	...	...
Esmolol HCl	●	...	...
Famotidine	●	...	...
Fentanyl citrate	●	...	...
Fluconazole	●	...	...
Furosemide	●	...	...
Gentamicin sulfate	●	...	...
Haloperidol lactate	●	...	...
Heparin sodium	●	...	...

Drugs	Compatible	Incompatible	Variable
Hydrocortisone sodium succinate	●	...	...
Hydromorphone HCl	●	...	...
Isoproterenol HCl	●	...	...
Labetalol HCl	●	...	...
Levofloxacin	●	...	...
Lidocaine HCl	●	...	...
Lorazepam	●	...	...
Magnesium sulfate	●	...	...
Mannitol	●	...	...
Meperidine HCl	●	...	...
Methylprednisolone sodium succinate	●	...	...
Metoclopramide HCl	●	...	...
Metronidazole	●	...	...
Midazolam HCl	●	...	...
Milrinone lactate	●	...	...
Morphine sulfate	●	...	...
Nalbuphine HCl	●	...	...
Nitroglycerin	●	...	...
Norepinephrine bitartrate	●	...	...
Phenylephrine HCl	●	...	...
Piperacillin sodium	●	...	...
Piperacillin sodium–tazobactam sodium	●	...	...
Potassium chloride	●	...	...
Procainamide HCl	●	...	...
Prochlorperazine edisylate	...	●	...
Promethazine HCl	●	...	...
Ranitidine HCl	●	...	...
Reteplase	...	●	...
Sodium bicarbonate	●	...	...
Sodium nitroprusside	●	...	...
Streptokinase	...	●	...
Sufentanil citrate	●	...	...
Theophylline	●	...	...
Thiopental sodium	●	...	...
Ticarcillin disodium–clavulanate potassium	●	...	...
Tirofiban HCl	●	...	...
Tobramycin sulfate	●	...	...
Trimethoprim–sulfamethoxazole	●	...	...
Vancomycin HCl	...	●	...
Verapamil HCl	●	...	...
Warfarin sodium	●	...	...

Bleomycin Sulfate

Handbook on Injectable Drugs pp. 213–218.

Description: A mixture of related cytotoxic antibiotics.

Products: Blenoxane; 15 and 30 units/vial. *pH:* From 4.5 to 6, depending on the diluent.

Preparation: For IM or SC use, reconstitute the 15-unit vial with 1 to 5 mL and the 30-unit vial with 2 to 10 mL of sterile water for injection, sodium chloride 0.9%, dextrose 5%, or bacteriostatic water for injection to yield a 3- to 15-unit/mL solution. For IV or intra-arterial injection, reconstitute the vials with sodium chloride 0.9% using a minimum of 5 mL for the 15-unit vial and 10 mL for the 30-unit vial.

Administration: Administer by IM, SC, or intrapleural injection or by IV or intra-arterial injection slowly over 10 minutes.

Stability: In sodium chloride 0.9%, bleomycin sulfate is stable for at least 24 hours at room temperature. No sorption to glass or plastic containers or to administration sets or filters has been noted.

Compatibility Table

Solutions	Compatible	Incompatible	Variable
Amino acids	...	●	...
Dextrose 5%	●	...	...
Sodium chloride 0.9%	●	...	...

Drugs			
Allopurinol sodium	●	...	...
Amifostine	●	...	...
Amikacin sulfate	●	...	...
Aminophylline	...	●	...
Ascorbic acid injection	...	●	...
Aztreonam	●	...	...
Cefazolin sodium	...	●	...
Cefepime HCl	●	...	...
Cisplatin	●	...	...
Cyclophosphamide	●	...	...

Drugs	Compatible	Incompatible	Variable
Dacarbazine	●	...	...
Dexamethasone sodium phosphate	●	...	...
Diazepam	...	●	...
Diphenhydramine HCl	●	...	...
Doxorubicin HCl	●	...	...
Doxorubicin HCl liposome injection	●	...	...
Droperidol	●	...	...
Etoposide phosphate	●	...	...
Filgrastim	●	...	...
Fludarabine phosphate	●	...	...
Fluorouracil	●	...	...
Furosemide	●	...	...
Gemcitabine HCl	●	...	...
Gentamicin sulfate	●	...	...
Granisetron HCl	●	...	...
Heparin sodium	●	...	...
Hydrocortisone sodium phosphate	●	...	...
Hydrocortisone sodium succinate	...	●	...
Leucovorin calcium	●	...	...
Melphalan HCl	●	...	...
Methotrexate sodium	...	...	●
Metoclopramide HCl	●	...	...
Mitomycin	...	...	●
Nafcillin sodium	...	●	...
Ondansetron HCl	●	...	...
Paclitaxel	●	...	...
Penicillin G sodium	...	●	...
Piperacillin sod.–tazobactam sod.	●	...	...
Sargramostim	●	...	...
Streptomycin sulfate	●	...	...
Teniposide	●	...	...
Terbutaline sulfate	...	●	...
Thiotepa	●	...	...
Tobramycin sulfate	●	...	...
Vinblastine sulfate	●	...	...
Vincristine sulfate	●	...	...
Vinorelbine sulfate	●	...	...

Butorphanol Tartrate

Handbook on Injectable Drugs pp. 233–237.

Description: A synthetic narcotic analgesic.

Products: Stadol; 1-mg/mL solution in 1-mL vials; 2-mg/mL solution in 1- and 2-mL single-use vials and 10-mL multiple-dose vials. *pH:* From 3.5 to 5.

Administration: Administer by IM or IV injection.

Stability: Store at room temperature and protect from light. Avoid freezing.

Compatibility Table

Drugs	Compatible	Incompatible	Variable
Allopurinol sodium	●	...	...
Amifostine	●	...	...
Amphotericin B cholesteryl sulfate complex	...	●	...
Atropine sulfate	●	...	...
Aztreonam	●	...	...
Bivalirudin	●	...	...
Cefepime HCl	●	...	...
Chlorpromazine HCl	●	...	...
Cimetidine HCl	●	...	...
Cisatracurium besylate	●	...	...
Cladribine	●	...	...
Dexmedetomidine HCl	●	...	...
Dimenhydrinate	...	●	...
Diphenhydramine HCl	●	...	...
Docetaxel	●	...	...
Doxorubicin HCl liposome injection	●	...	...
Droperidol	●	...	...
Enalaprilat	●	...	...
Esmolol HCl	●	...	...
Etoposide phosphate	●	...	...
Fenoldopam mesylate	●	...	...
Fentanyl citrate	●	...	...
Filgrastim	●	...	...

Drugs	Compatible	Incompatible	Variable
Fludarabine phosphate	●	...	...
Gemcitabine HCl	●	...	...
Granisetron HCl	●	...	...
Hextend	●	...	...
Hydroxyzine HCl	●	...	...
Labetalol HCl	●	...	...
Lansoprazole	...	●	...
Linezolid	●	...	...
Melphalan HCl	●	...	...
Meperidine HCl	●	...	...
Metoclopramide HCl	●	...	●
Midazolam HCl	...	...	●
Morphine sulfate	●	...	...
Nicardipine HCl	●	...	...
Oxaliplatin	●	...	...
Paclitaxel	●	...	...
Pemetrexed disodium	●	...	...
Pentazocine lactate	●	...	...
Pentobarbital sodium	...	●	...
Piperacillin sod.–tazobactam sod.	●	...	...
Prochlorperazine edisylate	●	...	...
Promethazine HCl	●	...	...
Propofol	●	...	...
Remifentanil HCl	●	...	...
Sargramostim	●	...	...
Scopolamine HBr	●	...	...
Teniposide	●	...	...
Thiethylperazine malate	●	...	...
Thiotepa	●	...	...
Vinorelbine sulfate	●	...	...

Butorphanol Tartrate

Calcium Chloride

Handbook on Injectable Drugs pp. 242–246.

Description: A calcium salt used in the prevention and treatment of calcium depletion.

Products: Available in 10-mL vials and prefilled syringes containing 1 g of calcium chloride, providing 270 mg (13.6 mEq) of calcium. *pH:* From 5.5 to 7.5.

Administration: Administer by direct IV injection or infusion at a rate not exceeding 0.7 to 1.8 mEq/min. It may also be injected into the ventricular cavity in cardiac resuscitation. Severe necrosis and sloughing may result if calcium chloride is injected IM or SC or leaks into the perivascular tissue.

Stability: Store intact containers at room temperature.

Compatibility Table

Solutions	Compatible	Incompatible	Variable
NOTE: Unrecognized calcium phosphate precipitation in a 3-in-1 parenteral nutrition mixture resulted in patient death.			
Fat emulsion 10%, IV	...	●	...
Calcium chloride is compatible in most common IV infusion solutions.			

Drugs			
Amikacin sulfate	●	...	...
Amiodarone HCl	●	...	...
Amphotericin B	...	●	...
Amphotericin B cholesteryl sulfate complex	...	●	...
Ascorbic acid injection	●	...	...
Cefamandole nafate	...	●	...
Chloramphenicol sodium succinate	●	...	...
Dobutamine HCl	...	...	●
Dopamine HCl	●	...	...
Doxapram HCl	●	...	...
Epinephrine HCl	●	...	...
Esmolol HCl	●	...	...
Hydrocortisone sodium succinate	●	...	...

Drugs	Compatible	Incompatible	Variable
Isoproterenol HCl	•	...	...
Lansoprazole	...	•	...
Lidocaine HCl	•	...	...
Magnesium sulfate	...	...	•
Milrinone lactate	•	...	...
Morphine sulfate	•	...	...
Norepinephrine bitartrate	•	...	...
Paclitaxel	•	...	...
Pantoprazole sodium	...	•	...
Penicillin G potassium	•	...	...
Penicillin G sodium	•	...	...
Pentobarbital sodium	•	...	...
Phenobarbital sodium	•	...	...
Potassium phosphates	...	...	•
Propofol	...	•	...
Sodium bicarbonate	...	...	•
Sodium nitroprusside	•	...	...
Sodium phosphate	...	...	•
Tobramycin sulfate	...	•	...
Verapamil HCl	•	...	...

Calcium Gluconate

Handbook on Injectable Drugs pp. 247–258.

Description: A calcium salt used in the prevention and treatment of calcium depletion.

Products: Available as a 10% solution in 10-, 50-, and 100-mL containers providing 94 or 98 mg/mL of calcium gluconate and 9.3 mg/mL (0.465 mEq/mL) of calcium. *pH:* From 6 to 8.2.

Administration: Administer by IV infusion or direct IV injection. IV administration should be performed slowly at a rate not exceeding 0.7 to 1.8 mEq/min. SC or IM injection should not be performed. Numerous reports indicate that tissue irritation and necrosis may result from SC or IM injection or extravasation from IV administration, especially in children.

Stability: Store intact containers at room temperature and protect from freezing.

Compatibility Table

Solutions	Compatible	Incompatible	Variable
NOTE: Unrecognized calcium phosphate precipitation in a 3-in-1 parenteral nutrition mixture resulted in patient death.			
Dextrose 5 & 10%	●	...	...
Dextrose 5% in Ringer's injection, lactated	●	...	...
Dextrose 5% in sodium chloride 0.2, 0.45, & 0.9%	●	...	...
Fat emulsion 10%, IV	...	●	...
Ringer's injection, lactated	●	...	...
Sodium chloride 0.9%	●	...	...

Drugs			
Aldesleukin	●	...	...
Allopurinol sodium	●	...	...
Amifostine	●	...	...
Amikacin sulfate	●	...	...
Aminophylline	●	...	...

Drugs	Compatible	Incompatible	Variable
Amiodarone HCl	●	...	...
Amphotericin B	...	●	...
Amphotericin B cholesteryl sulfate complex	...	●	...
Ampicillin sodium	...	...	●
Ascorbic acid injection	●	...	...
Aztreonam	●	...	...
Bivalirudin	●	...	...
Cefamandole nafate	...	●	...
Cefazolin sodium	...	...	●
Cefepime HCl	●	...	...
Chloramphenicol sod. succ.	●	...	...
Ciprofloxacin	●	...	...
Cisatracurium besylate	●	...	...
Cladribine	●	...	...
Clindamycin phosphate	...	●	...
Corticotropin	●	...	...
Dexmedetomidine HCl	●	...	...
Dimenhydrinate	●	...	...
Dobutamine HCl	...	...	●
Docetaxel	●	...	...
Doxapram HCl	●	...	...
Doxorubicin HCl liposome injection	●	...	...
Enalaprilat	●	...	...
Epinephrine HCl	●	...	...
Etoposide phosphate	●	...	...
Famotidine	●	...	...
Fenoldopam mesylate	●	...	...
Filgrastim	●	...	...
Fluconazole	...	●	...
Furosemide	●	...	...
Gemcitabine HCl	●	...	...
Granisetron HCl	●	...	...
Heparin sodium	●	...	...
Hextend	●	...	...
Hydrocortisone sodium succinate	●	...	...
Indomethacin sod. trihydrate	...	●	...
Labetalol HCl	●	...	...
Lansoprazole	...	●	...

Drugs	Compatible	Incompatible	Variable
Lidocaine HCl	●	…	…
Linezolid	●	…	…
Magnesium sulfate	…	…	●
Melphalan HCl	●	…	…
Meropenem	…	…	●
Methylprednisolone sod. succ.	…	●	…
Metoclopramide HCl	…	●	…
Midazolam HCl	●	…	…
Milrinone lactate	●	…	…
Nicardipine HCl	●	…	…
Norepinephrine bitartrate	●	…	…
Oxaliplatin	●	…	…
Pantoprazole sodium	…	●	…
Pemetrexed disodium	…	●	…
Penicillin G potassium and sodium	●	…	…
Phenobarbital sodium	●	…	…
Piperacillin sod.–tazobactam sod.	●	…	…
Potassium chloride	●	…	…
Potassium phosphates	…	…	●
Prochlorperazine edisylate	…	…	●
Propofol	●	…	…
Remifentanil HCl	●	…	…
Sargramostim	●	…	…
Sodium bicarbonate	…	…	●
Tacrolimus	●	…	…
Teniposide	●	…	…
Thiotepa	●	…	…
Tobramycin sulfate	…	…	●
Vancomycin sulfate	●	…	…
Verapamil HCl	●	…	…
Vinorelbine tartrate	●	…	…

Carboplatin

Handbook on Injectable Drugs pp. 258–262.

Description: A platinum-containing antineoplastic agent.

Products: Paraplatin; 50-, 150-, and 450-mg vials. Also, 10-mg/mL in 5-mL (50-mg), 15-mL (150-mg), 45-mL (450-mg), and 60-mL (600-mg) vials. *pH:* From 5 to 7.

Preparation: Reconstitute the dry powder vials with dextrose 5%, sodium chloride 0.9%, or sterile water for injection in the following amounts to yield a 10-mg/mL solution:

Vial Size	Diluent Volume
50 mg	5 mL
150 mg	15 mL
450 mg	45 mL

Administration: Administer by continuous or intermittent infusion over at least 15 minutes. The reconstituted solution may be diluted with dextrose 5% or sodium chloride 0.9% to a concentration as low as 0.5 mg/mL.

Stability: Store intact containers at room temperature and protect from light. Reconstituted solutions are clear and colorless and are stable for 24 hours at room temperature. No sorption to plastic bags or Silastic catheters has been noted.

Carboplatin may react with the metal aluminum to form a precipitate that results in a loss of potency. Therefore equipment (e.g., needles, syringes, catheters, etc.) containing aluminum should not be used for preparation and administration of carboplatin.

Compatibility Table

Solutions	Compatible	Incompatible	Variable
Dextrose 5%	●	...	...
Dextrose 5% in sodium chloride 0.2, 0.45, & 0.9%	●	...	...
Sodium bicarbonate	...	●	...
Sodium chloride 0.9%	●	...	...

Drugs	Compatible	Incompatible	Variable
Allopurinol sodium	●	...	...
Amifostine	●	...	...
Amphotericin B cholesteryl sulfate complex	...	●	...
Anidulafungin	●	...	...
Aztreonam	●	...	...
Cefepime HCl	●	...	...
Cisplatin	●	...	...
Cladribine	●	...	...
Doxorubicin HCl liposome injection	●	...	...
Etoposide	●	...	...
Etoposide phosphate	●	...	...
Filgrastim	●	...	...
Fludarabine phosphate	●	...	...
Fluorouracil	...	●	...
Gemcitabine HCl	●	...	...
Granisetron HCl	●	...	...
Ifosfamide	●	...	...
Lansoprazole	...	●	...
Linezolid	●	...	...
Melphalan HCl	●	...	...
Mesna	...	●	...
Ondansetron HCl	●	...	...
Oxaliplatin	●	...	...
Paclitaxel	●	...	...
Palonosetron HCl	●	...	...
Pemetrexed disodium	●	...	...
Piperacillin sod.–tazobactam sod.	●	...	...
Propofol	●	...	...
Sargramostim	●	...	...
Teniposide	●	...	...
Thiotepa	●	...	...
Topotecan HCl	●	...	...
Vinorelbine tartrate	●	...	...

Cefazolin Sodium

Handbook on Injectable Drugs pp. 273–283.

Description: A semisynthetic cephalosporin antibiotic.

Products: Ancef, Kefzol; 500-mg and 1-g vials and piggyback units and 10- and 20-g vials. *pH:* From 4.5 to 6 when reconstituted.

Preparation: Reconstitute the 500-mg vial with 2 mL and the 1-g vial with 2.5 mL of diluent to yield concentrations of 225 and 330 mg/mL, respectively. Sterile water for injection or bacteriostatic water for injection may be used for either the 500-mg or 1-g vials while sodium chloride 0.9% may be used only for the 500-mg vial. For direct IV injection, further dilute the reconstituted solution with 5 to 10 mL of sterile water for injection.

Administration: IM administration should be made deep into a large muscle mass. Direct IV injection should be given slowly over three to five minutes into the vein or the tubing of a running IV solution. Continuous or intermittent IV infusion in 50 to 100 mL of compatible diluent may be performed.

Stability: Store intact vials at room temperature and protect from light. The manufacturer recommends discarding the reconstituted solutions after 24 hours at room temperature or 10 days under refrigeration. Crystals may form in reconstituted solutions, especially if refrigerated.

Compatibility Table

Solutions	Compatible	Incompatible	Variable
Dextrose 5%	●	…	…
Dextrose 5% in Ringer's injection, lactated	●	…	…
Dextrose 5% in sodium chloride 0.2, 0.45, & 0.9%	●	…	…
Ringer's injection	●	…	…
Ringer's injection, lactated	●	…	…
Sodium chloride 0.9%	●	…	…

Drugs	Compatible	Incompatible	Variable
Acyclovir sodium	●	...	...
Allopurinol sodium	●	...	...
Amifostine	●	...	...
Amikacin sulfate	...	●	...
Amiodarone HCl	...	...	●
Amobarbital sodium	...	●	...
Amphotericin B cholesteryl sulfate complex	...	●	...
Anakinra	...	...	●
Anidulafungin	●	...	...
Ascorbic acid injection	...	●	...
Atracurium besylate	...	...	●
Aztreonam	●	...	...
Bivalirudin	●	...	...
Bleomycin sulfate	...	●	...
Calcium gluconate	...	...	●
Cimetidine HCl	...	...	●
Cisatracurium besylate	...	...	●
Clindamycin phosphate	●	...	...
Colistimethate sodium	...	●	...
Cyclophosphamide	●	...	...
Dexmedetomidine HCl	●	...	...
Diltiazem HCl	●	...	...
Dimenhydrinate	●	...	...
Docetaxel	●	...	...
Doxapram HCl	●	...	...
Doxorubicin HCl liposome injection	●	...	...
Enalaprilat	●	...	...
Esmolol HCl	●	...	...
Etoposide phosphate	●	...	...
Famotidine	●	...	...
Fenoldopam mesylate	●	...	...
Filgrastim	●	...	...
Fluconazole	●	...	...
Fludarabine phosphate	●	...	...
Foscarnet sodium	●	...	...
Gallium nitrate	●	...	...
Gemcitabine HCl	●	...	...
Granisetron HCl	●	...	...

Drugs	Compatible	Incompatible	Variable
Heparin sodium	●	…	…
Hetastarch in sodium chloride 0.9%	…	…	●
Hextend	●	…	…
Hydromorphone HCl	…	…	●
Idarubicin HCl	…	●	…
Insulin, regular	●	…	…
Labetalol HCl	●	…	…
Lansoprazole	…	●	…
Lidocaine HCl	…	…	●
Linezolid	●	…	…
Magnesium sulfate	●	…	…
Melphalan HCl	●	…	…
Meperidine HCl	●	…	…
Metronidazole	●	…	…
Midazolam HCl	●	…	…
Milrinone lactate	●	…	…
Morphine sulfate	●	…	…
Multivitamins	●	…	…
Nicardipine HCl	●	…	…
Ondansetron HCl	●	…	…
Pancuronium bromide	●	…	…
Pantoprazole sodium	…	…	●
Pemetrexed disodium	…	●	…
Pentamidine isethionate	…	●	…
Pentobarbital sodium	…	●	…
Promethazine HCl	…	…	●
Propofol	●	…	…
Ranitidine HCl	…	…	●
Remifentanil HCl	●	…	…
Sargramostim	●	…	…
Tacrolimus	●	…	…
Teniposide	●	…	…
Theophylline	●	…	…
Thiotepa	●	…	…
Vancomycin HCl	…	…	●
Vecuronium bromide	●	…	…
Verapamil HCl	●	…	…
Vinorelbine tartrate	…	●	…
Warfarin sodium	●	…	…

Cefepime Hydrochloride

Handbook on Injectable Drugs pp. 284–296.

Description: A semisynthetic cephalosporin antibiotic.

Products: **Maxipime**; 500-mg, 1- and 2-g vials, and 1- and 2-g infusion containers. *pH:* From 4 to 6 when reconstituted.

Preparation: For IM administration, reconstitute the 500-mg and 1-g vials with 1.3 and 2.4 mL, respectively, to yield 280 mg/mL. Use sterile water for injection, sodium chloride 0.9%, dextrose 5%, lidocaine hydrochloride 0.5 or 1%, or bacteriostatic water for injection for reconstitution.

For IV use, reconstitute the vials with a compatible infusion solution. The 500-mg and 1-g vials are reconstituted with 5 and 10 mL, respectively, to yield 100 mg/mL, and the 2-g vials are reconstituted with 10 mL to yield 160 mg/mL. The 1- and 2-g infusion containers should be reconstituted with 50 to 100 mL of a compatible infusion solution.

Administration: Administer by deep IM injection or intermittent IV infusion over approximately 30 minutes.

Stability: Store intact vials between 2 and 25 °C and protect from light. Solutions may range from colorless to amber. Reconstituted solutions in compatible diluents are stable for 24 hours at room temperatures of 20 to 25 °C and for seven days under refrigeration.

Compatibility Table

Solutions	Compatible	Incompatible	Variable
Dextrose 5 & 10%	●	...	...
Dextrose 5% in Ringer's injection, lactated	●	...	...
Dextrose 5% in sod. chloride 0.9% ...	●	...	...
Sodium chloride 0.9%	●	...	...

Drugs	Compatible	Incompatible	Variable
Acetylcysteine	...	●	...
Acyclovir sodium	...	●	...
Amikacin sulfate	●	...	...
Aminophylline	...	●	...
Amphotericin B	...	●	...
Amphotericin B cholesteryl sulfate complex	...	●	...
Ampicillin sodium	...	...	●
Ampicillin sod.–sulbactam sod.	●	...	...
Anidulafungin	●	...	...
Aztreonam	●	...	...
Bivalirudin	●	...	...
Bleomycin sulfate	●	...	...
Bumetanide	●	...	...
Buprenorphine HCl	●	...	...
Butorphanol tartrate	●	...	...
Calcium gluconate	●	...	...
Carboplatin	●	...	...
Carmustine	●	...	...
Chlordiazepoxide HCl	...	●	...
Chlorpromazine HCl	...	●	...
Cimetidine HCl	...	●	...
Ciprofloxacin	...	●	...
Cisplatin	...	●	...
Clindamycin phosphate	●	...	...
Cyclophosphamide	●	...	...
Cytarabine	●	...	...
Dacarbazine	...	●	...
Dactinomycin	●	...	...
Daunorubicin HCl	...	●	...
Dexamethasone sodium phosphate	●	...	...
Dexmedetomidine HCl	●	...	...
Diazepam	...	●	...
Diphenhydramine HCl	...	●	...
Dobutamine HCl	...	...	●
Docetaxel	●	...	...
Dopamine HCl	...	...	●
Doxorubicin HCl	...	●	...
Doxorubicin HCl liposome injection	●	...	...

Drugs	Compatible	Incompatible	Variable
Droperidol	...	●	...
Enalaprilat	...	●	...
Erythromycin lactobionate	...	●	...
Etoposide	...	●	...
Etoposide phosphate	...	●	...
Famotidine	...	●	...
Fenoldopam mesylate	●	...	...
Filgrastim	...	●	...
Floxuridine	...	●	...
Fluconazole	●	...	...
Fludarabine phosphate	●	...	...
Fluorouracil	●	...	...
Furosemide	●	...	...
Gallium nitrate	...	●	...
Ganciclovir sodium	...	●	...
Gentamicin sulfate	...	●	...
Granisetron HCl	●	...	...
Haloperidol lactate	...	●	...
Heparin sodium	●	...	...
Hextend	●	...	...
Hydrocortisone sodium phosphate	●	...	...
Hydrocortisone sodium succinate	●	...	...
Hydromorphone HCl	●	...	...
Hydroxyzine HCl	...	●	...
Idarubicin HCl	...	●	...
Ifosfamide	...	●	...
Imipenem–cilastatin sodium	●	...	...
Insulin, regular	●	...	...
Isosorbide dinitrate	●	...	...
Ketamine hydrochloride	●	...	...
Lansoprazole	...	●	...
Leucovorin calcium	●	...	...
Lorazepam	●	...	...
Magnesium sulfate	...	●	...
Mannitol	...	●	...
Mechlorethamine HCl	...	●	...
Melphalan	●	...	...
Meperidine HCl	...	●	...
Mesna	●	...	...
Methotrexate sodium	●	...	...

Drugs	Compatible	Incompatible	Variable
Methylprednisolone sod. succ.	●	...	...
Metoclopramide HCl	...	●	...
Metronidazole	...	...	●
Midazolam HCl	...	●	...
Milrinone lactate	●	...	...
Mitomycin	...	●	...
Mitoxantrone HCl	...	●	...
Morphine sulfate	...	●	...
Nalbuphine HCl	...	●	...
Nicardipine HCl	...	●	...
Ondansetron HCl	...	●	...
Paclitaxel	●	...	...
Phenytoin sodium	...	●	...
Piperacillin sod.–tazobactam sod.	●	...	...
Potassium chloride	●	...	...
Prochlorperazine edisylate	...	●	...
Promethazine HCl	...	●	...
Propofol	...	...	●
Ranitidine HCl	●	...	...
Remifentanil HCl	●	...	...
Sargramostim	●	...	...
Sodium bicarbonate	●	...	...
Streptozocin	...	●	...
Sufentanil citrate	●	...	...
Theophylline	...	...	●
Thiotepa	●	...	...
Ticarcillin disod.–clavulanate pot.	●	...	...
Tobramycin sulfate	...	...	●
Trimethoprim–sulfamethoxazole	●	...	...
Uradipil hydrochloride	●	...	...
Valproate sodium	●	...	...
Vancomycin HCl	...	...	●
Vinblastine sulfate	...	●	...
Vincristine sulfate	...	●	...
Zidovudine	●	...	...

Cefepime Hydrochloride

Cefotaxime Sodium

Handbook on Injectable Drugs pp. 296–303.

Description: A semisynthetic cephalosporin antibiotic.

Products: Claforan; 500-mg, 1- and 2-g vials, and 1- and 2-g infusion containers. *pH:* From 5 to 7.5 when reconstituted.

Preparation: For IV administration, reconstitute the 500-mg, 1-g, and 2-g vials with 10 mL of sterile water for injection to yield concentrations of 50, 95, and 180 mg/mL, respectively. For IM administration, reconstitute the 1-g vial with 3 mL and the 2-g vial with 5 mL of sterile or bacteriostatic water for injection to yield 300 and 330 mg/mL, respectively.

The 1- and 2-g infusion bottles may be reconstituted with 50 or 100 mL of dextrose 5% or sodium chloride 0.9%.

Administration: Administer by deep IM injection, direct IV injection over three to five minutes, or continuous or intermittent IV infusion over 20 to 30 minutes.

Stability: Solutions may range from light yellow to amber, and discoloration may indicate potency loss. Store at room temperature and protect dry material and solutions from elevated temperatures and excessive light.

Reconstituted solutions are stable for 24 hours at room temperature at concentrations of 10 to 95 mg/mL, for 12 hours at higher concentrations, and for at least seven days under refrigeration. Dilutions in dextrose 5% or sodium chloride 0.9% in plastic bags are stable for 24 hours at room temperature or five days under refrigeration. Frozen solutions are stable for 13 weeks.

Compatibility Table

Solutions	Compatible	Incompatible	Variable
Dextrose 5 & 10%	●	...	...
Dextrose 5% in sodium chloride 0.2, 0.45, & 0.9%	●	...	...
Ringer's injection, lactated	●	...	...
Sodium bicarbonate 5%	...	●	...
Sodium chloride 0.9%	●	...	...

Drugs	Compatible	Incompatible	Variable
Acyclovir sodium	●	...	...
Allopurinol sodium	...	●	...
Amifostine	●	...	...
Amikacin sulfate	...	...	●
Aminophylline	...	●	...
Anakinra	...	...	●
Azithromycin	...	●	...
Aztreonam	●	...	...
Bivalirudin	●	...	...
Caffeine citrate	●	...	...
Cisatracurium besylate	...	...	●
Clindamycin phosphate	●	...	...
Cyclophosphamide	●	...	...
Dexmedetomidine HCl	●	...	...
Diltiazem HCl	●	...	...
Dimenhydrinate	●	...	...
Docetaxel	●	...	...
Doxapram HCl	...	●	...
Etoposide phosphate	●	...	...
Famotidine	●	...	...
Fenoldopam mesylate	●	...	...
Filgrastim	...	●	...
Fluconazole	...	●	...
Fludarabine phosphate	●	...	...
Gemcitabine HCl	...	●	...
Gentamicin sulfate	...	...	●
Granisetron HCl	●	...	...
Heparin sodium	●	...	...
Hetastarch in sodium chloride 0.9%	...	●	...
Hextend	●	...	...
Hydromorphone HCl	●	...	...
Levofloxacin	●	...	...
Lorazepam	●	...	...
Magnesium sulfate	●	...	...
Meperidine HCl	●	...	...
Metronidazole	●	...	...
Midazolam HCl	●	...	...
Milrinone lactate	●	...	...
Morphine sulfate	●	...	...

Drugs	Compatible	Incompatible	Variable
Ondansetron HCl	●	...	...
Pantoprazole sodium	...	●	...
Pemetrexed disodium	...	●	...
Pentamidine isethionate	...	●	...
Propofol	●	...	...
Remifentanil HCl	●	...	...
Sargramostim	●	...	...
Sodium bicarbonate	...	●	...
Teniposide	●	...	...
Thiotepa	●	...	...
Vancomycin HCl	...	...	●
Verapamil HCl	●	...	...
Vinorelbine tartrate	●	...	...

Cefoxitin Sodium

Handbook on Injectable Drugs pp. 307–316.

Description: A semisynthetic cephamycin antibiotic.

Products: **Mefoxin**; 1- and 2-g vials, PVC bags, and infusion bottles. *pH:* From 4.2 to 7 when reconstituted.

Preparation: For IV administration, reconstitute the vials with sterile water for injection; the infusion bottles can be reconstituted with any compatible diluent.

Vial Size	Route	Diluent Volume	Approximate Concentration
1 g	IV	10 mL	95 mg/mL
(Inf. bottle)	IV	50 or 100 mL	20 or 10 mg/mL
2 g	IV	10 or 20 mL	180 or 95 mg/mL
(Inf. bottle)	IV	50 or 100 mL	40 or 20 mg/mL

Administration: Administer by IV infusion or direct IV injection over three to five minutes or into the tubing of a running IV solution.

Stability: Solutions may range from colorless to light amber and may darken during storage. Discoloration is stated not to affect potency adversely. Reconstituted solutions are stable for 48 hours at room temperature or at least seven days under refrigeration. Frozen solutions retain potency for at least 26 weeks. No sorption to plastic syringes, sets, or filters has been noted.

Compatibility Table

Solutions	Compatible	Incompatible	Variable
Dextrose 5 & 10%	●	...	...
Dextrose 5% in Ringer's injection, lactated	●	...	...
Dextrose 5% in sodium chloride 0.2, 0.45, & 0.9%	●	...	...
Invert sugar 5 & 10% in water	●	...	...
Ringer's injection	●	...	...
Ringer's injection, lactated	●	...	...
Sodium chloride 0.9%	●	...	...

Drugs	Compatible	Incompatible	Variable
Acyclovir sodium	●	...	...
Amifostine	●	...	...
Amikacin sulfate	...	...	●
Amphotericin B cholesteryl sulfate complex	●	...	...
Anakinra	...	...	●
Anidulafungin	●	...	...
Aztreonam	...	...	●
Bivalirudin	●	...	...
Cimetidine HCl	●	...	...
Cisatracurium besylate	...	...	●
Clindamycin phosphate	●	...	...
Cyclophosphamide	●	...	...
Dexmedetomidine HCl	●	...	...
Diltiazem HCl	●	...	...
Docetaxel	●	...	...
Doxorubicin HCl liposome injection	●	...	...
Etoposide phosphate	●	...	...
Famotidine	●	...	...
Fenoldopam mesylate	...	●	...
Filgrastim	...	●	...
Fluconazole	●	...	...
Foscarnet sodium	●	...	...
Gemcitabine HCl	●	...	...
Gentamicin sulfate	...	...	●
Granisetron HCl	●	...	...
Heparin sodium	●	...	...
Hetastarch in sodium chloride 0.9%	...	●	...
Hextend	●	...	...
Hydromorphone HCl	●	...	...
Kanamycin sulfate	●	...	...
Lansoprazole	...	●	...
Lidocaine HCl	●	...	...
Linezolid	●	...	...
Magnesium sulfate	●	...	...
Meperidine HCl	●	...	...
Metronidazole	...	...	●
Morphine sulfate	●	...	...

Drugs	Compatible	Incompatible	Variable
Ondansetron HCl	●	...	...
Pantoprazole sodium	...	●	...
Pemetrexed disodium	...	●	...
Pentamidine isethionate	...	●	...
Propofol	●	...	...
Ranitidine HCl	...	...	●
Remifentanil HCl	●	...	...
Sodium bicarbonate	●	...	...
Teniposide	●	...	...
Thiotepa	●	...	...
Tobramycin sulfate	...	...	●
Vancomycin HCl	...	...	●
Verapamil HCl	●	...	...

Cefoxitin Sodium

Ceftazidime

Handbook on Injectable Drugs pp. 316–329.

Description: A semisynthetic cephalosporin antibiotic.

Products: **Fortaz, Tazicef, Tazidime;** 500-mg and 1- and 2-g vials and infusion packs. *pH:* From 5 to 8.

Preparation: For IM use, reconstitute the 500-mg vial with 1.5 mL and the 1-g vial with 3 mL of bacteriostatic or sterile water for injection or lidocaine hydrochloride 0.5 to 1%. For direct IV injection, reconstitute the 500-mg, 1-g, and 2-g vials with 5, 10, and 10 mL, respectively, of compatible diluent such as sterile water for injection. Carbon dioxide forms during dissolution but clears in one to two minutes. The reconstituted solution may be added to a compatible IV solution for infusion.

Administration: Administer by deep IM injection, direct IV injection over three to five minutes, or intermittent IV infusion over 15 to 30 minutes.

Stability: Reconstituted solutions range from light yellow to amber and may darken during storage without affecting potency. Solution stability varies among the commercial products. Fortaz and Tazidime solutions of 95 to 280 mg/mL in sterile water for injection are stable for 24 hours at room temperature or seven days (Fortaz) or 10 days (Tazidime) under refrigeration. No loss due to sorption to plastic or glass containers has been found.

Compatibility Table

Solutions	Compatible	Incompatible	Variable
Dextrose 5 & 10%	●	...	...
Dextrose 5% in sodium chloride 0.2, 0.45, & 0.9%	●	...	...
Ringer's injection	●	...	...
Ringer's injection, lactated	●	...	...
Sodium chloride 0.9%	●	...	...

Drugs	Compatible	Incompatible	Variable
Acetylcysteine	...	●	...
Acyclovir sodium	●	...	...
Allopurinol sodium	●	...	...
Amifostine	●	...	...
Amikacin sulfate	...	...	●
Aminophylline	...	...	●
Amiodarone HCl	...	●	...
Amphotericin B cholesteryl sulfate complex	...	●	...
Anidulafungin	●	...	...
Azithromycin	...	●	...
Aztreonam	●	...	...
Bivalirudin	●	...	...
Cimetidine HCl	●	...	...
Ciprofloxacin	...	...	●
Cisatracurium besylate	...	...	●
Clindamycin phosphate	●	...	...
Daptomycin	●	...	...
Dexmedetomidine HCl	●	...	...
Diltiazem HCl	●	...	...
Dimenhydrinate	●	...	...
Docetaxel	●	...	...
Dobutamine HCl	...	...	●
Dopamine HCl	●	...	...
Doxapram HCl	●	...	...
Doxorubicin HCl liposome injection	...	●	...
Drotrecogin alfa (activated)	...	...	●
Enalaprilat	●	...	...
Epinephrine HCl	●	...	...
Erythromycin lactobionate	...	●	...
Esmolol HCl	●	...	...
Etoposide phosphate	●	...	...
Famotidine	●	...	...
Fenoldopam mesylate	●	...	...
Filgrastim	●	...	...
Fluconazole	...	...	●
Fludarabine phosphate	●	...	...
Foscarnet sodium	●	...	...
Furosemide	●	...	...

Drugs	Compatible	Incompatible	Variable
Gallium nitrate	●	...	...
Gemcitabine HCl	●	...	...
Gentamicin sulfate	...	...	●
Granisetron HCl	●	...	...
Heparin sodium	●	...	...
Hextend	●	...	...
Hydromorphone HCl	●	...	...
Idarubicin HCl	...	●	...
Insulin, regular	●	...	...
Isosorbide dinitrate	●	...	...
Ketamine HCl	●	...	...
Labetalol HCl	●	...	...
Lansoprazole	...	●	...
Linezolid	●	...	...
Melphalan HCl	●	...	...
Meperidine HCl	●	...	...
Methylprednisolone sod. succ.	●	...	...
Metronidazole	●	...	...
Midazolam HCl	...	●	...
Milrinone lactate	●	...	...
Morphine sulfate	●	...	...
Nicardipine HCl	...	...	●
Ondansetron HCl	●	...	...
Paclitaxel	●	...	...
Pantoprazole sodium	...	●	...
Pemetrexed disodium	...	●	...
Pentamidine isethionate	...	●	...
Phenytoin sodium	...	●	...
Potassium chloride	●	...	...
Propofol	...	...	●
Ranitidine HCl	...	...	●
Remifentanil HCl	●	...	...
Sargramostim	...	...	●
Sufentanil citrate	●	...	...
Tacrolimus	●	...	...
Theophylline	...	...	●
Thiotepa	●	...	...
Tobramycin sulfate	●	...	...
Uradipil HCl	●	...	...
Valproate sodium	●	...	...
Vancomycin HCl	...	...	●
Vinorelbine tartrate	●	...	...
Warfarin sodium	...	●	...
Zidovudine	●	...	...

Ceftizoxime Sodium

Handbook on Injectable Drugs pp. 329–334.

Description: A semisynthetic cephalosporin antibiotic.

Products: Cefizox; 500-mg, 1-g, and 2-g vials, and 1-g and 2-g piggyback bottles. *pH:* From 6 to 8 when reconstituted.

Preparation: For IM injection, reconstitute the 500-mg, 1-g, and 2-g vials with 1.5, 3, and 6 mL, respectively, of sterile water for injection. The resulting solutions have concentrations of 280, 270, and 270 mg/mL of ceftizoxime.

For IV use, reconstitute the 500-mg, 1-g, and 2-g vials with 5, 10, and 20 mL, respectively, of sterile water for injection. The resulting solutions have a ceftizoxime concentration of 95 mg/mL.

For IV use, reconstitute the piggyback bottles with 50 to 100 mL of sodium chloride 0.9% or other compatible diluent to yield concentrations of 20 to 10 mg/mL for the 1-g size and 40 to 20 mg/mL for the 2-g size.

Administration: Administer by deep IM injection, IV injection over at least three to five minutes, or IV infusion over 15 to 30 minutes. IM doses of 2 g should be divided between different large muscles.

Stability: Reconstituted solutions may range from colorless to amber in color, darkening on storage. The reconstituted solution at 95 mg/mL is stable for 24 hours at room temperature and four days refrigerated. Reconstituted solutions for IM use at 270 to 280 mg/mL are stable for 16 hours at room temperature. After dilution in a compatible diluent for IV infusion, the drug is stable for at least 24 hours at room temperature and four days refrigerated.

Compatibility Table

Solutions	Compatible	Incompatible	Variable
Dextrose 5%	●	...	...
Dextrose 5% in sodium chloride 0.2, 0.45, & 0.9%	●	...	...
Ringer's injection, lactated	●	...	...
Sodium chloride 0.9%	●	...	...

Drugs	Compatible	Incompatible	Variable
Acyclovir sodium	●	...	...
Allopurinol sodium	●	...	...
Amifostine	●	...	...
Amiodarone HCl	●	...	...
Amphotericin B cholesteryl sulfate complex	●	...	...
Anidulafungin	●	...	...
Aztreonam	●	...	...
Bivalirudin	●	...	...
Cisatracurium besylate	...	...	●
Clindamycin phosphate	●	...	...
Dexmedetomidine HCl	●	...	...
Docetaxel	●	...	...
Doxorubicin HCl liposome injection	●	...	...
Enalaprilat	●	...	...
Esmolol HCl	●	...	...
Etoposide phosphate	●	...	...
Famotidine	●	...	...
Fenoldopam mesylate	●	...	...
Filgrastim	...	●	...
Fludarabine phosphate	●	...	...
Foscarnet sodium	●	...	...
Gemcitabine HCl	●	...	...
Granisetron HCl	●	...	...
Hextend	●	...	...
Hydromorphone HCl	●	...	...
Labetalol HCl	●	...	...
Lansoprazole	...	●	...
Linezolid	●	...	...
Melphalan HCl	●	...	...
Meperidine HCl	●	...	...
Metronidazole	●	...	...
Morphine sulfate	●	...	...
Nicardipine HCl	●	...	...
Ondansetron HCl	●	...	...
Pemetrexed disodium	●	...	...
Promethazine HCl	...	...	●
Propofol	●	...	...
Ranitidine HCl	●	...	...
Remifentanil HCl	●	...	...

Drugs	Compatible	Incompatible	Variable
Sargramostim	●	...	...
Teniposide	●	...	...
Thiotepa	●	...	...
Vancomycin HCl	...	...	●
Vinorelbine tartrate	●	...	...

Ceftriaxone Sodium

Handbook on Injectable Drugs pp. 334–342.

Description: A semisynthetic cephalosporin antibiotic.

Products: **Rocephin;** 250-mg, 500-mg, 1-g, and 2-g vials and piggyback bottles. *pH:* A 1% solution has a pH of approximately 6.7.

Preparation: For IM use, reconstitute the 250- and 500-mg vials with 0.9 and 1.8 mL, respectively, and the 1- and 2-g vials with 3.6 and 7.2 mL, respectively, of compatible diluent to yield a 250-mg/mL solution. Alternatively, the 1- and 2-g vials may be reconstituted with 2.1 and 4.2 mL of compatible diluent to yield a 350-mg/mL concentration for IM use.

For IV use, reconstitute the 250- and 500-mg vials with 2.4 and 4.8 mL, respectively, and the 1- and 2-g vials with 9.6 and 19.2 mL, respectively, of compatible diluent to yield a 100-mg/mL solution.

Reconstitute the 1- and 2-g infusion bottles with 10 and 20 mL, respectively, of compatible diluent. Then dilute further to 50 to 100 mL.

Administration: Administer by IM injection deep into a large muscle or by intermittent IV infusion over 15 to 30 minutes in adults or 10 to 30 minutes in pediatric patients.

Stability: Store intact vials at room temperature and protect from light. Solutions vary from light yellow to amber. Reconstituted solutions of 250 mg/mL are stable for 24 hours at room temperature or three days under refrigeration. Solutions of 100 mg/mL in most diluents are stable for three days at room temperature or 10 days under refrigeration.

Compatibility Table

Solutions	Compatible	Incompatible	Variable
Dextrose 5 & 10%	●	...	...
Dextrose 5% in sodium chloride 0.45 & 0.9%	...	...	●
Ringer's injection, lactated	...	...	●
Sodium chloride 0.9%	●	...	...

Drugs	Compatible	Incompatible	Variable
Acyclovir sodium	●	...	...
Allopurinol sodium	●	...	...
Amikacin sulfate	●	...	...
Aminophylline	...	●	...
Amiodarone HCl	●	...	...
Amphotericin B cholesteryl sulfate complex	...	●	...
Anakinra	...	...	●
Anidulafungin	●	...	...
Azithromycin	...	●	...
Aztreonam	●	...	...
Bivalirudin	●	...	...
Cisatracurium besylate	●	...	...
Clindamycin phosphate	...	●	...
Daptomycin	●	...	...
Dexmedetomidine HCl	●	...	...
Diltiazem HCl	●	...	...
Docetaxel	●	...	...
Doxorubicin HCl liposome injection	●	...	...
Drotrecogin alfa (activated)	●	...	...
Etoposide phosphate	●	...	...
Famotidine	●	...	...
Fenoldopam mesylate	●	...	...
Filgrastim	...	●	...
Fluconazole	...	●	...
Fludarabine phosphate	●	...	...
Foscarnet sodium	●	...	...
Gallium nitrate	●	...	...
Gemcitabine HCl	●	...	...
Gentamicin sulfate	...	...	●
Granisetron HCl	●	...	...
Heparin sodium	●	...	...
Hextend	●	...	...
Labetalol HCl	...	●	...
Lansoprazole	●	...	...
Lidocaine HCl	...	...	●
Linezolid	...	...	●
Melphalan HCl	●	...	...
Meperidine HCl	●	...	...

Drugs	Compatible	Incompatible	Variable
Methotrexate sodium	●	...	...
Metronidazole	●	...	...
Morphine sulfate	●	...	...
Paclitaxel	●	...	...
Pantoprazole sodium	●	...	...
Pemetrexed disodium	●	...	...
Pentamidine isethionate	...	●	...
Propofol	●	...	...
Remifentanil HCl	●	...	...
Sargramostim	●	...	...
Sodium bicarbonate	●	...	...
Tacrolimus	●	...	...
Teniposide	●	...	...
Theophylline	...	...	●
Thiotepa	●	...	...
Vancomycin HCl	...	...	●
Vinorelbine tartrate	...	●	...
Warfarin sodium	●	...	...
Zidovudine	●	...	...

Cefuroxime Sodium

Handbook on Injectable Drugs pp. 343–349.

Description: A semisynthetic cephalosporin antibiotic.

Products: **Kefurox, Zinacef;** 750-mg and 1.5-g sizes. *pH:* From 6 to 8.5 when reconstituted.

Preparation: Reconstitute the vials with sterile water for injection or use any compatible solution for the infusion packs:

Vial Size	Route	Diluent Volume	Approximate Concentration
750 mg	IM	3 mL	220 mg/mL
	IV	8 mL	90 mg/mL
(Inf. pack)	IV	100 mL	7.5 mg/mL
1.5 g	IV	16 mL	90 mg/mL
(Inf. pack)	IV	100 mL	15 mg/mL

Administration: Administer by deep IM or direct IV injection over three to five minutes or by continuous or intermittent IV infusion over 15 to 60 minutes.

Stability: Store intact vials at room temperature and protect from light. Solutions range from light yellow to amber; powder and solutions may darken without loss of potency.

Reconstituted solutions are stable for 24 hours at room temperature or 48 hours under refrigeration. Dilutions in dextrose 5% or sodium chloride 0.9% are stable for 48 hours at room temperature.

Compatibility Table

Solutions	Compatible	Incompatible	Variable
Dextrose 5 & 10%	●	...	...
Dextrose 5% in sodium chloride 0.2, 0.45, & 0.9%	●	...	...
Ringer's injection	●	...	...
Ringer's injection, lactated	●	...	...
Sodium chloride 0.9%	●	...	...

Drugs	Compatible	Incompatible	Variable
Acyclovir sodium	●	...	...
Allopurinol sodium	●	...	...
Amifostine	●	...	...
Amiodarone HCl	●	...	...
Anidulafungin	●	...	...
Atracurium besylate	●	...	...
Azithromycin	...	●	...
Aztreonam	●	...	...
Bivalirudin	●	...	...
Ciprofloxacin	...	●	...
Cisatracurium besylate	...	...	●
Clindamycin phosphate	●	...	...
Cyclophosphamide	●	...	...
Dexmedetomidine HCl	●	...	...
Diltiazem HCl	●	...	...
Dimenhydrinate	●	...	...
Docetaxel	●	...	...
Doxapram HCl	...	●	...
Etoposide phosphate	●	...	...
Famotidine	●	...	...
Fenoldopam mesylate	●	...	...
Filgrastim	...	●	...
Fluconazole	...	●	...
Fludarabine phosphate	●	...	...
Foscarnet sodium	●	...	...
Furosemide	●	...	...
Gemcitabine HCl	●	...	...
Gentamicin sulfate	...	...	●
Granisetron HCl	●	...	...
Heparin sodium	●	...	...
Hextend	●	...	...
Hydromorphone HCl	●	...	...
Linezolid	●	...	...
Melphalan HCl	●	...	...
Meperidine HCl	●	...	...
Metronidazole	●	...	...
Midazolam HCl	...	...	●
Milrinone lactate	●	...	...
Morphine sulfate	●	...	...
Ondansetron HCl	●	...	...

Drugs	Compatible	Incompatible	Variable
Pancuronium bromide	●	...	...
Pantoprazole sodium	...	●	...
Pemetrexed disodium	●	...	...
Potassium chloride	●	...	...
Propofol	●	...	...
Ranitidine HCl	...	...	●
Remifentanil HCl	●	...	...
Sargramostim	●	...	...
Sodium bicarbonate	...	...	●
Tacrolimus	●	...	...
Teniposide	●	...	...
Thiotepa	●	...	...
Vancomycin HCl	...	...	●
Vecuronium bromide	●	...	...
Vinorelbine tartrate	...	●	...

Chlorpromazine Hydrochloride

Handbook on Injectable Drugs pp. 363–370.

Description: A phenothiazine tranquilizer and antiemetic.

Products: **Thorazine;** 25-mg/mL solution in 1- and 2-mL ampuls and 10-mL multiple-dose vials. *pH:* From 3 to 5.

Preparation: For direct IV injection, dilute with sodium chloride 0.9% to a concentration not more than 1 mg/mL. For IV infusion, dilute in 500 to 1000 mL of sodium chloride 0.9%.

Administration: Administer by IM injection deep into a large muscle mass or by direct IV injection (when diluted) at 1 mg/min (adults) or 0.5 mg/min (children). It may be administered by slow IV infusion for intractable hiccups.

Stability: Protect from light to prevent discoloration. A slightly yellowed solution does not indicate potency loss, but a markedly discolored solution should be discarded. Alkaline solutions may cause oxidation and precipitation. Sorption to plastic bags and sets may occur.

Compatibility Table

Solutions	Compatible	Incompatible	Variable
Dextrose 5%	●	...	...
Dextrose 5% in Ringer's injection, lactated	●	...	...
Dextrose 5% in sodium chloride 0.2, 0.45, & 0.9%	●	...	...
Ringer's injection, lactated	●	...	...
Sodium chloride 0.45 & 0.9%	●	...	...

Drugs			
Allopurinol sodium	...	●	...
Amifostine	...	●	...
Aminophylline	...	●	...
Amphotericin B	...	●	...
Amphotericin B cholesteryl sulfate complex	...	●	...

Drugs	Compatible	Incompatible	Variable
Ampicillin sodium	...	●	...
Atropine sulfate	●	...	...
Aztreonam	...	●	...
Bivalirudin	...	●	...
Butorphanol tartrate	●	...	...
Cefepime HCl	...	●	...
Chlorothiazide sodium	...	●	...
Cimetidine HCl	...	●	...
Cisatracurium besylate	●	...	...
Cisplatin	●	...	...
Cladribine	●	...	...
Cloxacillin sodium	...	●	...
Cyclophosphamide	●	...	...
Cytarabine	●	...	...
Dexmedetomidine HCl	●	...	...
Dimenhydrinate	...	...	●
Diphenhydramine HCl	●	...	...
Docetaxel	●	...	...
Doxapram HCl	●	...	...
Doxorubicin HCl	●	...	...
Doxorubicin HCl liposome injection	●	...	...
Droperidol	●	...	...
Etoposide phosphate	...	●	...
Famotidine	●	...	...
Fenoldopam mesylate	●	...	...
Fentanyl citrate	●	...	...
Filgrastim	●	...	...
Fluconazole	●	...	...
Fludarabine phosphate	...	●	...
Furosemide	...	●	...
Gemcitabine HCl	●	...	...
Glycopyrrolate	●	...	...
Granisetron HCl	●	...	...
Heparin sodium	...	...	●
Hextend	●	...	...
Hydrocortisone sodium succinate	●	...	...
Hydromorphone HCl	●	...	...
Hydroxyzine HCl	●	...	...
Lansoprazole	...	●	...

Drugs	Compatible	Incompatible	Variable
Linezolid	●	…	…
Melphalan HCl	…	●	…
Meperidine HCl	●	…	…
Methohexital sodium	…	●	…
Methotrexate sodium	…	●	…
Metoclopramide HCl	●	…	…
Midazolam HCl	●	…	…
Morphine sulfate	…	…	●
Ondansetron HCl	●	…	…
Oxaliplatin	●	…	…
Paclitaxel	…	●	…
Pantoprazole sodium	…	●	…
Pemetrexed disodium	…	●	…
Penicillin G potassium & sodium	…	●	…
Pentazocine lactate	●	…	…
Pentobarbital sodium	…	●	…
Phenobarbital sodium	…	●	…
Piperacillin sod.–tazobactam sod.	…	●	…
Potassium chloride	●	…	…
Prochlorperazine edisylate	●	…	…
Promethazine HCl	●	…	…
Propofol	●	…	…
Ranitidine HCl	…	…	●
Remifentanil HCl	…	…	●
Sargramostim	…	●	…
Scopolamine HBr	●	…	…
Teniposide	●	…	…
Theophylline	●	…	…
Thiopental sodium	…	●	…
Vinorelbine tartrate	●	…	…

Cimetidine Hydrochloride

Handbook on Injectable Drugs pp. 372–386.

Description: A histamine H_2 receptor antagonist.

Products: **Tagamet;** 150-mg/mL solution in 2-mL single-dose vials and 8-mL multiple-dose vials as well as a premixed infusion of 300 mg/50 mL in sodium chloride 0.9%. *pH:* From 3.8 to 6.

Preparation: For direct IV injection, dilute the dose to 20 mL with sodium chloride 0.9% or another compatible diluent. For intermittent IV infusion, dilute the dose in at least 50 mL of compatible diluent, or for continuous IV infusion, dilute in 100 to 1000 mL of compatible diluent.

Administration: Administer by IM injection, direct IV injection (when diluted) over five minutes or longer, or intermittent IV infusion over 15 to 20 minutes.

Stability: Store intact vials at room temperature protected from light and excessive heat. Exposure to cold may result in precipitation, but the drug can be redissolved by warming. Frozen IV admixtures are stable for 30 days. No sorption to plastic bags, sets, or syringes has been noted.

Compatibility Table

Solutions	Compatible	Incompatible	Variable
Dextrose 5%	●	...	...
Dextrose 5% in Ringer's injection, lactated	●	...	...
Dextrose 5% in sodium chloride 0.2, 0.45, & 0.9%	●	...	...
Ringer's injection	●	...	...
Ringer's injection, lactated	●	...	...
Sodium chloride 0.9%	●	...	...

Drugs			
Acetazolamide sodium	●	...	...
Acyclovir sodium	●	...	...
Allopurinol sodium	...	●	...
Amifostine	●	...	...
Amikacin sulfate	●	...	...

Drugs	Compatible	Incompatible	Variable
Aminophylline	●	...	...
Amphotericin B	...	●	...
Amphotericin B cholesteryl sulfate complex	...	●	...
Ampicillin sodium	...	...	●
Anakinra	●	...	...
Anidulafungin	●	...	...
Atracurium besylate	●	...	...
Atropine sulfate	●	...	...
Aztreonam	●	...	...
Bivalirudin	●	...	...
Butorphanol tartrate	●	...	...
Caffeine citrate	●	...	...
Cefamandole nafate	...	...	●
Cefazolin sodium	...	...	●
Cefepime HCl	...	●	...
Cefoxitin sodium	●	...	...
Chlorothiazide sodium	●	...	...
Chlorpromazine HCl	...	●	...
Ciprofloxacin	●	...	...
Cisatracurium besylate	●	...	...
Cisplatin	●	...	...
Cladribine	●	...	...
Clindamycin phosphate	●	...	...
Colistimethate sodium	●	...	...
Cyclophosphamide	●	...	...
Cytarabine	●	...	...
Dexamethasone sodium succinate	●	...	...
Dexmedetomidine HCl	●	...	...
Diazepam	●	...	...
Digoxin	●	...	...
Diltiazem HCl	●	...	...
Diphenhydramine HCl	●	...	...
Docetaxel	●	...	...
Doxapram HCl	●	...	...
Doxorubicin HCl	●	...	...
Doxorubicin HCl liposome inj.	●	...	...
Droperidol	●	...	...
Enalaprilat	●	...	...
Epinephrine HCl	●	...	...

Drugs	Compatible	Incompatible	Variable
Erythromycin lactobionate	●	...	...
Esmolol HCl	●	...	...
Ethacrynate sodium	●	...	...
Etoposide phosphate	●	...	...
Fenoldopam mesylate	●	...	...
Fentanyl citrate	●	...	...
Filgrastim	●	...	...
Fluconazole	●	...	...
Fludarabine phosphate	●	...	...
Flumazenil	●	...	...
Foscarnet sodium	●	...	...
Furosemide	●	...	...
Gallium nitrate	●	...	...
Gemcitabine HCl	●	...	...
Gentamicin sulfate	●	...	...
Glycopyrrolate	●	...	...
Granisetron HCl	●	...	...
Haloperidol lactate	●	...	...
Heparin sodium	●	...	...
Hetastarch in sodium chloride 0.9%	●	...	...
Hextend	●	...	...
Hydromorphone HCl	●	...	...
Hydroxyzine HCl	●	...	...
Idarubicin HCl	●	...	...
Indomethacin sod. trihydrate	...	●	...
Insulin, regular	●	...	...
Isoproterenol HCl	●	...	...
Labetalol HCl	●	...	...
Lansoprazole	...	●	...
Levofloxacin	●	...	...
Linezolid	●	...	...
Lidocaine HCl	●	...	...
Lincomycin HCl	●	...	...
Lorazepam	●	...	...
Melphalan HCl	●	...	...
Meperidine HCl	●	...	...
Meropenem	●	...	...
Methotrexate sodium	●	...	...
Methylprednisolone sod. succ.	●	...	...
Metoclopramide HCl	...	...	●

Drugs	Compatible	Incompatible	Variable
Midazolam HCl	●	...	...
Milrinone lactate	●	...	...
Morphine sulfate	●	...	...
Nafcillin sodium	●	...	...
Nalbuphine HCl	●	...	...
Nicardipine HCl	●	...	...
Norepinephrine bitartrate	●	...	...
Ondansetron HCl	●	...	...
Oxaliplatin	●	...	...
Paclitaxel	●	...	...
Pancuronium bromide	●	...	...
Pemetrexed disodium	●	...	...
Penicillin G pot. & sod.	●	...	...
Pentazocine lactate	●	...	...
Pentobarbital sodium	...	●	...
Phytonadione	●	...	...
Piperacillin sod.–tazobactam sod.	●	...	...
Polymyxin B sulfate	●	...	...
Potassium chloride	●	...	...
Prochlorperazine edisylate	●	...	...
Promethazine HCl	●	...	...
Propofol	●	...	...
Protamine sulfate	●	...	...
Quinidine gluconate	●	...	...
Remifentanil HCl	●	...	...
Sargramostim	●	...	...
Scopolamine HBr	●	...	...
Sodium acetate	●	...	...
Sodium lactate	●	...	...
Sodium nitroprusside	●	...	...
Tacrolimus	●	...	...
Teniposide	●	...	...
Theophylline	●	...	...
Thiotepa	●	...	...
Topotecan HCl	●	...	...
Vancomycin HCl	●	...	...
Vecuronium bromide	●	...	...
Verapamil HCl	●	...	...
Vinorelbine tartrate	●	...	...
Warfarin sodium	...	●	...
Zidovudine	●	...	...

Ciprofloxacin

Handbook on Injectable Drugs pp. 386–395.

Description: A synthetic quinolone anti-infective.

Products: **Cipro I.V.;** 10 mg/mL in 20- and 40-mL vials and also premixed, ready-to-use, 2 mg/mL in 100- and 200-mL containers. *pH:* Vials, 3.3 to 3.9; bags, 3.5 to 4.6.

Preparation: For IV use, dilute to a final concentration of 1 or 2 mg/mL with a compatible diluent.

Administration: Administer by intermittent IV infusion slowly into a large vein over 60 minutes.

Stability: The solution is clear and colorless to slightly yellow. It should be protected from excessive heat and freezing. No sorption to plastic bags or sets has been noted.

Compatibility Table

Solutions	Compatible	Incompatible	Variable
Dextrose 5 & 10%	●	…	…
Dextrose 5% in sodium chloride 0.2 & 0.45%	●	…	…
Ringer's injection	●	…	…
Ringer's injection, lactated	●	…	…
Sodium chloride 0.9%	●	…	…

Drugs	Compatible	Incompatible	Variable
Amifostine	●	…	…
Amikacin sulfate	●	…	…
Aminophylline	…	●	…
Amiodarone HCl	●	…	…
Amphotericin B	…	●	…
Ampicillin sod.–sulbactam sod.	…	●	…
Anidulafungin	●	…	…
Atracurium besylate	●	…	…
Azithromycin	…	●	…
Aztreonam	●	…	…
Bivalirudin	●	…	…
Calcium gluconate	●	…	…
Cefepime HCl	…	●	…
Ceftazidime	…	…	●
Cefuroxime sodium	…	●	…

Drugs	Compatible	Incompatible	Variable
Cimetidine HCl	●	...	...
Cisatracurium besylate	●	...	...
Clindamycin phosphate	...	●	...
Cyclosporine	●	...	...
Dexamethasone sodium phosphate ...	...	●	...
Dexmedetomidine HCl	●	...	...
Digoxin	●	...	...
Diltiazem HCl	●	...	...
Dimenhydrinate	●	...	...
Diphenhydramine HCl	●	...	...
Dobutamine HCl	●	...	...
Docetaxel	●	...	...
Dopamine HCl	●	...	...
Doxorubicin HCl liposome injection	●	...	...
Drotrecogin alfa (activated)	...	●	...
Etoposide phosphate	●	...	...
Fenoldopam mesylate	●	...	...
Fluconazole	●	...	...
Furosemide	...	●	...
Gallium nitrate	●	...	...
Gemcitabine HCl	●	...	...
Gentamicin sulfate	●	...	...
Heparin sodium	...	●	...
Hextend	●	...	...
Hydrocortisone sodium succinate	...	●	...
Hydroxyzine HCl	●	...	...
Lansoprazole	...	●	...
Lidocaine HCl	●	...	...
Linezolid	●	...	...
Lorazepam	●	...	...
Magnesium sulfate	...	...	●
Methylprednisolone sod. succ.	...	●	...
Metoclopramide HCl	●	...	...
Metronidazole	●	...	...
Metronidazole HCl	...	●	...
Midazolam HCl	●	...	...
Milrinone lactate	●	...	...
Norepinephrine bitartrate	●	...	...
Pancuronium bromide	●	...	...

Drugs	Compatible	Incompatible	Variable
Pantoprazole sodium	...	●	...
Pemetrexed disodium	...	●	...
Phenytoin sodium	...	●	...
Piperacillin sodium	...	...	●
Potassium acetate & chloride	●	...	...
Potassium phosphates	...	●	...
Promethazine HCl	●	...	...
Propofol	...	●	...
Quinupristin–dalfopristin	●	...	...
Ranitidine HCl	●	...	...
Remifentanil HCl	●	...	...
Sodium bicarbonate	...	...	●
Sodium phosphates	...	...	●
Tacrolimus	●	...	...
Teniposide	●	...	...
Thiotepa	●	...	...
Ticarcillin disodium–clavulanate potassium	...	...	●
Tobramycin sulfate	●	...	...
Vecuronium bromide	●	...	...
Verapamil HCl	●	...	...
Warfarin sodium	...	●	...

Ciprofloxacin

Cisatracurium Besylate

Handbook on Injectable Drugs pp. 395–403.

Description: A synthetic, nondepolarizing, neuromuscular blocking agent.

Products: **Nimbex;** 2 mg/mL in 5- and 10-mL vials and 10 mg/mL in 20-mL vials. *pH:* From 3.25 to 3.65.

Administration: Administer intravenously only. Both bolus doses and continuous infusion have been used. The rate of administration depends on the drug concentration, desired dose, and patient weight.

Stability: The clear slightly yellow or greenish-yellow solution should be stored under refrigeration and protected from light and freezing. Losses of 5% per month are stated to occur when stored at room temperature; use within 21 days is recommended if the vials are warmed to room temperature. However, research studies indicate the potency is retained through 45 days at room temperature. Cisatracurium besylate is stable for at least 24 hours in compatible infusion solutions at concentrations as low as 0.1 mg/mL. Contact with alkaline drugs and solutions should be avoided during administration.

Compatibility Table

Solutions	Compatible	Incompatible	Variable
Dextrose 5%	●	...	...
Dextrose 5% in lactated Ringer's injection	...	...	●
Dextrose 5% in sodium chloride 0.9%	●	...	...
Sodium chloride 0.9%	●	...	...

Drugs	Compatible	Incompatible	Variable
Acyclovir sodium	...	...	●
Alfentanil HCl	●	...	...
Amikacin sulfate	●	...	...
Aminophylline	...	...	●
Amphotericin B	...	...	●
Amphotericin B cholesteryl sulfate complex	...	●	...
Ampicillin sodium	...	...	●
Ampicillin sod.–sulbactam sod.	...	...	●
Aztreonam	●	...	...

Drugs	Compatible	Incompatible	Variable
Bumetanide	●	...	...
Buprenorphine HCl	●	...	...
Butorphanol tartrate	●	...	...
Calcium gluconate	●	...	...
Cefazolin sodium	...	...	●
Cefotaxime sodium	...	...	●
Cefotetan disodium	...	...	●
Cefoxitin sodium	...	...	●
Ceftazidime	...	...	●
Ceftizoxime sodium	...	...	●
Ceftriaxone sodium	●	...	...
Cefuroxime sodium	...	...	●
Chlorpromazine HCl	●	...	...
Cimetidine HCl	●	...	...
Ciprofloxacin	●	...	...
Clindamycin phosphate	●	...	...
Dexamethasone sodium phosphate ...	●	...	...
Dexmedetomidine HCl	●	...	...
Diazepam	...	...	●
Digoxin	●	...	...
Diphenhydramine HCl	●	...	...
Dobutamine HCl	●	...	...
Dopamine HCl	●	...	...
Doxycycline hyclate	●	...	...
Droperidol	●	...	...
Drotrecogin alfa (activated)	●	...	...
Enalaprilat	●	...	...
Epinephrine HCl	●	...	...
Esmolol HCl	●	...	...
Famotidine	●	...	...
Fenoldopam mesylate	●	...	...
Fentanyl citrate	●	...	...
Fluconazole	●	...	...
Furosemide	...	...	●
Ganciclovir sodium	...	...	●
Gentamicin sulfate	●	...	...
Haloperidol lactate	●	...	...
Heparin sodium	...	...	●
Hextend	●	...	...
Hydrocortisone sodium succinate	●	...	...

Drugs	Compatible	Incompatible	Variable
Hydromorphone HCl	●	...	...
Hydroxyzine HCl	●	...	...
Imipenem–cilastatin sodium	●	...	...
Isoproterenol HCl	●	...	...
Ketorolac tromethamine	...	...	●
Lidocaine HCl	●	...	...
Linezolid	●	...	...
Lorazepam	●	...	...
Magnesium sulfate	●	...	...
Mannitol	●	...	...
Meperidine HCl	●	...	...
Methylprednisolone sod. succ.	...	...	●
Metoclopramide HCl	●	...	...
Metronidazole	●	...	...
Midazolam HCl	●	...	...
Morphine sulfate	●	...	...
Nalbuphine HCl	●	...	...
Nitroglycerin	●	...	...
Norepinephrine HCl	●	...	...
Ondansetron HCl	●	...	...
Phenylephrine HCl	●	...	...
Piperacillin sodium	...	...	●
Piperacillin sod.–tazobactam sod.	...	...	●
Potassium chloride	●	...	...
Procainamide HCl	●	...	...
Prochlorperazine edisylate	●	...	...
Promethazine HCl	●	...	...
Propofol	...	●	...
Ranitidine HCl	●	...	...
Remifentanil HCl	●	...	...
Sodium bicarbonate	...	...	●
Sodium nitroprusside	...	...	●
Sufentanil citrate	●	...	...
Theophylline	●	...	...
Thiopental sodium	...	...	●
Ticarcillin disod.–clavulanate pot.	...	...	●
Tobramycin sulfate	●	...	...
Trimethoprim–sulfamethoxazole	...	...	●
Vancomycin HCl	●	...	...
Zidovudine	●	...	...

Cisplatin

Handbook on Injectable Drugs pp. 404–413.

Description: A platinum-containing antineoplastic agent.

Products: **Platinol-AQ;** 1 mg/mL in 50-, 100-, and 200-mL vials. *pH:* From 3.9 to 5.0.

Preparation: For IV infusion, dilute the dose in 1 to 2 L of compatible infusion solution containing mannitol 18.75 g/L. NOTE: Because of possible skin reactions, gloves should be worn during preparation.

Administration: Administer by IV infusion in 1 to 2 L of compatible infusion solution over variable time periods from one or two hours up to several days, depending on the regimen, with adequate hydration.

Stability: The injection is clear and colorless and should be stored at room temperature and protected from light. Do not refrigerate because of possible precipitation. To be stable in aqueous solutions, cisplatin requires at least 0.2% sodium chloride. Decomposition occurs in solutions having a lower chloride content.

Cisplatin may react with the metal aluminum to form a black precipitate. Therefore equipment (e.g., needles, syringes, catheters, etc.) containing aluminum should not be used for preparation and administration of cisplatin.

Compatibility Table

Solutions	Compatible	Incompatible	Variable
Dextrose 5%	...	●	...
Dextrose 5% in sodium chloride 0.2, 0.45, & 0.9%	●	...	...
Sodium bicarbonate	...	●	...
Sodium chloride 0.2, 0.3, 0.45, & 0.9%	●	...	...

Drugs			
Allopurinol sodium	●	...	...
Amifostine	...	●	...
Amphotericin B cholesteryl sulfate complex	...	●	...
Aztreonam	●	...	...

Drugs	Compatible	Incompatible	Variable
Bleomycin sulfate	●	…	…
Cefepime HCl	…	●	…
Chlorpromazine HCl	●	…	…
Cimetidine HCl	●	…	…
Cladribine	●	…	…
Cyclophosphamide	●	…	…
Dexamethasone sodium phosphate	●	…	…
Diphenhydramine HCl	●	…	…
Doxapram HCl	●	…	…
Doxorubicin HCl	●	…	…
Doxorubicin HCl liposome injection	●	…	…
Droperidol	●	…	…
Etoposide	…	…	●
Etoposide phosphate	●	…	…
Famotidine	●	…	…
Filgrastim	●	…	…
Fludarabine phosphate	●	…	…
Fluorouracil	…	…	●
Furosemide	●	…	…
Gallium nitrate	…	●	…
Ganciclovir sodium	●	…	…
Gemcitabine HCl	●	…	…
Granisetron HCl	●	…	…
Heparin sodium	●	…	…
Hydromorphone HCl	●	…	…
Hydroxyzine HCl	●	…	…
Ifosfamide	●	…	…
Lansoprazole	…	●	…
Leucovorin calcium	●	…	…
Linezolid	●	…	…
Lorazepam	●	…	…
Magnesium sulfate	●	…	…
Mannitol	…	…	●
Melphalan HCl	●	…	…
Mesna	…	●	…
Methotrexate sodium	●	…	…
Methylprednisolone sod. succ.	●	…	…
Metoclopramide HCl	●	…	…
Mitomycin	●	…	…

Drugs	Compatible	Incompatible	Variable
Morphine sulfate	●	...	...
Ondansetron HCl	●	...	...
Paclitaxel	...	...	●
Palonosetron HCl	●	...	...
Pemetrexed disodium	●	...	...
Piperacillin sod.–tazobactam sod.	...	●	...
Prochlorperazine edisylate	●	...	...
Promethazine HCl	●	...	...
Propofol	●	...	...
Ranitidine HCl	●	...	...
Sulfites	...	●	...
Teniposide	●	...	...
Thiotepa	...	●	...
Topotecan HCl	●	...	...
Vinblastine sulfate	●	...	...
Vincristine sulfate	●	...	...
Vinorelbine tartrate	●	...	...

Cladribine

Handbook on Injectable Drugs pp. 413–417.

Description: A synthetic purine nucleoside antineoplastic agent.

Products: **Leustatin;** 1 mg/mL in 10-mL vials. *pH:* From 5.5 to 8.

Preparation: The injection is a concentrate that must be diluted. Daily doses are diluted in 500 mL of sodium chloride 0.9% for administration. Do not use dextrose 5%. For a continuous single infusion over seven days, cladribine may be diluted in 100 mL of bacteriostatic sodium chloride 0.9% containing benzyl alcohol 0.9%, adding both drug and diluent through 0.22-μm filters.

Administration: Administer by continuous IV infusion after dilution.

Stability: Store under refrigeration protected from light. The drug is a clear, colorless solution. A precipitate may form upon low-temperature storage; it may be redissolved by warming to room temperature with vigorous shaking. Heating is not recommended. Freezing does not adversely affect product stability.

Admixtures in sodium chloride 0.9% are stable for at least 24 hours at room temperature exposed to fluorescent light. Use of dextrose 5% results in increased rates of decomposition. At a concentration of 0.15 to 0.3 mg/mL in bacteriostatic sodium chloride 0.9% preserved with benzyl alcohol, cladribine is stable for at least 14 days.

Compatibility Table

Solutions	Compatible	Incompatible	Variable
Dextrose 5%	...	●	...
Sodium chloride 0.9%	●	...	...

Drugs			
Aminophylline	●	...	...
Bumetanide	●	...	...
Buprenorphine HCl	●	...	...
Butorphanol tartrate	●	...	...
Calcium gluconate	●	...	...

Drugs	Compatible	Incompatible	Variable
Carboplatin	●	...	...
Chlorpromazine HCl	●	...	...
Cimetidine HCl	●	...	...
Cisplatin	●	...	...
Cyclophosphamide	●	...	...
Cytarabine	●	...	...
Dexamethasone sodium phosphate	●	...	...
Diphenhydramine HCl	●	...	...
Dobutamine HCl	●	...	...
Dopamine HCl	●	...	...
Doxorubicin HCl	●	...	...
Droperidol	●	...	...
Enalaprilat	●	...	...
Etoposide	●	...	...
Famotidine	●	...	...
Furosemide	●	...	...
Gallium nitrate	●	...	...
Granisetron HCl	●	...	...
Haloperidol lactate	●	...	...
Heparin sodium	●	...	...
Hydrocortisone sodium phosphate	●	...	...
Hydrocortisone sodium succinate	●	...	...
Hydromorphone HCl	●	...	...
Hydroxyzine HCl	●	...	...
Idarubicin HCl	●	...	...
Leucovorin calcium	●	...	...
Lorazepam	●	...	...
Mannitol	●	...	...
Meperidine HCl	●	...	...
Mesna	●	...	...
Methylprednisolone sod. succ.	●	...	...
Metoclopramide HCl	●	...	...
Mitoxantrone HCl	●	...	...
Morphine sulfate	●	...	...
Nalbuphine HCl	●	...	...
Ondansetron HCl	●	...	...
Paclitaxel	●	...	...
Potassium chloride	●	...	...
Prochlorperazine edisylate	●	...	...
Promethazine HCl	●	...	...
Ranitidine HCl	●	...	...
Sodium bicarbonate	●	...	...
Teniposide	●	...	...
Vincristine sulfate	●	...	...

Clindamycin Phosphate

Handbook on Injectable Drugs pp. 420–431.

Description: A semisynthetic antibiotic derived from lincomycin.

Products: Cleocin Phosphate; 150-mg/mL solution in 2-, 4-, and 6-mL vials and in premixed 50-mL minibags of 300, 600, and 900 mg in dextrose 5%. *pH:* From 5.5 to 7.

Preparation: For intermittent IV infusion, dilute with a compatible diluent to a concentration of 18 mg/mL or less.

Administration: Administer IM or by IV infusion. Do not administer as an IV bolus. For a single IM injection, no more than 600 mg is recommended. For IV infusion, administer at a rate not exceeding 30 mg/min. Clindamycin phosphate also may be administered by continuous infusion.

Stability: Store intact vials at room temperature. Crystallization may occur during refrigeration. The crystals resolubilize upon warming to room temperature. Frozen solutions are reported to be stable for up to eight weeks. No sorption to plastic bags has been noted.

Compatibility Table

Solutions	Compatible	Incompatible	Variable
Dextrose 5 & 10%	●	...	...
Dextrose 5% in Ringer's injection	●	...	...
Dextrose 5% in sodium chloride 0.45 & 0.9%	●	...	...
Ringer's injection, lactated	●	...	...
Sodium chloride 0.9%	●	...	...

Drugs	Compatible	Incompatible	Variable
Acyclovir sodium	●	...	...
Allopurinol sodium	...	●	...
Amifostine	●	...	...
Amikacin sulfate	●	...	...
Aminophylline	...	●	...
Amiodarone HCl	●	...	...
Amphotericin B cholesteryl sulfate complex	●	...	...
Ampicillin sodium	...	...	●
Anakinra	●	...	...

Drugs	Compatible	Incompatible	Variable
Azithromycin	...	●	...
Aztreonam	●	...	...
Barbiturates	...	●	...
Bivalirudin	●	...	...
Caffeine citrate	●	...	...
Calcium gluconate	...	●	...
Cefamandole nafate	●	...	...
Cefazolin sodium	●	...	...
Cefepime HCl	●	...	...
Cefotaxime sodium	●	...	...
Cefoxitin sodium	●	...	...
Ceftazidime	●	...	...
Ceftizoxime sodium	●	...	...
Ceftriaxone sodium	...	●	...
Cefuroxime sodium	●	...	...
Cimetidine HCl	●	...	...
Ciprofloxacin	...	●	...
Cisatracurium besylate	●	...	...
Cyclophosphamide	●	...	...
Dexmedetomidine HCl	●	...	...
Diltiazem HCl	●	...	...
Dimenhydrinate	●	...	...
Docetaxel	●	...	...
Doxapram HCl	...	●	...
Doxorubicin HCl liposome injection	●	...	...
Drotrecogin alfa (activated)	...	...	●
Enalaprilat	●	...	...
Esmolol HCl	●	...	...
Etoposide phosphate	●	...	...
Fenoldopam mesylate	●	...	...
Filgrastim	...	●	...
Fluconazole	...	...	●
Fludarabine phosphate	●	...	...
Foscarnet sodium	●	...	...
Gemcitabine HCl	●	...	...
Gentamicin sulfate	...	...	●
Granisetron HCl	●	...	...
Heparin sodium	●	...	...
Hextend	●	...	...
Hydrocortisone sodium succinate	●	...	...

Drugs	Compatible	Incompatible	Variable
Hydromorphone HCl	●	...	...
Idarubicin HCl	...	●	...
Kanamycin sulfate	●	...	...
Labetalol HCl	●	...	...
Lansoprazole	...	●	...
Levofloxacin	●	...	...
Linezolid	●	...	...
Magnesium sulfate	...	...	●
Melphalan HCl	●	...	...
Meperidine HCl	●	...	...
Methylprednisolone sod. succ.	●	...	...
Metoclopramide HCl	●	...	...
Metronidazole	●	...	...
Midazolam HCl	●	...	...
Milrinone lactate	●	...	...
Morphine sulfate	●	...	...
Multivitamins	●	...	...
Nicardipine HCl	●	...	...
Ondansetron HCl	●	...	...
Pantoprazole sodium	...	●	...
Pemetrexed disodium	●	...	...
Phenytoin sodium	...	●	...
Piperacillin sodium	●	...	...
Piperacillin sod.–tazobactam sod.	●	...	...
Potassium chloride	●	...	...
Propofol	●	...	...
Ranitidine HCl	...	...	●
Remifentanil HCl	●	...	...
Sargramostim	●	...	...
Sodium bicarbonate	●	...	...
Tacrolimus	●	...	...
Teniposide	●	...	...
Theophylline	●	...	...
Thiotepa	●	...	...
Tobramycin sulfate	...	...	●
Verapamil HCl	●	...	...
Vinorelbine tartrate	●	...	...
Zidovudine	●	...	...

Cyclophosphamide

Handbook on Injectable Drugs pp. 450–458.

Description: An antineoplastic related to nitrogen mustard which acts as an alkylating agent after metabolic conversion.

Products: **Cytoxan, Neosar;** 100-, 200-, and 500-mg and 1- and 2-g vials in lyophilized form. *pH:* From 3 to 9 when reconstituted.

Preparation: Reconstitute with sterile water for injection or bacteriostatic water for injection (paraben preserved only) in the amounts noted on the label. Shake to dissolve the powder. The solutions contain cyclophosphamide 20 to 25 mg/mL.

Administration: Administer by direct IV injection or continuous or intermittent infusion, IM, intraperitoneally, or intrapleurally.

Stability: Store the vials at 25 °C or less. Reconstituted solutions should be used within 24 hours if stored at room temperature or within six days if refrigerated. Frozen storage results in a 0 to 3% loss in four weeks and a 4 to 8% loss in 19 weeks.

Compatibility Table

Solutions	Compatible	Incompatible	Variable
Dextrose 5%	●	…	…
Dextrose 5% in Ringer's injection	●	…	…
Dextrose 5% in sodium chloride 0.9%	●	…	…
Ringer's injection, lactated	●	…	…
Sodium chloride 0.45 & 0.9%	●	…	…

Drugs			
Allopurinol sodium	●	…	…
Amifostine	●	…	…
Amikacin sulfate	●	…	…
Amphotericin B cholesteryl sulfate complex	…	●	…
Ampicillin sodium	●	…	…
Aztreonam	●	…	…
Bleomycin sulfate	●	…	…
Cefamandole nafate	●	…	…
Cefazolin sodium	●	…	…

Drugs	Compatible	Incompatible	Variable
Cefepime HCl	●	...	...
Cefotaxime sodium	●	...	...
Cefoxitin sodium	●	...	...
Cefuroxime sodium	●	...	...
Chloramphenicol sodium succinate	●	...	...
Chlorpromazine HCl	●	...	...
Cimetidine HCl	●	...	...
Cisplatin	●	...	...
Cladribine	●	...	...
Clindamycin phosphate	●	...	...
Dacarbazine	●	...	...
Dexamethasone sodium phosphate	●	...	...
Diphenhydramine HCl	●	...	...
Doxapram HCl	●	...	...
Doxorubicin HCl	●	...	...
Doxorubicin HCl liposome injection	●	...	...
Doxycycline hyclate	●	...	...
Droperidol	●	...	...
Erythromycin lactobionate	●	...	...
Etoposide phosphate	●	...	...
Famotidine	●	...	...
Filgrastim	●	...	...
Fludarabine phosphate	●	...	...
Fluorouracil	●	...	...
Furosemide	●	...	...
Gallium nitrate	●	...	...
Ganciclovir sodium	●	...	...
Gemcitabine HCl	●	...	...
Gentamicin sulfate	●	...	...
Granisetron HCl	●	...	...
Heparin sodium	●	...	...
Hydromorphone HCl	●	...	...
Hydroxyzine HCl	●	...	...
Idarubicin HCl	●	...	...
Kanamycin sulfate	●	...	...
Lansoprazole	...	●	...
Leucovorin sodium	●	...	...
Linezolid	●	...	...
Lorazepam	●	...	...

Drugs	Compatible	Incompatible	Variable
Melphalan HCl	•	...	...
Mesna	...	...	•
Methotrexate sodium	•	...	...
Methylprednisolone sod. succ.	•	...	...
Metoclopramide HCl	•	...	...
Metronidazole	•	...	...
Mitomycin	•	...	...
Mitoxantrone HCl	•	...	...
Morphine sulfate	•	...	...
Nafcillin sodium	•	...	...
Ondansetron HCl	•	...	...
Oxacillin sodium	•	...	...
Oxaliplatin	•	...	...
Paclitaxel	•	...	...
Pemetrexed disodium	•	...	...
Penicillin G potassium	•	...	...
Piperacillin sodium	•	...	...
Piperacillin sod.–tazobactam sod.	•	...	...
Prochlorperazine edisylate	•	...	...
Promethazine HCl	•	...	...
Propofol	•	...	...
Ranitidine HCl	•	...	...
Sargramostim	•	...	...
Sodium bicarbonate	•	...	...
Teniposide	•	...	...
Thiotepa	•	...	...
Ticarcillin disod.–clavulanate pot.	•	...	...
Tobramycin sulfate	•	...	...
Topotecan HCl	•	...	...
Trimethoprim–sulfamethoxazole	•	...	...
Vancomycin HCl	•	...	...
Vinblastine sulfate	•	...	...
Vincristine sulfate	•	...	...
Vinorelbine tartrate	•	...	...

Cytarabine

Handbook on Injectable Drugs pp. 461–467.

Description: A synthetic nucleoside antineoplastic agent.

Products: **Cytosar-U;** 100-mg, 500-mg, 1-g, and 2-g multiple-dose vials. *pH:* 4 to 6 (lyophilized); 7 to 9 (commercial solution).

Preparation: Reconstitute with bacteriostatic water for injection containing benzyl alcohol. (Do not use this diluent for intrathecal use.) Use 5 mL for the 100-mg vial to yield a 20-mg/mL solution. Use 10 mL for the 500-mg vial to yield a 50-mg/mL solution. Reconstitute the 1- and 2-g vials with 10 and 20 mL, respectively, to yield a 100-mg/mL solution. For IV infusion, the dose may be further diluted in a compatible diluent such as dextrose 5% or sodium chloride 0.9%.

Administration: Administer by direct IV injection, IV infusion, IM or SC injection, or intrathecal injection.

Stability: Store intact vials at room temperature. Reconstituted solutions are stable for at least 48 hours at room temperature. Solutions with a haze should be discarded. No sorption to plastic containers has been found.

Compatibility Table

Solutions	Compatible	Incompatible	Variable
Dextrose 5%	●	...	...
Dextrose 5% in Ringer's injection, lactated	●	...	...
Dextrose 5% in sodium chloride 0.2 & 0.9%	●	...	...
Ringer's injection, lactated	●	...	...
Sodium chloride 0.9%	●	...	...

Drugs			
Allopurinol sodium	...	●	...
Amifostine	●	...	...
Amphotericin B cholesteryl sulfate complex	...	●	...
Aztreonam	●	...	...

Drugs	Compatible	Incompatible	Variable
Cefepime HCl	●	...	...
Chlorpromazine HCl	●	...	...
Cimetidine HCl	●	...	...
Cladribine	●	...	...
Daunorubicin HCl	●	...	...
Dexamethasone sodium phosphate	●	...	...
Diphenhydramine HCl	●	...	...
Doxorubicin HCl liposome injection	●	...	...
Droperidol	●	...	...
Etoposide	●	...	...
Etoposide phosphate	●	...	...
Famotidine	●	...	...
Filgrastim	●	...	...
Fludarabine phosphate	●	...	...
Fluorouracil	...	●	...
Furosemide	●	...	...
Gallium nitrate	...	●	...
Ganciclovir sodium	...	●	...
Gemcitabine HCl	●	...	...
Gentamicin sulfate	...	...	●
Granisetron HCl	●	...	...
Heparin sodium	...	...	●
Hydrocortisone sodium succinate	...	...	●
Hydromorphone HCl	●	...	...
Hydroxyzine HCl	●	...	...
Idarubicin HCl	●	...	...
Insulin, regular	...	●	...
Lansoprazole	...	●	...
Lincomycin HCl	●	...	...
Linezolid	●	...	...
Lorazepam	●	...	...
Melphalan HCl	●	...	...
Methotrexate sodium	●	...	...
Methylprednisolone sod. succ.	...	...	●
Metoclopramide HCl	●	...	...
Mitoxantrone HCl	●	...	...
Morphine sulfate	●	...	...
Nafcillin sodium	...	●	...
Ondansetron HCl	●	...	...

Cytarabine

Drugs	Compatible	Incompatible	Variable
Oxacillin sodium	...	●	...
Paclitaxel	●	...	...
Pemetrexed disodium	●	...	...
Penicillin G sodium	...	●	...
Piperacillin sod.–tazobactam sod.	●	...	...
Potassium chloride	●	...	...
Prochlorperazine edisylate	●	...	...
Promethazine HCl	●	...	...
Propofol	●	...	...
Ranitidine HCl	●	...	...
Sargramostim	●	...	...
Sodium bicarbonate	●	...	...
Teniposide	●	...	...
Thiotepa	●	...	...
Vincristine sulfate	●	...	...
Vinorelbine tartrate	●	...	...

Daptomycin

Handbook on Injectable Drugs pp. 474–475.

Description: A cyclic lipopeptide antibiotic generally used in the treatment of skin infections caused by susceptible gram-positive bacteria.

Products: Cubicin; 250- and 500-mg vials.

Preparation: Reconstitute with 5 or 10 mL of sodium chloride 0.9% for the 250- and 500-mg vials, respectively. Dilute in sodium chloride 0.9% to a concentration not exceeding 20 mg/mL.

Administration: Administer by intravenous infusion over 30 minutes.

Stability: Store under refrigeration at 2 to 8 °C. Daptomycin reconstituted as directed is stable for 12 hours at room temperature and 48 hours under refrigeration. Diluted for infusion in a compatible diluent, daptomycin is also stable for 12 hours at room temperature and 48 hours under refrigeration. However, the time after reconstitution in the vial and after dilution for infusion in the bag together should not exceed a combined time of 12 hours at room temperature and 48 hours under refrigeration. Daptomycin is incompatible with dextrose-containing solutions.

Compatibility Table

Solutions	Compatible	Incompatible	Variable
Dextrose 5%	...	●	...
Ringer's injection, lactated	●	...	...
Sodium chloride 0.9%	●	...	...

Drugs	Compatible	Incompatible	Variable
Aztreonam	●	...	...
Ceftazidime	●	...	...
Ceftriaxone sodium	●	...	...
Dopamine HCl	●	...	...
Fluconazole	●	...	...
Gentamicin sulfate	●	...	...
Heparin sodium	●	...	...
Levofloxacin	●	...	...
Lidocaine HCl	●	...	...

Dexamethasone Sodium Phosphate

Handbook on Injectable Drugs pp. 479–489.

Description: A synthetic adrenocortical steroid.

Products: **Decadron;** 4, 10, and 24 mg/mL in a variety of container sizes. *pH:* From 7 to 8.5.

Administration: The 4-mg/mL concentration may be given IM, IV, by intra-articular injection, intrasynovial, intralesional, or by soft tissue infiltration. The 10-mg/mL concentration is administered by IM and IV injection only. The 24-mg/mL concentration is for IV use only. IV administration may be performed as a direct injection over one to several minutes or as a continuous or intermittent injection.

Stability: The solution is clear and colorless to light yellow. The drug must be protected from light and freezing, and it must not be autoclaved because it is heat labile. No sorption to plastic bags, sets, or filters has been noted.

Compatibility Table

Solutions	Compatible	Incompatible	Variable
Dextrose 5%	●	...	...
Sodium chloride 0.9%	●	...	...

Drugs			
Acyclovir sodium	●	...	...
Allopurinol sodium	●	...	...
Amifostine	●	...	...
Amikacin sulfate	...	...	●
Aminophylline	●	...	...
Amphotericin B cholesteryl sulfate complex	●	...	...
Aztreonam	●	...	...
Bivalirudin	●	...	...
Bleomycin sulfate	●	...	...

Drugs	Compatible	Incompatible	Variable
Caffeine citrate	●	...	...
Cefepime HCl	●	...	...
Cimetidine HCl	●	...	...
Ciprofloxacin	...	●	...
Cisatracurium besylate	●	...	...
Cisplatin	●	...	...
Cladribine	●	...	...
Cyclophosphamide	●	...	...
Cytarabine	●	...	...
Daunorubicin HCl	...	●	...
Dexmedetomidine HCl	●	...	...
Dimenhydrinate	●	...	...
Diphenhydramine HCl	...	...	●
Docetaxel	●	...	...
Doxapram HCl	...	●	...
Doxorubicin HCl	●	...	...
Doxorubicin HCl liposome injection	●	...	...
Etoposide phosphate	●	...	...
Famotidine	●	...	...
Fenoldopam mesylate	...	●	...
Fentanyl citrate	●	...	...
Filgrastim	●	...	...
Fluconazole	●	...	...
Fludarabine phosphate	●	...	...
Foscarnet sodium	●	...	...
Furosemide	●	...	...
Gallium nitrate	●	...	...
Gemcitabine HCl	●	...	...
Glycopyrrolate	...	●	...
Granisetron HCl	●	...	...
Heparin sodium	●	...	...
Hextend	●	...	...
Hydromorphone HCl	...	...	●
Idarubicin HCl	...	●	...
Lansoprazole	●	...	...
Levofloxacin	●	...	...
Lidocaine HCl	●	...	...
Linezolid	●	...	...
Lorazepam	●	...	...

Drugs	Compatible	Incompatible	Variable
Meperidine HCl	●	. . .	. . .
Meropenem	●	. . .	. . .
Methadone HCl	●	. . .	. . .
Methotrexate sodium	. . .	. . .	●
Metoclopramide HCl	●	. . .	. . .
Midazolam HCl	. . .	. . .	●
Milrinone lactate	●	. . .	. . .
Mitomycin	●	. . .	. . .
Morphine sulfate	●	. . .	. . .
Nafcillin sodium	●	. . .	. . .
Ondansetron HCl	. . .	. . .	●
Oxaliplatin	●	. . .	. . .
Oxycodone HCl	●	. . .	. . .
Paclitaxel	●	. . .	. . .
Palonosetron HCl	●	. . .	. . .
Pantoprazole sodium	. . .	●	. . .
Pemetrexed disodium	●	. . .	. . .
Piperacillin sod.–tazobactam sod.	●	. . .	. . .
Potassium chloride	●	. . .	. . .
Prochlorperazine edisylate	. . .	. . .	●
Propofol	●	. . .	. . .
Ranitidine HCl	●	. . .	. . .
Remifentanil HCl	●	. . .	. . .
Sargramostim	●	. . .	. . .
Sodium bicarbonate	●	. . .	. . .
Sufentanil citrate	●	. . .	. . .
Tacrolimus	●	. . .	. . .
Teniposide	●	. . .	. . .
Theophylline	●	. . .	. . .
Thiotepa	●	. . .	. . .
Topotecan HCl	●	. . .	. . .
Vancomycin HCl	. . .	●	. . .
Verapamil HCl	●	. . .	. . .
Vinorelbine tartrate	●	. . .	. . .
Zidovudine	●	. . .	. . .

Dexmedetomidine Hydrochloride

Handbook on Injectable Drugs pp. 489–495.

Description: An α_2-adrenergic agonist used as a sedative.

Products: **Precedex;** 100-mcg/mL concentrate in 2-mL single-use vials. *pH:* From 4.5 to 7.0.

Preparation: The concentrate must be diluted with a compatible infusion solution for use. To prepare a 4-mcg/mL dilution of the drug for administration, the manufacturer recommends adding 2 mL of the injection to 48 mL of sodium chloride 0.9% and shaking gently to mix.

Administration: Administer by slow IV infusion using a controlled infusion device over periods not exceeding 24 hours.

Stability: The clear, colorless injection should be stored at room temperature.

Compatibility Table

Solutions	Compatible	Incompatible	Variable
Dextrose 5%	●	…	…
Ringer's injection, lactated	●	…	…
Sodium chloride 0.9%	●	…	…

Drugs			
Alfentanil HCl	●	…	…
Amikacin sulfate	●	…	…
Aminophylline	●	…	…
Amiodarone HCl	●	…	…
Amphotericin B	…	●	…
Ampicillin sodium	●	…	…
Ampicillin sodium–sulbactam sodium	●	…	…
Atracurium besylate	●	…	…
Atropine sulfate	●	…	…
Azithromycin	●	…	…
Aztreonam	●	…	…
Bumetanide	●	…	…
Butorphanol tartrate	●	…	…
Calcium gluconate	●	…	…

Drugs	Compatible	Incompatible	Variable
Cefazolin sodium	●	...	...
Cefepime HCl	●	...	...
Cefotaxime sodium	●	...	...
Cefotetan disodium	●	...	...
Cefoxitin sodium	●	...	...
Ceftazidime	●	...	...
Ceftizoxime sodium	●	...	...
Ceftriaxone sodium	●	...	...
Cefuroxime sodium	●	...	...
Chlorpromazine HCl	●	...	...
Cimetidine HCl	●	...	...
Ciprofloxacin	●	...	...
Cisatracurium besylate	●	...	...
Clindamycin phosphate	●	...	...
Dexamethasone sodium phosphate ...	●	...	...
Diazepam	...	●	...
Digoxin	●	...	...
Diltiazem HCl	●	...	...
Diphenhydramine HCl	●	...	...
Dobutamine HCl	●	...	...
Dolasetron mesylate	●	...	...
Dopamine HCl	●	...	...
Doxycycline HCl	●	...	...
Droperidol	●	...	...
Enalaprilat	●	...	...
Ephedrine sulfate	●	...	...
Epinephrine HCl	●	...	...
Erythromycin lactobionate	●	...	...
Esmolol HCl	●	...	...
Etomidate	●	...	...
Famotidine	●	...	...
Fenoldopam mesylate	●	...	...
Fentanyl citrate	●	...	...
Fluconazole	●	...	...
Furosemide	●	...	...
Gentamicin sulfate	●	...	...
Glycopyrrolate	●	...	...
Granisetron HCl	●	...	...
Haloperidol lactate	●	...	...
Heparin sodium	●	...	...

Drugs	Compatible	Incompatible	Variable
Hydromorphone HCl	●	...	...
Hydroxyzine HCl	●	...	...
Isoproterenol HCl	●	...	...
Ketorolac tromethamine	●	...	...
Labetalol HCl	●	...	...
Levofloxacin	●	...	...
Lidocaine IICl	●	...	...
Linezolid	●	...	...
Lorazepam	●	...	...
Magnesium sulfate	●	...	...
Meperidine HCl	●	...	...
Methylprednisolone sodium succinate	●	...	...
Metoclopramide HCl	●	...	...
Metronidazole	●	...	...
Midazolam HCl	●	...	...
Milrinone lactate	●	...	...
Mivacurium chloride	●	...	...
Morphine sulfate	●	...	...
Nalbuphine HCl	●	...	...
Nitroglycerin	●	...	...
Norepinephrine bitartrate	●	...	...
Ondansetron HCl	●	...	...
Pancuronium bromide	●	...	...
Phenylephrine HCl	●	...	...
Piperacillin sodium	●	...	...
Piperacillin sodium–tazobactam sodium	●	...	...
Potassium chloride	●	...	...
Procainamide HCl	●	...	...
Prochlorperazine edisylate	●	...	...
Promethazine HCl	●	...	...
Propofol	●	...	...
Ranitidine HCl	●	...	...
Remifentanil HCl	●	...	...
Rocuronium bromide	●	...	...
Sodium bicarbonate	●	...	...
Sodium nitroprusside	●	...	...
Succinylcholine chloride	●	...	...
Sufentanil citrate	●	...	...

Drugs	Compatible	Incompatible	Variable
Theophylline	●	...	...
Thiopental sodium	●	...	...
Ticarcillin disodium–clavulanate potassium	●	...	...
Tobramycin sulfate	●	...	...
Trimethoprim–sulfamethoxazole	●	...	...
Vancomycin HCl	●	...	...
Vecuronium bromide	●	...	...
Verapamil HCl	●	...	...

Diazepam

Handbook on Injectable Drugs pp. 508–517.

Description: A benzodiazepine tranquilizer.

Products: Valium; 5-mg/mL solution in 2-mL ampuls, 10-mL vials, and 2-mL disposable syringes. *pH:* From 6.2 to 6.9.

Administration: Administer by direct IV injection slowly at a rate not exceeding 5 mg/min in adults. In children, administration should be over not less than 3 minutes. Avoid extravasation.

Stability: Store at room temperature and protect from light.

Diazepam infusions, delivered over seven hours through 0.2-μm membrane filters, lost 7 to 17% over the first hour but subsequently returned to normal concentrations.

The manufacturer recommends that diazepam not be mixed with other solutions or drugs or be added to IV infusion solutions. However, it is stated that the drug may be injected slowly through infusion tubing as close to the vein insertion as possible.

Studies have shown that diazepam may indeed be compatible at some concentrations in some IV fluids. In dilutions of 1:40 to 1:100 in IV solutions in glass bottles, diazepam was both compatible and stable for 24 hours. As the solutions became more concentrated, haziness and precipitation were noted in varying time periods.

In addition, diazepam undergoes significant absorption into PVC IV fluid bags and administration sets and tubing. When added to solutions in PVC bags, drug losses of about 25 to 55% have been reported to occur in the first 30 to 120 minutes. Losses due to sorption also have been found with storage of diazepam in plastic syringes.

Compatibility Table

Solutions	Compatible	Incompatible	Variable
Dextrose 5%	...	...	●
Ringer's injection	...	...	●
Ringer's injection, lactated	...	...	●
Sodium chloride 0.9%	...	...	●

Drugs	Compatible	Incompatible	Variable
Amphotericin B cholesteryl sulfate complex	...	●	...
Atracurium besylate	...	●	...
Bivalirudin	...	●	...
Bleomycin sulfate	...	●	...
Buprenorphine HCl	...	●	...
Cefepime HCl	...	●	...
Cimetidine HCl	●	...	...
Cisatracurium besylate	...	...	●
Dexmedetomidine HCl	...	●	...
Diltiazem HCl	...	●	...
Dimenhydrinate	...	●	...
Dobutamine HCl	...	...	●
Doxapram HCl	...	●	...
Doxorubicin HCl	...	●	...
Fenoldopam mesylate	...	●	...
Fentanyl citrate	●	...	...
Fluconazole	...	●	...
Fluorouracil	...	●	...
Foscarnet sodium	...	●	...
Furosemide	...	●	...
Glycopyrrolate	...	●	...
Heparin sodium	...	●	...
Hextend	...	●	...
Hydromorphone HCl	...	●	...
Ketorolac tromethamine	...	...	●
Lansoprazole	...	●	...
Linezolid	...	●	...
Meropenem	...	●	...
Methadone HCl	●	...	...
Morphine sulfate	●	...	...
Nafcillin sodium	●	...	...
Nalbuphine HCl	...	●	...
Oxaliplatin	...	●	...
Pancuronium bromide	...	●	...
Pantoprazole sodium	...	●	...
Potassium chloride	...	●	...
Propofol	...	●	...
Quinidine gluconate	●	...	...
Ranitidine HCl	...	...	●

Drugs	Compatible	Incompatible	Variable
Remifentanil HCl	...	●	...
Sufentanil citrate	...	...	●
Tirofiban HCl	...	●	...
Vecuronium bromide	...	●	...
Verapamil HCl	●	...	...

Digoxin

Handbook on Injectable Drugs pp. 518–522.

Description: A cardiac glycoside.

Products: Lanoxin; 0.25 mg/mL in 1- and 2-mL ampuls and 0.1 mg/mL (pediatric) in 1-mL ampuls. *pH:* From 6.8 to 7.2.

Preparation: For direct IV injection, the drug may be given undiluted or diluted with a four-fold or greater volume of sterile water for injection, dextrose 5%, or sodium chloride 0.9%.

Administration: Administer by direct IV injection or, rarely, by IM injection. Because of pain, IM injection should be limited to not more than 2 mL and made deep into the muscle and followed by massage. Direct IV injection should be done slowly over one to five minutes.

Stability: Store at room temperature protected from light. Hydrolysis occurs in solutions with pH less than 3. Variable losses of digoxin due to sorption to filter materials have occurred. Digoxin does not leach plasticizer from PVC bags.

Compatibility Table

Solutions	Compatible	Incompatible	Variable
Dextrose 5%	●	…	…
Ringer's injection, lactated	●	…	…
Sodium chloride 0.45%	●	…	…
Sodium chloride 0.9%	●	…	…

Drugs	Compatible	Incompatible	Variable
Amiodarone HCl	…	●	…
Amphotericin B cholesteryl sulfate complex	…	●	…
Bivalirudin	●	…	…
Cimetidine HCl	●	…	…
Ciprofloxacin	●	…	…
Cisatracurium besylate	●	…	…
Dexmedetomidine HCl	●	…	…
Diltiazem HCl	●	…	…
Dimenhydrinate	●	…	…

Drugs	Compatible	Incompatible	Variable
Dobutamine HCl	...	●	...
Doxapram HCl	...	●	...
Famotidine	●	...	...
Fenoldopam mesylate	●	...	...
Fluconazole	...	●	...
Foscarnet sodium	...	●	...
Furosemide	●	...	...
Heparin sodium	●	...	...
Hextend	●	...	...
Insulin	...	...	●
Lansoprazole	...	●	...
Linezolid	●	...	...
Lidocaine HCl	●	...	...
Meperidine HCl	●	...	...
Meropenem	●	...	...
Midazolam HCl	●	...	...
Milrinone lactate	●	...	...
Morphine sulfate	●	...	...
Pantoprazole sodium	...	●	...
Potassium chloride	●	...	...
Propofol	...	●	...
Ranitidine HCl	●	...	...
Remifentanil HCl	●	...	...
Tacrolimus	●	...	...
Verapamil HCl	●	...	...

Diltiazem Hydrochloride

Handbook on Injectable Drugs pp. 522–528.

Description: A calcium-channel blocking agent.

Products: Cardizem; 5 mg/mL in 5-mL (25-mg), 10-mL (50-mg), and 25-mL (125-mg) vials. *pH:* From 3.7 to 4.1.

Preparation: Dilute in 100 to 500 mL of a compatible diluent for IV infusion.

Administration: Administer undiluted by direct IV injection or administer by IV infusion following dilution.

Stability: Diltiazem hydrochloride injection should be stored under refrigeration and protected from freezing. Intact vials may be stored for up to one month at room temperature but should then be destroyed. The powder for injection should be stored at controlled room temperature and protected from freezing. Reconstituted solutions are stable for 24 hours at room temperature. Some loss due to sorption to PVC may occur, especially at neutral or alkaline pH.

Compatibility Table

Solutions	Compatible	Incompatible	Variable
Dextrose 5%	●	...	...
Dextrose 5% in sodium chloride 0.45%	●	...	...
Sodium chloride 0.9%	●	...	...

Drugs			
Acetazolamide sodium	...	...	●
Acyclovir sodium	...	...	●
Albumin	●	...	...
Amikacin sulfate	●	...	...
Aminophylline	...	...	●
Amphotericin B	●	...	...
Ampicillin sodium	...	...	●
Ampicillin sodium–sulbactam sodium	...	...	●
Argatroban	●	...	...

Drugs	Compatible	Incompatible	Variable
Aztreonam	●	...	...
Bivalirudin	●	...	...
Bumetanide	●	...	...
Cefamandole nafate	...	...	●
Cefazolin sodium	●	...	...
Cefotaxime sodium	●	...	...
Cefotetan disodium	●	...	...
Cefoxitin sodium	●	...	...
Ceftazidime	●	...	...
Ceftriaxone sodium	●	...	...
Cefuroxime sodium	●	...	...
Cimetidine HCl	●	...	...
Ciprofloxacin	●	...	...
Clindamycin phosphate	●	...	...
Dexmedetomidine HCl	●	...	...
Diazepam	...	●	...
Digoxin	●	...	...
Dobutamine HCl	●	...	...
Dopamine HCl	●	...	...
Doxycycline hyclate	●	...	...
Epinephrine HCl	●	...	...
Erythromycin lactobionate	●	...	...
Esmolol HCl	●	...	...
Fenoldopam mesylate	●	...	...
Fentanyl citrate	●	...	...
Fluconazole	●	...	...
Furosemide	...	●	...
Gentamicin sulfate	●	...	...
Heparin sodium	...	...	●
Hetastarch in sodium chloride 0.9%	●	...	...
Hextend	●	...	...
Hydrocortisone sodium succinate	...	...	●
Hydromorphone HCl	●	...	...
Imipenem–cilastatin sodium	●	...	...
Insulin, regular	...	...	●
Labetalol HCl	●	...	...
Lansoprazole	...	●	...
Lidocaine HCl	●	...	...
Lorazepam	●	...	...
Meperidine HCl	●	...	...

Diltiazem Hydrochloride

123

Drugs	Compatible	Incompatible	Variable
Methylprednisolone sod. succ.	...	...	●
Metoclopramide HCl	●	...	...
Metronidazole	●	...	...
Midazolam HCl	●	...	...
Milrinone lactate	●	...	...
Morphine sulfate	●	...	...
Multivitamins	●	...	...
Nafcillin sodium	...	...	●
Nicardipine HCl	●	...	...
Nitroglycerin	●	...	...
Norepinephrine bitartrate	●	...	...
Oxacillin sodium	●	...	...
Penicillin G potassium	●	...	...
Pentamidine isethionate	●	...	...
Phenytoin sodium	...	●	...
Piperacillin sodium	●	...	...
Potassium chloride	●	...	...
Potassium phosphates	●	...	...
Procainamide HCl	...	...	●
Ranitidine HCl	●	...	...
Rifampin	...	●	...
Sodium bicarbonate	...	...	●
Sodium nitroprusside	●	...	...
Theophylline	●	...	...
Thiopental sodium	...	●	...
Ticarcillin disod.–clavulanate pot.	●	...	...
Tobramycin sulfate	●	...	...
Trimethoprim–sulfamethoxazole	●	...	...
Vancomycin HCl	●	...	...
Vasopressin	●	...	...
Vecuronium bromide	●	...	...

Diphenhydramine Hydrochloride

Handbook on Injectable Drugs pp. 535–544.

Description: A potent antihistamine with anticholinergic, anti-emetic, and sedative effects.

Products: Benadryl; 10-mg/mL solution in 30-mL vials; 50-mg/mL solution in 1-mL ampuls, vials, and disposable syringes and 10-mL vials. *pH:* From 5 to 6.

Administration: Administer by deep IM or slow direct IV injection or continuous or intermittent IV infusion.

Stability: Store in light-resistant containers at room temperature. Freezing should be avoided.

Compatibility Table

Solutions	Compatible	Incompatible	Variable
Dextrose 5%	●	...	...
Dextrose 5% in Ringer's injection	●	...	...
Dextrose 5% in Ringer's injection, lactated	●	...	...
Dextrose 5% in sodium chloride 0.2, 0.45, & 0.9%	●	...	...
Ringer's injection	●	...	...
Ringer's injection, lactated	●	...	...
Sodium chloride 0.45 & 0.9%	●	...	...

Drugs	Compatible	Incompatible	Variable
Abciximab	●	...	...
Acyclovir sodium	●	...	...
Aldesleukin	●	...	...
Allopurinol sodium	...	●	...
Amifostine	●	...	...
Amikacin sulfate	●	...	...
Aminophylline	●	...	...
Amobarbital sodium	...	●	...
Amphotericin B	...	●	...
Amphotericin B cholesteryl sulfate complex	...	●	...

Drugs	Compatible	Incompatible	Variable
Argatroban	●	...	...
Ascorbic acid injection	●	...	...
Atropine sulfate	●	...	...
Azithromycin	●	...	...
Aztreonam	●	...	...
Bivalirudin	●	...	...
Bleomycin sulfate	●	...	...
Buprenorphine HCl	●	...	...
Butorphanol tartrate	●	...	...
Cefepime HCl	...	●	...
Chlorpromazine HCl	●	...	...
Cimetidine HCl	●	...	...
Ciprofloxacin	●	...	...
Cisatracurium besylate	●	...	...
Cisplatin	●	...	...
Cladribine	●	...	...
Colistimethate sodium	●	...	...
Cyclophosphamide	●	...	...
Cytarabine	●	...	...
Dexamethasone sodium phosphate	...	...	●
Dexmedetomidine HCl	●	...	...
Diatrizoate meglumine & sodium	...	...	●
Dimenhydrinate	●	...	...
Docetaxel	●	...	...
Doxorubicin HCl	●	...	...
Doxorubicin HCl liposome injection	●	...	...
Droperidol	●	...	...
Erythromycin lactobionate	●	...	...
Etoposide phosphate	●	...	...
Famotidine	●	...	...
Fenoldopam mesylate	●	...	...
Fentanyl citrate	●	...	...
Filgrastim	●	...	...
Fluconazole	●	...	...
Fludarabine phosphate	●	...	...
Fluphenazine HCl	●	...	...
Foscarnet sodium	...	●	...
Gallium nitrate	●	...	...
Gemcitabine HCl	●	...	...

Drugs	Compatible	Incompatible	Variable
Glycopyrrolate	●	...	...
Granisetron HCl	●	...	...
Haloperidol lactate	...	●	...
Heparin sodium	●	...	...
Hextend	●	...	...
Hydrocortisone sodium succinate	...	...	●
Hydromorphone HCl	●	...	...
Hydroxyzine HCl	●	...	...
Idarubicin HCl	●	...	...
Iodipamide meglumine	...	●	...
Iothalamate meglumine & sodium	...	...	●
Ioxaglate meglumine & sodium	...	●	...
Lansoprazole	...	●	...
Lidocaine HCl	●	...	...
Linezolid	●	...	...
Melphalan HCl	●	...	...
Meperidine HCl	●	...	...
Meropenem	●	...	...
Methadone HCl	●	...	...
Methotrexate sodium	●	...	...
Methyldopate HCl	●	...	...
Metoclopramide HCl	●	...	...
Midazolam HCl	●	...	...
Morphine sulfate	●	...	...
Nafcillin sodium	●	...	...
Nalbuphine HCl	●	...	...
Ondansetron HCl	●	...	...
Oxaliplatin	●	...	...
Paclitaxel	●	...	...
Pantoprazole sodium	...	●	...
Pemetrexed disodium	●	...	...
Penicillin G potassium	●	...	...
Penicillin G sodium	●	...	...
Pentazocine lactate	●	...	...
Pentobarbital sodium	...	●	...
Phenobarbital sodium	...	●	...
Phenytoin sodium	...	●	...
Piperacillin sod.–tazobactam sod.	●	...	...
Polymyxin B sulfate	●	...	...
Potassium chloride	●	...	...

Drugs	Compatible	Incompatible	Variable
Prochlorperazine edisylate	●	...	...
Promethazine HCl	●	...	...
Propofol	●	...	...
Ranitidine HCl	●	...	...
Remifentanil HCl	●	...	...
Sargramostim	●	...	...
Scopolamine HBr	●	...	...
Sufentanil citrate	●	...	...
Tacrolimus	●	...	...
Teniposide	●	...	...
Thiopental sodium	...	...	●
Thiotepa	●	...	...
Vinorelbine tartrate	●	...	...

Dobutamine Hydrochloride

Handbook on Injectable Drugs pp. 544–555.

Description: A synthetic sympathomimetic drug structurally related to dopamine.

Products: **Dobutrex;** 12.5 mg/mL in a variety of vial sizes. Also, 0.5, 1, 2, and 4 mg/mL premixed in plastic bags for infusion. *pH:* From 2.5 to 5.5.

Preparation: Dobutamine hydrochloride must be diluted to a concentration of not more than 5 mg/mL before use.

To prepare infusion solutions, dilute 250 mg with a compatible diluent. Dilution with 1000 mL yields a 250-mcg/mL solution, 500 mL yields a 500-mcg/mL solution, and 250 mL yields a 1000-mcg/mL solution.

Administration: Administer by IV infusion using an infusion pump to control the flow rate.

Stability: Store intact containers at room temperature and protect from freezing and excessive heat. Infusion solutions should be used within 24 hours. A pink discoloration may form due to slight oxidation of the drug. However, there is no significant drug loss within recommended times. No loss due to sorption to plastic or glass containers has been found.

Compatibility Table

Solutions	Compatible	Incompatible	Variable
Dextrose 5%	●	...	...
Dextrose 5% in Ringer's injection, lactated	●	...	...
Dextrose 5% in sodium chloride 0.45 & 0.9%	●	...	...
Ringer's injection, lactated	●	...	...
Sodium chloride 0.45 & 0.9%	●	...	...

Drugs	Compatible	Incompatible	Variable
Acyclovir sodium	...	●	...
Alteplase	...	●	...
Amifostine	●	...	...
Aminophylline	...	●	...
Amiodarone HCl	●	...	...
Amphotericin B cholesteryl sulfate complex	...	●	...
Argatroban	●	...	...
Atracurium besylate	●	...	...
Atropine sulfate	●	...	...
Aztreonam	●	...	...
Bivalirudin	●	...	...
Bumetanide	...	●	...
Caffeine citrate	●	...	...
Calcium chloride & gluconate	...	...	●
Cefepime HCl	...	...	●
Ceftazidime	...	...	●
Ciprofloxacin	●	...	...
Cisatracurium besylate	●	...	...
Cladribine	●	...	...
Dexmedetomidine HCl	●	...	...
Diazepam	...	...	●
Digoxin	...	●	...
Diltiazem HCl	●	...	...
Dimenhydrinate	●	...	...
Docetaxel	●	...	...
Dopamine HCl	●	...	...
Doxapram HCl	...	●	...
Doxorubicin HCl liposome injection	●	...	...
Drotrecogin alfa (activated)	...	...	●
Enalaprilat	●	...	...
Epinephrine HCl	●	...	...
Etoposide phosphate	●	...	...
Famotidine	●	...	...
Fenoldopam mesylate	●	...	...
Fentanyl citrate	●	...	...
Fluconazole	●	...	...
Flumazenil	●	...	...
Foscarnet sodium	...	●	...

Drugs	Compatible	Incompatible	Variable
Furosemide	...	●	...
Gemcitabine HCl	●	...	...
Granisetron HCl	●	...	...
Haloperidol lactate	●	...	...
Heparin sodium	...	...	●
Hextend	●	...	...
Hydralazine HCl	●	...	...
Hydromorphone HCl	●	...	...
Indomethacin sodium trihydrate	...	●	...
Insulin, regular	...	●	...
Isoproterenol HCl	●	...	...
Labetalol HCl	●	...	...
Lansoprazole	...	●	...
Levofloxacin	●	...	...
Lidocaine HCl	●	...	...
Linezolid	●	...	...
Lorazepam	●	...	...
Magnesium sulfate	...	...	●
Meperidine HCl	●	...	...
Meropenem	●	...	...
Midazolam HCl	...	...	●
Milrinone lactate	●	...	...
Morphine sulfate	●	...	...
Nicardipine HCl	●	...	...
Nitroglycerin	●	...	...
Norepinephrine bitartrate	●	...	...
Oxaliplatin	●	...	...
Pancuronium bromide	●	...	...
Pantoprazole sodium	...	●	...
Pemetrexed disodium	...	●	...
Phenylephrine HCl	●	...	...
Phenytoin sodium	...	●	...
Phytonadione	...	●	...
Piperacillin sod.–tazobactam sod.	...	●	...
Potassium chloride	...	...	●
Potassium phosphates	...	●	...
Procainamide HCl	●	...	...
Propofol	●	...	...
Propranolol HCl	●	...	...
Ranitidine HCl	●	...	...

Dobutamine Hydrochloride

Drugs	Compatible	Incompatible	Variable
Remifentanil HCl	●	...	...
Sodium bicarbonate	...	●	...
Sodium nitroprusside	...	...	●
Streptokinase	●	...	...
Tacrolimus	●	...	...
Theophylline	●	...	...
Thiopental sodium	...	●	...
Thiotepa	●	...	...
Tirofiban HCl	●	...	...
Vasopressin	●	...	...
Vecuronium bromide	●	...	...
Verapamil HCl	...	...	●
Warfarin sodium	...	●	...
Zidovudine	●	...	...

Docetaxel

Handbook on Injectable Drugs pp. 555–562.

Description: A semisynthetic taxoid antineoplastic agent.

Products: Taxotere; 40-mg/mL solution (as concentrate) in 0.5-mL (20-mg) and 2-mL (80-mg) vials packaged with special diluent.

Preparation: Allow the docetaxel vials to warm to room temperature. Add the accompanying special diluent to each vial of concentrate and gently rotate for about 15 seconds to mix, forming a clear 10-mg/mL solution. Add the proper amount of docetaxel to a 250-mL (or larger) glass bottle or polyolefin (not PVC) container of dextrose 5% or sodium chloride 0.9% to produce a final concentration of 0.3 to 0.74 mg/mL. Rotate the admixture to mix.

Administration: Administer by IV infusion over one hour to patients that have been adequately premedicated.

Stability: Store intact vials under refrigeration or at room temperature; freezing does not adversely affect the concentrate. The initial diluted solution (10 mg/mL) is stable for at least eight hours under refrigeration or at room temperature. Fully diluted admixtures (0.3 to 0.74 mg/mL) should be used within four hours including the one-hour administration time.

The surfactant present in the formulation leaches plasticizer from PVC containers and administration sets. The use of inline filters is not recommended.

Compatibility Table

Solutions	Compatible	Incompatible	Variable
Dextrose 5%	●	...	...
Sodium chloride 0.9%	●	...	...

Drugs	Compatible	Incompatible	Variable
Acyclovir sodium	●	...	...
Amifostine	●	...	...
Amikacin sulfate	●	...	...
Aminophylline	●	...	...
Amphotericin B	...	●	...

Drugs	Compatible	Incompatible	Variable
Ampicillin sodium	●	...	...
Ampicillin sod.–sulbactam sod.	●	...	...
Aztreonam	●	...	...
Bumetanide	●	...	...
Buprenorphine HCl	●	...	...
Butorphanol tartrate	●	...	...
Calcium gluconate	●	...	...
Cefazolin sodium	●	...	...
Cefepime HCl	●	...	...
Cefotaxime sodium	●	...	...
Cefotetan disodium	●	...	...
Cefoxitin sodium	●	...	...
Ceftazidime	●	...	...
Ceftizoxime sodium	●	...	...
Ceftriaxone sodium	●	...	...
Cefuroxime sodium	●	...	...
Chlorpromazine HCl	●	...	...
Cimetidine HCl	●	...	...
Ciprofloxacin	●	...	...
Clindamycin phosphate	●	...	...
Dexamethasone sodium phosphate	●	...	...
Diphenhydramine HCl	●	...	...
Dobutamine HCl	●	...	...
Dopamine HCl	●	...	...
Doxorubicin HCl liposome injection	...	●	...
Doxycycline hyclate	●	...	...
Droperidol	●	...	...
Enalaprilat	●	...	...
Famotidine	●	...	...
Fluconazole	●	...	...
Furosemide	●	...	...
Ganciclovir sodium	●	...	...
Gemcitabine HCl	●	...	...
Gentamicin sulfate	●	...	...
Granisetron HCl	●	...	...
Haloperidol lactate	●	...	...
Heparin sodium	●	...	...
Hydrocortisone sodium phosphate	●	...	...
Hydrocortisone sodium succinate	●	...	...
Hydromorphone HCl	●	...	...

Drugs	Compatible	Incompatible	Variable
Hydroxyzine HCl	●	...	...
Imipenem–cilastatin sodium	●	...	...
Leucovorin calcium	●	...	...
Lorazepam	●	...	...
Magnesium sulfate	●	...	...
Mannitol	●	...	...
Meperidine HCl	●	...	...
Meropenem	●	...	...
Mesna	●	...	...
Methylprednisolone sod. succ.	...	●	...
Metoclopramide HCl	●	...	...
Metronidazole	●	...	...
Morphine sulfate	●	...	...
Nalbuphine HCl	...	●	...
Ondansetron HCl	●	...	...
Oxaliplatin	●	...	...
Palonosetron HCl	●	...	...
Pemetrexed disodium	●	...	...
Piperacillin sodium	●	...	...
Piperacillin sod.–tazobactam sod.	●	...	...
Potassium chloride	●	...	...
Prochlorperazine edisylate	●	...	...
Promethazine HCl	●	...	...
Ranitidine HCl	●	...	...
Sodium bicarbonate	●	...	...
Ticarcillin disod.–clavulanate pot.	●	...	...
Tobramycin sulfate	●	...	...
Trimethoprim-sulfamethoxazole	●	...	...
Vancomycin HCl	●	...	...
Zidovudine	●	...	...

Dopamine Hydrochloride

Handbook on Injectable Drugs pp. 563–573.

Description: A naturally occurring catecholamine precursor of norepinephrine.

Products: 200-mg (40 mg/mL), 400-mg (80 mg/mL), and 800-mg (160 mg/mL) sizes. Also available in premixed infusions. *pH:* About 3.3.

Preparation: The concentrated solution must be diluted for use. Dilution of 200 mg in 250- or 500-mL bottles forms 800- or 400-mcg/mL solutions, respectively. Addition of 400 mg to 250- or 500-mL bottles forms 1600- or 800-mcg/mL solutions, respectively.

Administration: Administer by IV infusion only using an infusion control device, into a large vein if possible. Avoid extravasation. The drug must be diluted before use. The concentration used depends on the patient's dosage and fluid requirements.

Stability: Store intact containers at room temperature and protect from freezing and excessive heat. Stable at pH 4 to 6.4. Dopamine hydrochloride decomposes to highly colored materials. Discolored solutions should not be used. No loss due to sorption to plastic containers has been found.

Compatibility Table

Solutions	Compatible	Incompatible	Variable
Dextrose 5 & 10%	●	…	…
Dextrose 5% in Ringer's injection, lactated	●	…	…
Dextrose 5% in sodium chloride 0.45 & 0.9%	●	…	…
Ringer's injection, lactated	●	…	…
Sodium bicarbonate 5%	…	●	…
Sodium chloride 0.9%	●	…	…

Drugs	Compatible	Incompatible	Variable
Acyclovir sodium	...	●	...
Aldesleukin	...	...	●
Alteplase	...	●	...
Amifostine	●	...	...
Aminophylline	●	...	...
Amiodarone HCl	●	...	...
Amphotericin B	...	●	...
Amphotericin B cholesteryl sulfate complex	...	●	...
Ampicillin sodium	...	●	...
Argatroban	●	...	...
Atracurium besylate	●	...	...
Aztreonam	●	...	...
Bivalirudin	●	...	...
Caffeine citrate	●	...	...
Calcium chloride	●	...	...
Cefepime HCl	...	...	●
Ceftazidime	●	...	...
Chloramphenicol sodium succinate	●	...	...
Ciprofloxacin	●	...	...
Cisatracurium besylate	●	...	...
Cladribine	●	...	...
Daptomycin	●	...	...
Dexmedetomidine HCl	●	...	...
Diltiazem HCl	●	...	...
Dobutamine HCl	●	...	...
Docetaxel	●	...	...
Doxapram HCl	●	...	...
Doxorubicin HCl liposome injection	●	...	...
Drotrecogin alfa (activated)	...	...	●
Enalaprilat	●	...	...
Epinephrine HCl	●	...	...
Esmolol HCl	●	...	...
Etoposide phosphate	●	...	...
Famotidine	●	...	...
Fenoldopam mesylate	●	...	...
Fentanyl citrate	●	...	...
Fluconazole	●	...	...
Flumazenil	●	...	...

Dopamine Hydrochloride

Drugs	Compatible	Incompatible	Variable
Foscarnet sodium	●	. . .	. . .
Furosemide	. . .	. . .	●
Gemcitabine HCl	●	. . .	. . .
Gentamicin sulfate	. . .	. . .	●
Granisetron HCl	●	. . .	. . .
Haloperidol lactate	●	. . .	. . .
Heparin sodium	. . .	. . .	●
Hextend	●	. . .	. . .
Hydrocortisone sodium succinate	●	. . .	. . .
Hydromorphone HCl	●	. . .	. . .
Indomethacin sodium trihydrate	. . .	●	. . .
Insulin, regular	. . .	●	. . .
Kanamycin sulfate	●	. . .	. . .
Labetalol HCl	●	. . .	. . .
Lansoprazole	. . .	●	. . .
Levofloxacin	●	. . .	. . .
Lidocaine HCl	●	. . .	. . .
Linezolid	●	. . .	. . .
Lorazepam	●	. . .	. . .
Meperidine HCl	●	. . .	. . .
Meropenem	●	. . .	. . .
Methylprednisolone sod. succ.	●	. . .	. . .
Metronidazole	●	. . .	. . .
Midazolam HCl	●	. . .	. . .
Milrinone lactate	●	. . .	. . .
Morphine sulfate	●	. . .	. . .
Nicardipine HCl	●	. . .	. . .
Nitroglycerin	●	. . .	. . .
Norepinephrine HCl	●	. . .	. . .
Ondansetron HCl	●	. . .	. . .
Oxacillin sodium	●	. . .	. . .
Oxaliplatin	●	. . .	. . .
Pancuronium bromide	●	. . .	. . .
Pantoprazole sodium	. . .	. . .	●
Pemetrexed disodium	●	. . .	. . .
Penicillin G potassium	. . .	●	. . .
Piperacillin sod.–tazobactam sod.	●	. . .	. . .
Potassium chloride	●	. . .	. . .
Propofol	●	. . .	. . .
Ranitidine HCl	●	. . .	. . .

Drugs	Compatible	Incompatible	Variable
Remifentanil HCl	●	...	...
Sargramostim	●	...	...
Sodium nitroprusside	●	...	...
Streptokinase	●	...	...
Tacrolimus	●	...	...
Theophylline	●	...	...
Thiopental sodium	...	●	...
Thiotepa	●	...	...
Tirofiban HCl	●	...	...
Vasopressin	●	...	...
Vecuronium bromide	●	...	...
Verapamil HCl	●	...	...
Warfarin sodium	●	...	...
Zidovudine	●	...	...

Dopamine Hydrochloride

Doxorubicin Hydrochloride

Handbook on Injectable Drugs pp. 576–586.

Description: An anthracycline antineoplastic antibiotic.

Products: Adriamycin; 10-, 20-, 50-, and 200-mg vials. *pH:* From 3.8 to 6.5 when reconstituted. The solution product has a pH of 3.

Preparation: Reconstitute the rapid-dissolution formula with sodium chloride 0.9%. Add 5 mL per 10 mg of drug to yield a 2-mg/mL solution. Do not use bacteriostatic diluents because of possible discoloration and precipitation. The preservative-free solution is supplied ready to administer.

Administration: Administer IV into the tubing of a running infusion of dextrose 5% or sodium chloride 0.9%. The rate of injection depends on the dose and size of the vein but should not be over less than three to five minutes. Avoid extravasation because of local tissue necrosis.

Stability: Store intact containers at room temperature (lyophilized) or under refrigeration (liquid) and protect from light. Reconstituted Adriamycin RDF is stable for seven days at room temperature or 15 days under refrigeration. The drug is unstable at pH less than 3 or above 7. In alkaline solutions, a color change to deep purple indicates decomposition.

Little or no loss of drug has been noted after filtration. Contact with aluminum (such as aluminum needle hubs) may result in darkening, precipitation, and an increased rate of drug loss.

Compatibility Table

Solutions	Compatible	Incompatible	Variable
Dextrose 5%	●	...	...
Ringer's injection, lactated	●	...	...
Sodium chloride 0.9%	●	...	...

Drugs	Compatible	Incompatible	Variable
Allopurinol sodium	...	●	...
Amifostine	●	...	...
Aminophylline	...	●	...
Amphotericin B cholesteryl sulfate complex	...	●	...
Aztreonam	●	...	...
Bleomycin sulfate	●	...	...
Cefepime HCl	...	●	...
Chlorpromazine HCl	●	...	...
Cimetidine HCl	●	...	...
Cisplatin	●	...	...
Cladribine	●	...	...
Cyclophosphamide	●	...	...
Dexamethasone sodium phosphate ...	●	...	...
Diazepam	...	●	...
Diphenhydramine HCl	●	...	...
Droperidol	●	...	...
Etoposide phosphate	●	...	...
Famotidine	●	...	...
Filgrastim	●	...	...
Fludarabine phosphate	●	...	...
Fluorouracil	...	●	...
Furosemide	...	...	●
Gallium nitrate	...	●	...
Ganciclovir sodium	...	●	...
Gemcitabine HCl	●	...	...
Granisetron HCl	●	...	...
Heparin sodium	...	...	●
Hydromorphone HCl	●	...	...
Lansoprazole	...	●	...
Leucovorin calcium	●	...	...
Linezolid	●	...	...
Lorazepam	●	...	...
Melphalan HCl	●	...	...
Methotrexate sodium	●	...	...
Methylprednisolone sod. succ.	●	...	...
Metoclopramide HCl	●	...	...
Mitomycin	●	...	...
Morphine sulfate	●	...	...
Ondansetron HCl	●	...	...

Doxorubicin Hydrochloride

Drugs	Compatible	Incompatible	Variable
Oxaliplatin	●	...	...
Paclitaxel	●	...	...
Pemetrexed disodium	...	●	...
Piperacillin sod.–tazobactam sod.	...	●	...
Prochlorperazine edisylate	●	...	...
Promethazine HCl	●	...	...
Propofol	...	●	...
Ranitidine HCl	●	...	...
Sargramostim	●	...	...
Teniposide	●	...	...
Thiotepa	●	...	...
Topotecan HCl	●	...	...
Vinblastine sulfate	...	...	●
Vincristine sulfate	●	...	...
Vinorelbine tartrate	●	...	...

Doxorubicin Hydrochloride Liposome Injection

Handbook on Injectable Drugs pp. 587–593.

Description: A liposomal formulation of the anthracycline antineoplastic antibiotic doxorubicin hydrochloride.

Products: **Doxil**; 2 mg/mL in 10- and 25-mL vials. *pH:* Approximately 6.5.

Preparation: The dose should be diluted in 250 mL of dextrose 5% for IV administration.

Administration: Administer by IV infusion after proper dilution. Do not give undiluted, by rapid bolus injection, or by other routes. Extravasation should be avoided because the product is extremely irritating to tissues. CAUTION: Ensure that the correct drug product, dose, and administration procedure are used; do not confuse with other products.

Stability: The vials should be stored under refrigeration and protected from freezing. When diluted appropriately for administration in dextrose 5%, the admixture should be stored under refrigeration and administered within 24 hours. Filtration, including inline filtration, should not be performed on this liposomal dispersion.

Compatibility Table

Solutions	Compatible	Incompatible	Variable
Dextrose 5%	●	...	...

Drugs			
Acyclovir sodium	●	...	...
Allopurinol sodium	●	...	...
Aminophylline	●	...	...
Amphotericin B	...	●	...
Amphotericin B cholesteryl sulfate complex	...	●	...

Drugs	Compatible	Incompatible	Variable
Ampicillin sodium	●	...	...
Aztreonam	●	...	...
Bleomycin sulfate	●	...	...
Buprenorphine HCl	...	●	...
Butorphanol tartrate	●	...	...
Calcium gluconate	●	...	...
Carboplatin	●	...	...
Cefazolin sodium	●	...	...
Cefepime HCl	●	...	...
Cefoxitin sodium	●	...	...
Ceftazidime	...	●	...
Ceftizoxime sodium	●	...	...
Ceftriaxone sodium	●	...	...
Chlorpromazine HCl	●	...	...
Cimetidine HCl	●	...	...
Ciprofloxacin	●	...	...
Cisplatin	●	...	...
Clindamycin phosphate	●	...	...
Cyclophosphamide	●	...	...
Cytarabine	●	...	...
Dacarbazine	●	...	...
Dexamethasone sodium phosphate ...	●	...	...
Diphenhydramine HCl	●	...	...
Dobutamine HCl	●	...	...
Docetaxel	...	●	...
Dopamine HCl	●	...	...
Droperidol	●	...	...
Enalaprilat	●	...	...
Etoposide	●	...	...
Famotidine	●	...	...
Fluconazole	●	...	...
Fluorouracil	●	...	...
Furosemide	●	...	...
Ganciclovir sodium	●	...	...
Gentamicin sulfate	●	...	...
Granisetron HCl	●	...	...
Haloperidol lactate	●	...	...
Heparin sodium	●	...	...
Hydrocortisone sodium succinate	●	...	...
Hydromorphone HCl	●	...	...

Drugs	Compatible	Incompatible	Variable
Hydroxyzine HCl	...	●	...
Ifosfamide	●	...	...
Leucovorin calcium	●	...	...
Lorazepam	●	...	...
Magnesium sulfate	●	...	...
Mannitol	...	●	...
Meperidine HCl	...	●	...
Mesna	●	...	...
Methotrexate sodium	●	...	...
Methylprednisolone sod. succ.	●	...	...
Metoclopramide HCl	...	●	...
Metronidazole	●	...	...
Mitoxantrone HCl	...	●	...
Morphine sulfate	...	●	...
Ondansetron HCl	●	...	...
Paclitaxel	...	●	...
Piperacillin sodium	●	...	...
Piperacillin sod.–tazobactam sod.	...	●	...
Potassium chloride	●	...	...
Prochlorperazine edisylate	●	...	...
Promethazine HCl	...	●	...
Ranitidine HCl	●	...	...
Sodium bicarbonate	...	●	...
Ticarcillin disod.–clavulanate pot.	●	...	...
Tobramycin sulfate	●	...	...
Trimethoprim–sulfamethoxazole	●	...	...
Vancomycin HCl	●	...	...
Vinblastine sulfate	●	...	...
Vincristine sulfate	●	...	...
Vinorelbine tartrate	●	...	...
Zidovudine	●	...	...

Droperidol

Handbook on Injectable Drugs pp. 597–605.

Description: A neuroleptic which produces marked tranquilization and sedation as well as an antiemetic effect.

Products: **Inapsine;** 2.5-mg/mL solution in 1- and 2-mL containers. *pH:* From 3 to 3.8.

Administration: Administer IM or slowly IV.

Stability: Store at room temperature and protect from light.

No sorption to plastic bags was observed from dextrose 5% and sodium chloride 0.9% infusion solutions. In Ringer's injection, lactated, a possible loss due to sorption was noted.

Compatibility Table

Solutions	Compatible	Incompatible	Variable
Dextrose 5%	●	...	...
Ringer's injection, lactated	...	...	●
Sodium chloride 0.9%	●	...	...

Drugs	Compatible	Incompatible	Variable
Allopurinol sodium	...	●	...
Amifostine	●	...	...
Amphotericin B cholesteryl sulfate complex	...	●	...
Atropine sulfate	●	...	...
Azithromycin	●	...	...
Aztreonam	●	...	...
Barbiturates	...	●	...
Bivalirudin	●	...	...
Bleomycin sulfate	●	...	...
Buprenorphine HCl	●	...	...
Butorphanol tartrate	●	...	...
Cefepime HCl	...	●	...
Chlorpromazine HCl	●	...	...
Cimetidine HCl	●	...	...
Cisatracurium besylate	●	...	...
Cisplatin	●	...	...
Cladribine	●	...	...
Cyclophosphamide	●	...	...
Cytarabine	●	...	...

Drugs	Compatible	Incompatible	Variable
Dexmedetomidine HCl	●	...	...
Dimenhydrinate	●	...	...
Diphenhydramine HCl	●	...	...
Docetaxel	●	...	...
Doxorubicin HCl	●	...	...
Doxorubicin HCl liposome injection	●	...	...
Etoposide phosphate	●	...	...
Famotidine	●	...	...
Fenoldopam mesylate	●	...	...
Fentanyl citrate	●	...	...
Filgrastim	●	...	...
Fluconazole	●	...	...
Fludarabine phosphate	●	...	...
Fluorouracil	...	●	...
Foscarnet sodium	...	●	...
Furosemide	...	●	...
Gemcitabine HCl	●	...	...
Glycopyrrolate	●	...	...
Granisetron HCl	●	...	...
Heparin sodium	...	●	...
Hextend	●	...	...
Hydrocortisone sodium succinate	●	...	...
Hydroxyzine HCl	●	...	...
Idarubicin HCl	●	...	...
Lansoprazole	...	●	...
Leucovorin calcium	...	●	...
Linezolid	●	...	...
Melphalan HCl	●	...	...
Meperidine HCl	●	...	...
Methotrexate sodium	...	...	●
Metoclopramide HCl	●	...	...
Midazolam HCl	●	...	...
Mitomycin	●	...	...
Morphine sulfate	●	...	...
Nafcillin sodium	...	●	...
Nalbuphine HCl	●	...	...
Ondansetron HCl	...	...	●
Oxaliplatin	●	...	...
Paclitaxel	●	...	...

Drugs	Compatible	Incompatible	Variable
Pemetrexed disodium	...	●	...
Pentazocine lactate	●	...	...
Pentobarbital sodium	...	●	...
Piperacillin sod.–tazobactam sod.	...	●	...
Potassium chloride	●	...	...
Prochlorperazine edisylate	●	...	...
Promethazine HCl	●	...	...
Propofol	●	...	...
Remifentanil HCl	●	...	...
Sargramostim	●	...	...
Scopolamine HBr	●	...	...
Teniposide	●	...	...
Thiotepa	●	...	...
Vinblastine sulfate	●	...	...
Vincristine sulfate	●	...	...
Vinorelbine tartrate	●	...	...

Enalaprilat

Handbook on Injectable Drugs pp. 610–616.

Description: An antihypertensive inhibitor of angiotensin-converting enzyme (ACE).

Products: **Vasotec I.V.;** 1.25 mg/mL in 1- and 2-mL vials.

Preparation: For IV infusion, the dose may be diluted in up to 50 mL of compatible diluent.

Administration: Administer IV undiluted slowly over at least five minutes or by IV infusion in up to 50 mL of diluent.

Stability: The solution is clear and colorless and should be stored below 30 °C.

Compatibility Table

Solutions	Compatible	Incompatible	Variable
Dextrose 5%	●	…	…
Dextrose 5% in Ringer's injection, lactated	●	…	…
Dextrose 5% in sodium chloride 0.9%	●	…	…
Sodium chloride 0.9%	●	…	…

Drugs	Compatible	Incompatible	Variable
Allopurinol sodium	●	…	…
Amifostine	●	…	…
Amikacin sulfate	●	…	…
Aminophylline	●	…	…
Amphotericin B	…	●	…
Amphotericin B cholesteryl sulfate complex	…	●	…
Ampicillin sodium	●	…	…
Ampicillin sod.–sulbactam sod.	●	…	…
Aztreonam	●	…	…
Bivalirudin	●	…	…
Butorphanol tartrate	●	…	…
Calcium gluconate	●	…	…
Cefazolin sodium	●	…	…
Cefepime HCl	…	●	…

Drugs	Compatible	Incompatible	Variable
Ceftazidime	●	...	...
Ceftizoxime sodium	●	...	...
Chloramphenicol sod. succ.	●	...	...
Cimetidine HCl	●	...	...
Cisatracurium besylate	●	...	...
Cladribine	●	...	...
Clindamycin phosphate	●	...	...
Dexmedetomidine HCl	●	...	...
Dobutamine HCl	●	...	...
Docetaxel	●	...	...
Dopamine HCl	●	...	...
Doxorubicin HCl liposome injection	●	...	...
Erythromycin lactobionate	●	...	...
Esmolol HCl	●	...	...
Famotidine	●	...	...
Fenoldopam mesylate	●	...	...
Fentanyl citrate	●	...	...
Ganciclovir sodium	●	...	...
Gemcitabine HCl	●	...	...
Gentamicin sulfate	●	...	...
Granisetron HCl	●	...	...
Heparin sodium	●	...	...
Hetastarch in sodium chloride 0.9%	●	...	...
Hextend	●	...	...
Hydrocortisone sodium succinate	●	...	...
Labetalol HCl	●	...	...
Lansoprazole	...	●	...
Lidocaine HCl	●	...	...
Linezolid	●	...	...
Meropenem	●	...	...
Methylprednisolone sod. succ.	●	...	...
Metronidazole	●	...	...
Morphine sulfate	●	...	...
Nafcillin sodium	●	...	...
Nicardipine HCl	●	...	...
Nitroglycerin	●	...	...
Oxaliplatin	●	...	...
Pantoprazole sodium	...	●	...

Drugs	Compatible	Incompatible	Variable
Pemetrexed disodium	●	...	...
Penicillin G potassium	●	...	...
Phenobarbital sodium	●	...	...
Phenytoin sodium	...	●	...
Piperacillin sodium	●	...	...
Piperacillin sod.–tazobactam sod.	●	...	...
Potassium chloride & phosphate	●	...	...
Propofol	●	...	...
Ranitidine HCl	●	...	...
Remifentanil HCl	●	...	...
Sodium nitroprusside	●	...	...
Teniposide	●	...	...
Thiotepa	●	...	...
Tobramycin sulfate	●	...	...
Trimethoprim–sulfamethoxazole	●	...	...
Vancomycin HCl	●	...	...
Vinorelbine tartrate	●	...	...

Enalaprilat

Epinephrine Hydrochloride

Handbook on Injectable Drugs pp. 619–626.

Description: An endogenous catecholamine which is the active principle of the adrenal medulla and acts as a sympathomimetic.

Products: **Adrenalin Chloride;** 0.1 (1:10,000), 0.5, and 1 mg/mL (1:1000) in a variety of containers. *pH:* From 2.2 to 5.

Administration: Administer by SC, IM, IV, or intracardiac injection. Avoid IM injection into the buttocks.

Stability: Epinephrine hydrochloride is sensitive to light and air. Do not remove ampuls from the carton until ready for use. As epinephrine oxidizes, it changes from colorless to pink to brown. Discolored solutions or those with a precipitate should not be used.

The primary determinant of stability in solution is pH. Epinephrine hydrochloride is unstable above pH 5.5. Significant decomposition may occur in solutions with no visually apparent color changes.

Resterilization of the ampuls did not result in loss of drug when autoclaved at 121 °C for 15 minutes or 115 °C for 30 minutes.

Compatibility Table

Solutions	Compatible	Incompatible	Variable
Dextrose 5%	●	...	...
Dextrose 5% in Ringer's injection	●	...	...
Dextrose 5% in Ringer's injection, lactated	●	...	...
Dextrose 5% in sodium chloride 0.2, 0.45, & 0.9%	●	...	...
Ionosol T with dextrose 5%	...	●	...
Ringer's injection	●	...	...
Ringer's injection, lactated	●	...	...
Sodium bicarbonate 5%	...	●	...
Sodium chloride 0.9%	●	...	...

Drugs	Compatible	Incompatible	Variable
Amikacin sulfate	●	...	...
Aminophylline	...	●	...
Amiodarone HCl	●	...	...
Ampicillin sodium	...	●	...
Bivalirudin	●	...	...
Caffeine citrate	●	...	...
Calcium chloride & gluconate	●	...	...
Ceftazidime	●	...	...
Cimetidine HCl	●	...	...
Cisatracurium besylate	●	...	...
Dexmedetomidine HCl	●	...	...
Diltiazem HCl	●	...	...
Dobutamine HCl	●	...	...
Dopamine HCl	●	...	...
Doxapram HCl	●	...	...
Drotrecogin alfa (activated)	...	...	●
Famotidine	●	...	...
Fenoldopam mesylate	●	...	...
Fentanyl citrate	●	...	...
Furosemide	●	...	...
Heparin sodium	●	...	...
Hextend	●	...	...
Hyaluronidase	...	●	...
Hydrocortisone sodium succinate	●	...	...
Hydromorphone HCl	●	...	...
Labetalol HCl	●	...	...
Levofloxacin	●	...	...
Lidocaine HCl	...	●	...
Lorazepam	●	...	...
Midazolam HCl	●	...	...
Milrinone lactate	●	...	...
Morphine sulfate	●	...	...
Nicardipine HCl	●	...	...
Nitroglycerin	●	...	...
Norepinephrine bitartrate	●	...	...
Pancuronium bromide	●	...	...
Pantoprazole sodium	...	...	●
Phytonadione	●	...	...
Potassium chloride	●	...	...
Propofol	●	...	...

Drugs	Compatible	Incompatible	Variable
Ranitidine HCl	●	...	...
Remifentanil HCl	●	...	...
Sodium bicarbonate	...	...	●
Sodium nitroprusside	●	...	...
Thiopental sodium	...	●	...
Tirofiban HCl	●	...	...
Vasopressin	●	...	...
Vecuronium bromide	●	...	...
Verapamil HCl	●	...	...
Warfarin sodium	●	...	...

Ertapenem

Handbook on Injectable Drugs pp. 631–633.

Description: A synthetic carbapenem antibiotic.

Products: **Invanz;** 1-g vials as the sodium salt. *pH:* 7.5.

Preparation: For IV administration, reconstitute the 1-g vial with 10 mL of sterile water for injection, bacteriostatic water for injection, or sodium chloride 0.9% and shake well. Upon dissolution, immediately transfer the reconstituted solution to 50 mL of sodium chloride 0.9%.

For IM injection, reconstitute the 1-g vial with 3.2 mL of lidocaine hydrochloride 1% (without epinephrine) and shake well. Upon dissolution, administer within one hour. Do NOT administer the reconstituted intramuscular injection intravenously.

Administration: By IV infusion diluted in sodium chloride 0.9%, administer over 30 minutes. By deep IM injection into a large muscle mass such as the gluteal muscle or the lateral part of the thigh.

Stability: Store at controlled room temperature. The reconstituted drug solution for IV administration should be immediately diluted in sodium chloride 0.9%. The drug diluted for infusion may be stored and used within six hours at room temperature or may be stored for 24 hours under refrigeration and used within four hours after removal from refrigeration. The drug prepared for IM administration should be used within one hour. Solutions of ertapenem should not be frozen.

Compatibility Table

Solutions	Compatible	Incompatible	Variable
Dextrose 5%	…	●	…
Dextrose 5% in sodium chloride 0.225 & 0.9%	…	●	…
Mannitol 5 & 20%	…	●	…
Ringer's injection*	…	…	●
Ringer's injection, lactated	…	●	…
Sodium bicarbonate 5%	…	●	…
Sodium chloride 0.225 & 0.9%*	…	…	●
Sodium lactate 1/6 M	…	●	…

*Stability in these solutions is insufficient to be considered truly compatible but recommended for dilution of ertapenem with use in shorter periods of time.

Drugs	Compatible	Incompatible	Variable
Dextran 40	●	...	...
Dextran 70	●	...	...
Heparin sodium	●	...	...
Hetastarch in sodium chloride 0.9%	●	...	...
Potassium chloride	●	...	...

Erythromycin Lactobionate

Handbook on Injectable Drugs pp. 633–639.

Description: A macrolide antibiotic.

Products: **Erythrocin Lactobionate-I.V., Erythrocin Piggyback;** 1-g and 500-mg vials. *pH:* From 6.5 to 7.5.

Preparation: Reconstitute the vials with sterile water for injection (no preservatives). Use at least 20 mL for the 1-g vial and 10 mL for the 500-mg vial. Reconstitute the 500-mg piggyback containers with 100 mL of sodium chloride 0.9%, Ringer's injection, lactated, or Normosol R.

Administration: To minimize venous irritation, slow continuous infusion at 1 mg/mL or intermittent infusion of one-fourth the total daily dose may be given every six hours over 20 to 60 minutes. Concentrations of 1 to 5 mg/mL should be used for intermittent infusions.

Stability: Do not use sodium chloride 0.9% or other solutions containing inorganic ions in the initial reconstitution of the vials because a precipitate will form. (This does not apply to the piggyback containers.) Reconstituted solutions are stable for 14 days under refrigeration or 24 hours at room temperature. The reconstituted piggyback containers should be used within eight hours when at room temperature or 24 hours when under refrigeration. The pH range of maximum stability is 6 to 8.

Compatibility Table

NOTE: If the pH of the solution is less than approximately 5 to 6, unacceptable potency loss may occur. Such solutions should be buffered to neutrality to ensure adequate stability.

Solutions	Compatible	Incompatible	Variable
Dextrose 5%	...	...	●
Dextrose 5% in sodium chloride 0.9%	...	...	●
Dextrose 10%	...	●	...
Ringer's injection	...	●	...
Ringer's injection, lactated	...	...	●
Sodium chloride 0.9%	●	...	...

Drugs	Compatible	Incompatible	Variable
Acyclovir sodium	●	...	...
Aminophylline	●	...	...
Amiodarone HCl	●	...	...
Ampicillin sodium	...	...	●
Bivalirudin	●	...	...
Cefepime HCl	...	●	...
Ceftazidime	...	●	...
Cimetidine HCl	●	...	...
Cloxacillin sodium	...	●	...
Colistimethate sodium	...	●	...
Cyclophosphamide	●	...	...
Dexmedetomidine HCl	●	...	...
Diltiazem HCl	●	...	...
Diphenhydramine HCl	●	...	...
Doxapram HCl	●	...	...
Enalaprilat	●	...	...
Esmolol HCl	●	...	...
Famotidine	●	...	...
Fenoldopam mesylate	●	...	...
Furosemide	...	●	...
Heparin sodium	...	...	●
Hextend	●	...	...
Hydrocortisone sodium succinate	●	...	...
Hydromorphone HCl	●	...	...
Idarubicin HCl	●	...	...
Labetalol HCl	●	...	...
Lidocaine HCl	●	...	...
Linezolid	...	●	...
Lorazepam	●	...	...
Magnesium sulfate	●	...	...
Meperidine HCl	●	...	...
Metoclopramide HCl	...	●	...
Midazolam HCl	●	...	...
Morphine sulfate	●	...	...
Nicardipine HCl	●	...	...
Penicillin G potassium	●	...	...
Penicillin G sodium	●	...	...
Pentobarbital sodium	●	...	...
Polymyxin B sulfate	●	...	...
Potassium chloride	●	...	...

Drugs	Compatible	Incompatible	Variable
Prochlorperazine edisylate	●	...	...
Ranitidine HCl	●	...	...
Sodium bicarbonate	●	...	...
Tacrolimus	●	...	...
Theophylline	●	...	...
Verapamil HCl	●	...	...
Zidovudine	●	...	...

Esmolol Hydrochloride

Handbook on Injectable Drugs pp. 640–644.

Description: A short-acting β_1-selective adrenergic blocker.

Products: Brevibloc; 250-mg/mL concentrate in 10-mL ampuls and 10-mg/mL ready-to-use formulation in 10-mL vials and 250-mL bags. *pH:* Concentrate, 3.5 to 5.5; ready-to-use, 4.5 to 5.5.

Preparation: The concentrate must be diluted before use. Add two ampuls (total 5 g) to 500 mL or one ampul (2.5 g) to 250 mL of compatible solution to yield a 10-mg/mL solution. Concentrations exceeding 10 mg/mL are not recommended.

Administration: Administer by IV infusion at a concentration of 10 mg/mL, usually with an infusion control device.

Stability: Esmolol hydrochloride is a colorless to light yellow solution. Store at room temperature; freezing does not affect the product adversely. It is relatively stable at neutral pH but undergoes rapid hydrolysis in strongly acidic or basic solutions. It is stable for 24 hours diluted in a compatible infusion solution.

Compatibility Table

Solutions	Compatible	Incompatible	Variable
Dextrose 5%	●	…	…
Dextrose 5% in sodium chloride 0.45 & 0.9%	●	…	…
Ringer's injection, lactated	●	…	…
Sodium bicarbonate 5%	…	…	●
Sodium chloride 0.45 & 0.9%	●	…	…

Drugs			
Amikacin sulfate	●	…	…
Aminophylline	●	…	…
Amiodarone HCl	●	…	…
Amphotericin B cholesteryl sulfate complex	…	●	…

Drugs	Compatible	Incompatible	Variable
Ampicillin sodium	●	...	...
Atracurium besylate	●	...	...
Bivalirudin	●	...	...
Butorphanol tartrate	●	...	...
Calcium chloride	●	...	...
Cefazolin sodium	●	...	...
Ceftazidime	●	...	...
Ceftizoxime sodium	●	...	...
Chloramphenicol sodium succinate	●	...	...
Cimetidine HCl	●	...	...
Cisatracurium besylate	●	...	...
Clindamycin phosphate	●	...	...
Dexmedetomidine HCl	●	...	...
Diazepam	...	●	...
Diltiazem HCl	●	...	...
Dopamine HCl	●	...	...
Enalaprilat	●	...	...
Erythromycin lactobionate	●	...	...
Famotidine	●	...	...
Fenoldopam mesylate	●	...	...
Fentanyl citrate	●	...	...
Furosemide	...	●	...
Gentamicin sulfate	●	...	...
Heparin sodium	●	...	...
Hextend	●	...	...
Hydrocortisone sodium succinate	●	...	...
Insulin, regular	●	...	...
Labetalol HCl	●	...	...
Lansoprazole	...	●	...
Linezolid	●	...	...
Magnesium sulfate	●	...	...
Methyldopate HCl	●	...	...
Metronidazole	●	...	...
Midazolam HCl	●	...	...
Morphine sulfate	●	...	...
Nafcillin sodium	●	...	...
Nicardipine HCl	●	...	...
Nitroglycerin	●	...	...
Norepinephrine HCl	●	...	...

Drugs	Compatible	Incompatible	Variable
Pancuronium bromide	●	...	...
Pantoprazole sodium	...	●	...
Penicillin G potassium	●	...	...
Piperacillin sodium	●	...	...
Polymyxin B sulfate	●	...	...
Potassium chloride & phosphate	●	...	...
Procainamide HCl	...	●	...
Propofol	●	...	...
Ranitidine HCl	●	...	...
Remifentanil HCl	●	...	...
Sodium acetate	●	...	...
Sodium nitroprusside	●	...	...
Streptomycin sulfate	●	...	...
Tacrolimus	●	...	...
Thiopental sodium	...	●	...
Tobramycin sulfate	●	...	...
Trimethoprim–sulfamethoxazole	●	...	...
Vancomycin HCl	●	...	...
Vecuronium bromide	●	...	...
Warfarin sodium	...	●	...

Etoposide Phosphate

Handbook on Injectable Drugs pp. 654–661.

Description: A semisynthetic podophyllotoxin-derived antineoplastic agent.

Products: Etopophos; 100-mg vials. *pH:* Approximately pH 2.9 at 1 mg/mL.

Preparation: Reconstitute the 100-mg vials with 5 or 10 mL of compatible diluent to yield a 20- or 10-mg/mL solution, respectively. Sterile water for injection, dextrose 5%, sodium chloride 0.9%, bacteriostatic water for injection (benzyl alcohol preserved), and bacteriostatic sodium chloride 0.9% (benzyl alcohol preserved) may be used for reconstitution.

Administration: Administer by IV infusion over periods from 5 to 210 minutes. The reconstituted drug may be given without further dilution or may be diluted to as low as 0.1 mg/mL with dextrose 5% or sodium chloride 0.9%.

Stability: The white to off-white powder in intact vials should be stored under refrigeration and protected from light. The reconstituted solution is stable for 24 hours at room temperature and seven days under refrigeration according to the manufacturer. However, other research of the drug's stability indicates little or no loss occurs within 31 days at room temperature or under refrigeration.

This phosphate ester form of etoposide is very water soluble (>100 mg/mL) and does not exhibit the high potential for precipitation from aqueous media that the organic-solvent-based formulation has. Similarly, the stability and compatibility characteristics of etoposide phosphate cannot be extended to conventional etoposide formulated in the organic solvent vehicle.

Compatibility Table

Solutions	Compatible	Incompatible	Variable
Dextrose 5%	●	...	...
Sodium chloride 0.9%	●	...	...

Drugs	Compatible	Incompatible	Variable
Acyclovir sodium	●	...	...
Amikacin sulfate	●	...	...
Aminophylline	●	...	...
Amphotericin B	...	●	...
Ampicillin sodium	●	...	...
Ampicillin sod.–sulbactam sod.	●	...	...
Aztreonam	●	...	...
Bleomycin sulfate	●	...	...
Bumetanide	●	...	...
Buprenorphine HCl	●	...	...
Butorphanol tartrate	●	...	...
Calcium gluconate	●	...	...
Carboplatin	●	...	...
Carmustine	●	...	...
Cefazolin sodium	●	...	...
Cefepime HCl	...	●	...
Cefotaxime sodium	●	...	...
Cefotetan disodium	●	...	...
Cefoxitin sodium	●	...	...
Ceftazidime	●	...	...
Ceftizoxime sodium	●	...	...
Ceftriaxone sodium	●	...	...
Cefuroxime sodium	●	...	...
Chlorpromazine HCl	...	●	...
Cimetidine HCl	●	...	...
Ciprofloxacin	●	...	...
Cisplatin	●	...	...
Clindamycin phosphate	●	...	...
Cyclophosphamide	●	...	...
Cytarabine	●	...	...
Dacarbazine	●	...	...
Dactinomycin	●	...	...
Daunorubicin HCl	●	...	...
Dexamethasone sodium phosphate ...	●	...	...
Diphenhydramine HCl	●	...	...
Dobutamine HCl	●	...	...
Dopamine HCl	●	...	...
Doxorubicin HCl	●	...	...
Doxycycline hyclate	●	...	...
Droperidol	●	...	...

Drugs	Compatible	Incompatible	Variable
Enalaprilat	●	...	...
Famotidine	●	...	...
Fluconazole	●	...	...
Fludarabine phosphate	●	...	...
Fluorouracil	●	...	...
Furosemide	●	...	...
Ganciclovir sodium	●	...	...
Gemcitabine HCl	●	...	...
Gentamicin sulfate	●	...	...
Granisetron HCl	●	...	...
Haloperidol lactate	●	...	...
Heparin sodium	●	...	...
Hydrocortisone sodium phosphate	●	...	...
Hydrocortisone sodium succinate	●	...	...
Hydromorphone HCl	●	...	...
Hydroxyzine HCl	●	...	...
Idarubicin HCl	●	...	...
Ifosfamide	●	...	...
Imipenem–cilastatin sodium	...	●	...
Lansoprazole	...	●	...
Leucovorin calcium	●	...	...
Linezolid	●	...	...
Lorazepam	●	...	...
Magnesium sulfate	●	...	...
Mannitol	●	...	...
Meperidine HCl	●	...	...
Mesna	●	...	...
Methotrexate sodium	●	...	...
Methylprednisolone sod. succ.	...	●	...
Metoclopramide HCl	●	...	...
Metronidazole	●	...	...
Mitomycin	...	●	...
Mitoxantrone HCl	●	...	...
Morphine sulfate	●	...	...
Nalbuphine HCl	●	...	...
Ondansetron HCl	●	...	...
Oxaliplatin	●	...	...
Paclitaxel	●	...	...
Piperacillin sodium	●	...	...
Piperacillin sod.–tazobactam sod.	●	...	...

Drugs	Compatible	Incompatible	Variable
Potassium chloride	●	...	...
Prochlorperazine edisylate	...	●	...
Promethazine HCl	●	...	...
Ranitidine HCl	●	...	...
Sodium bicarbonate	●	...	...
Streptozocin	●	...	...
Teniposide	●	...	...
Thiotepa	●	...	...
Ticarcillin disod.–clavulanate pot.	●	...	...
Tobramycin sulfate	●	...	...
Trimethoprim–sulfamethoxazole	●	...	...
Vancomycin HCl	●	...	...
Vinblastine sulfate	●	...	...
Vincristine sulfate	●	...	...
Zidovudine	●	...	...

Famotidine

Handbook on Injectable Drugs pp. 662–669.

Description: A histamine H$_2$ receptor antagonist.

Products: Pepcid; 10 mg/mL in 2-mL single-dose and 4- and 20-mL multiple-dose vials. Premixed solution of 20 mg/50 mL. *pH:* From 5 to 5.6 (vials); from 5.7 to 6.4 (premixed solution).

Preparation: A 20-mg dose should be diluted in 5 to 10 mL of sodium chloride 0.9% for IV injection or 100 mL of compatible diluent for IV infusion.

Administration: Administer by slow IV injection at a rate no faster than 10 mg/min or by IV infusion over 15 to 30 minutes.

Stability: Famotidine is a clear, colorless solution. Store intact vials under refrigeration with protection from freezing and temperatures over 40 °C. If freezing occurs, thaw famotidine at room temperature or under warm water; be sure that complete solubilization has occurred. Store premixed solutions at room temperature and protect from excessive heat. The drug is stable for up to 26 weeks at room temperatures not exceeding 25 °C.

Compatibility Table

Solutions	Compatible	Incompatible	Variable
Dextrose 5 & 10%	●	...	...
Fat emulsion 10%, IV	●	...	...
Ringer's injection, lactated	●	...	...
Sodium bicarbonate 5%	●	...	...
Sodium chloride 0.9%	●	...	...

Drugs	Compatible	Incompatible	Variable
Acyclovir sodium	●	...	...
Allopurinol sodium	●	...	...
Amifostine	●	...	...
Aminophylline	●	...	...
Amiodarone HCl	●	...	...
Amphotericin B cholesteryl sulfate complex	...	●	...
Ampicillin sodium	●	...	...
Ampicillin sod.–sulbactam sod.	●	...	...
Anakinra	●	...	...

Drugs	Compatible	Incompatible	Variable
Atropine sulfate	●	...	...
Azithromycin	...	●	...
Aztreonam	●	...	...
Bivalirudin	●	...	...
Calcium gluconate	●	...	...
Cefazolin sodium	●	...	...
Cefepime HCl	...	●	...
Cefotaxime sodium	●	...	...
Cefotetan disodium	●	...	...
Cefoxitin sodium	●	...	...
Ceftazidime	●	...	...
Ceftizoxime sodium	●	...	...
Ceftriaxone sodium	●	...	...
Cefuroxime sodium	●	...	...
Chlorpromazine HCl	●	...	...
Cisatracurium besylate	●	...	...
Cisplatin	●	...	...
Cladribine	●	...	...
Cyclophosphamide	●	...	...
Cytarabine	●	...	...
Dexamethasone sodium phosphate	●	...	...
Dexmedetomidine HCl	●	...	...
Digoxin	●	...	...
Diphenhydramine HCl	●	...	...
Dobutamine HCl	●	...	...
Docetaxel	●	...	...
Dopamine HCl	●	...	...
Doxorubicin HCl	●	...	...
Doxorubicin HCl liposome injection	●	...	...
Droperidol	●	...	...
Enalaprilat	●	...	...
Epinephrine HCl	●	...	...
Erythromycin lactobionate	●	...	...
Esmolol HCl	●	...	...
Etoposide phosphate	●	...	...
Fenoldopam mesylate	●	...	...
Filgrastim	●	...	...
Fluconazole	●	...	...
Fludarabine phosphate	●	...	...

Drugs	Compatible	Incompatible	Variable
Flumazenil	●	...	...
Folic acid	●	...	...
Furosemide	●	...	...
Gemcitabine HCl	●	...	...
Gentamicin sulfate	●	...	...
Granisetron HCl	●	...	...
Haloperidol lactate	●	...	...
Heparin sodium	●	...	...
Hextend	●	...	...
Hydrocortisone sodium succinate	●	...	...
Hydromorphone HCl	●	...	...
Hydroxyzine HCl	●	...	...
Imipenem–cilastatin sodium	●	...	...
Insulin, regular	●	...	...
Isoproterenol HCl	●	...	...
Labetalol HCl	●	...	...
Lansoprazole	...	●	...
Lidocaine HCl	●	...	...
Linezolid	●	...	...
Lorazepam	●	...	...
Magnesium sulfate	●	...	...
Melphalan HCl	●	...	...
Meperidine HCl	●	...	...
Methotrexate sodium	●	...	...
Methylprednisolone sod. succ.	●	...	...
Metoclopramide HCl	●	...	...
Midazolam HCl	●	...	...
Morphine sulfate	●	...	...
Nafcillin sodium	●	...	...
Nicardipine HCl	●	...	...
Nitroglycerin	●	...	...
Norepinephrine bitartrate	●	...	...
Ondansetron HCl	●	...	...
Oxacillin sodium	●	...	...
Oxaliplatin	●	...	...
Paclitaxel	●	...	...
Pemetrexed disodium	●	...	...
Phenylephrine HCl	●	...	...
Phenytoin sodium	●	...	...
Phytonadione	●	...	...

Drugs	Compatible	Incompatible	Variable
Piperacillin sodium	●	...	...
Piperacillin sod.–tazobactam sod.	...	●	...
Potassium chloride	●	...	...
Potassium phosphates	●	...	...
Procainamide HCl	●	...	...
Propofol	●	...	...
Remifentanil HCl	●	...	...
Sargramostim	●	...	...
Sodium bicarbonate	●	...	...
Sodium nitroprusside	●	...	...
Teniposide	●	...	...
Theophylline	●	...	...
Thiamine HCl	●	...	...
Thiotepa	●	...	...
Ticarcillin disod.–clavulanate pot.	●	...	...
Tirofiban HCl	●	...	...
Vancomycin HCl	●	...	...
Verapamil HCl	●	...	...
Vinorelbine tartrate	●	...	...

Fenoldopam Mesylate

Handbook on Injectable Drugs pp. 691–698.

Description: A dopamine agonist used in the short-term management of severe hypertension.

Products: **Corlopam**; 10-mg/mL concentrate in 1- and 2-mL ampuls. *pH:* From 2.8 to 3.8.

Preparation: The concentrate must be diluted with dextrose 5% or sodium chloride 0.9% for use; a 40-mcg/mL concentration is recommended.

Administration: After dilution, administer by slow IV infusion using a controlled infusion device. Bolus doses should not be given.

Stability: The injection should be stored at room temperature or under refrigeration. After dilution in dextrose 5% or sodium chloride 0.9%, fenoldopam mesylate is stable for at least 72 hours under normal ambient light and temperature and under refrigeration.

Compatibility Table

Solutions	Compatible	Incompatible	Variable
Dextrose 5%	●	...	...
Sodium chloride 0.9%	●	...	...

Drugs			
Alfentanil HCl	●	...	...
Amikacin sulfate	●	...	...
Aminocaproic acid	●	...	...
Aminophylline	...	●	...
Amiodarone HCl	●	...	...
Amphotericin B	...	●	...
Ampicillin sodium	...	●	...
Ampicillin sodium–sulbactam sodium	●	...	...
Argatroban	●	...	...
Atracurium besylate	●	...	...
Atropine sulfate	●	...	...
Aztreonam	●	...	...
Bumetanide	...	●	...
Butorphanol tartrate	●	...	...

Drugs	Compatible	Incompatible	Variable
Calcium gluconate	●	...	...
Cefazolin sodium	●	...	...
Cefepime HCl	●	...	...
Cefotaxime sodium	●	...	...
Cefotetan disodium	●	...	...
Cefoxitin sodium	...	●	...
Ceftazidime	●	...	...
Ceftizoxime sodium	●	...	...
Ceftriaxone sodium	●	...	...
Cefuroxime sodium	●	...	...
Chlorpromazine HCl	●	...	...
Cimetidine HCl	●	...	...
Ciprofloxacin	●	...	...
Cisatracurium besylate	●	...	...
Clindamycin phosphate	●	...	...
Dexamethasone sodium phosphate ...	...	●	...
Dexmedetomidine HCl	●	...	...
Diazepam	...	●	...
Digoxin	●	...	...
Diltiazem HCl	●	...	...
Diphenhydramine HCl	●	...	...
Dobutamine HCl	●	...	...
Dolasetron mesylate	●	...	...
Dopamine HCl	●	...	...
Doxycycline hyclate	●	...	...
Droperidol	●	...	...
Enalaprilat	●	...	...
Ephedrine sulfate	●	...	...
Epinephrine HCl	●	...	...
Erythromycin lactobionate	●	...	...
Esmolol HCl	●	...	...
Famotidine	●	...	...
Fentanyl citrate	●	...	...
Fluconazole	●	...	...
Fosphenytoin sodium	...	●	...
Furosemide	...	●	...
Gentamicin sulfate	●	...	...
Granisetron HCl	●	...	...
Haloperidol lactate	●	...	...
Heparin sodium	●	...	...

Drugs	Compatible	Incompatible	Variable
Hextend	●	...	...
Hydrocortisone sodium succinate	●	...	...
Hydromorphone HCl	●	...	...
Hydroxyzine HCl	●	...	...
Iodixanol	●	...	...
Iohexol	●	...	...
Iopamidol	●	...	...
Ioxaglate meglumine–ioxaglate sodium	●	...	...
Isoproterenol HCl	●	...	...
Ketorolac tromethamine	...	●	...
Labetalol HCl	●	...	...
Levofloxacin	●	...	...
Lidocaine HCl	●	...	...
Linezolid	●	...	...
Lorazepam	●	...	...
Magnesium sulfate	●	...	...
Mannitol	●	...	...
Meperidine HCl	●	...	...
Methohexital sodium	...	●	...
Methylprednisolone sodium succinate	...	●	...
Metoclopramide HCl	●	...	...
Metronidazole	●	...	...
Midazolam HCl	●	...	...
Milrinone lactate	●	...	...
Mivacurium chloride	●	...	...
Morphine sulfate	●	...	...
Nalbuphine HCl	●	...	...
Naloxone HCl	●	...	...
Nicardipine HCl	●	...	...
Nitroglycerin	●	...	...
Norepinephrine bitartrate	●	...	...
Ondansetron HCl	●	...	...
Pancuronium bromide	●	...	...
Pentobarbital sodium	...	●	...
Phenylephrine HCl	●	...	...
Phenytoin sodium	...	●	...
Piperacillin sodium	●	...	...
Piperacillin sodium–tazobactam sodium	●	...	...

173

Drugs	Compatible	Incompatible	Variable
Potassium chloride	●	...	...
Procainamide HCl	●	...	...
Prochlorperazine edisylate	...	●	...
Promethazine HCl	●	...	...
Propofol	●	...	...
Propranolol HCl	●	...	...
Quinupristin–dalfopristin	●	...	...
Ranitidine HCl	●	...	...
Remifentanil HCl	●	...	...
Rocuronium bromide	●	...	...
Sodium bicarbonate	...	●	...
Sufentanil citrate	●	...	...
Theophylline	●	...	...
Thiopental sodium	...	●	...
Ticarcillin disodium–clavulanate potassium	●	...	...
Tobramycin sulfate	●	...	...
Trimethoprim–sulfamethoxazole	●	...	...
Vancomycin HCl	●	...	...
Vecuronium bromide	●	...	...
Verapamil HCl	●	...	...

Fentanyl Citrate

Handbook on Injectable Drugs pp. 699–707.

Description: A synthetic potent narcotic analgesic.

Products: Sublimaze; 2-, 5-, 10-, and 20-mL ampuls containing 50 mcg (0.05 mg) of fentanyl (as citrate) in each milliliter. *pH:* From 4 to 7.5.

Administration: Administer IM or IV.

Stability: Intact ampuls should be stored at room temperature protected from light. The drug is most stable between pH 3.5 and 7.5. No loss due to sorption to plastic bags occurs at normal pH. However, if mixed with alkaline solutions, up to 50% losses due to sorption occur in one hour.

Compatibility Table

Solutions	Compatible	Incompatible	Variable
Dextrose 5%	●	...	...
Sodium chloride 0.9%	●	...	...

Drugs	Compatible	Incompatible	Variable
Abciximab	●	...	...
Amiodarone HCl	●	...	...
Amphotericin B cholesteryl sulfate complex	●	...	...
Argatroban	●	...	...
Atracurium besylate	●	...	...
Atropine sulfate	●	...	...
Azithromycin	...	●	...
Bivalirudin	●	...	...
Bupivacaine HCl	●	...	...
Butorphanol tartrate	●	...	...
Caffeine citrate	●	...	...
Chlorpromazine HCl	●	...	...
Cimetidine HCl	●	...	...
Cisatracurium besylate	●	...	...
Clonidine HCl	●	...	...
Dexamethasone sodium phosphate	●	...	...
Diazepam	●	...	...
Diltiazem HCl	●	...	...
Dimenhydrinate	●	...	...

Drugs	Compatible	Incompatible	Variable
Diphenhydramine HCl	●	...	...
Dobutamine HCl	●	...	...
Dopamine HCl	●	...	...
Doxapram HCl	●	...	...
Droperidol	●	...	...
Enalaprilat	●	...	...
Epinephrine HCl	●	...	...
Esmolol HCl	●	...	...
Fenoldopam mesylate	●	...	...
Fluorouracil	...	●	...
Haloperidol lactate	●	...	...
Heparin sodium	●	...	...
Hextend	●	...	...
Hydrocortisone sodium succinate	●	...	...
Hydromorphone HCl	●	...	...
Hydroxyzine HCl	●	...	...
Ketorolac tromethamine	●	...	...
Labetalol HCl	●	...	...
Lansoprazole	●	...	...
Levofloxacin	●	...	...
Lidocaine HCl	...	...	●
Linezolid	●	...	...
Lorazepam	●	...	...
Meperidine HCl	●	...	...
Methohexital sodium	...	●	...
Metoclopramide HCl	●	...	...
Midazolam HCl	●	...	...
Milrinone lactate	●	...	...
Morphine sulfate	●	...	...
Nafcillin sodium	●	...	...
Nicardipine HCl	●	...	...
Nitroglycerin	●	...	...
Norepinephrine bitartrate	●	...	...
Ondansetron HCl	●	...	...
Oxaliplatin	●	...	...
Pancuronium bromide	●	...	...
Pantoprazole sodium	...	●	...
Pentazocine lactate	●	...	...
Pentobarbital sodium	...	●	...
Phenobarbital sodium	●	...	...

Drugs	Compatible	Incompatible	Variable
Phenytoin sodium	...	●	...
Potassium chloride	●	...	...
Prochlorperazine edisylate	●	...	...
Promethazine HCl	●	...	...
Propofol	●	...	...
Ranitidine HCl	●	...	...
Remifentanil HCl	●	...	...
Ropivacaine HCl	●	...	...
Sargramostim	●	...	...
Scopolamine HBr	●	...	...
Thiopental sodium	...	...	●
Vecuronium bromide	●	...	...

Fentanyl Citrate

Filgrastim

Handbook on Injectable Drugs pp. 707–714.

Description: A recombinant human granulocyte colony stimulating factor.

Products: Neupogen; 300- and 480-mcg sizes in vials and syringes. *pH:* 4.

Preparation: Dilute in a suitable amount of dextrose 5% for IV infusion. For continuous SC infusion, dilute the dose in 10 to 50 mL of dextrose 5%. Add normal human serum albumin 0.2% to filgrastim concentrations of 5 to 15 mcg/mL. Do not dilute to less than 5 mcg/mL.

Administration: Administer by SC or IV injection or SC or IV infusion. Use a controlled infusion device for extended infusion.

Stability: Store the clear, colorless solution under refrigeration with protection from direct sunlight, freezing, and temperatures above 30 °C. The product is stable for up to 24 hours at 9 to 30 °C. Do not shake the solution.

Addition of normal human serum albumin 0.2% to filgrastim concentrations of 5 to 15 mcg/mL is necessary to minimize sorption to containers and equipment. At concentrations above 15 mcg/mL, albumin is unnecessary. Do not dilute to less than 5 mcg/mL.

Compatibility Table

Solutions	Compatible	Incompatible	Variable
Dextrose 5%	●	...	...
Sodium chloride 0.9%	...	●	...

Drugs	Compatible	Incompatible	Variable
Acyclovir sodium	●	...	...
Allopurinol sodium	●	...	...
Amikacin sulfate	●	...	...
Aminophylline	●	...	...
Amphotericin B	...	●	...
Ampicillin sodium	●	...	...
Ampicillin sod.–sulbactam sod.	●	...	...
Aztreonam	●	...	...
Bleomycin sulfate	●	...	...
Bumetanide	●	...	...

Drugs	Compatible	Incompatible	Variable
Buprenorphine HCl	●	...	...
Butorphanol tartrate	●	...	...
Calcium gluconate	●	...	...
Carboplatin	●	...	...
Carmustine	●	...	...
Cefazolin sodium	●	...	...
Cefepime HCl	...	●	...
Cefotaxime sodium	...	●	...
Cefotetan disodium	●	...	...
Cefoxitin sodium	...	●	...
Ceftazidime	●	...	...
Ceftizoxime sodium	...	●	...
Ceftriaxone sodium	...	●	...
Cefuroxime sodium	...	●	...
Chlorpromazine HCl	●	...	...
Cimetidine HCl	●	...	...
Cisplatin	●	...	...
Clindamycin phosphate	...	●	...
Cyclophosphamide	●	...	...
Cytarabine	●	...	...
Dacarbazine	●	...	...
Dactinomycin	...	●	...
Daunorubicin HCl	●	...	...
Dexamethasone sodium phosphate	●	...	...
Diphenhydramine HCl	●	...	...
Doxorubicin HCl	●	...	...
Doxycycline hyclate	●	...	...
Droperidol	●	...	...
Enalaprilat	●	...	...
Etoposide	...	●	...
Famotidine	●	...	...
Floxuridine	●	...	...
Fluconazole	●	...	...
Fludarabine phosphate	●	...	...
Fluorouracil	...	●	...
Furosemide	...	●	...
Gallium nitrate	●	...	...
Ganciclovir sodium	●	...	...
Gentamicin sulfate	...	...	●
Granisetron HCl	●	...	...

Drugs	Compatible	Incompatible	Variable
Haloperidol lactate	●	…	…
Heparin sodium	…	●	…
Hydrocortisone sodium phosphate . . .	●	…	…
Hydrocortisone sodium succinate	●	…	…
Hydromorphone HCl	●	…	…
Hydroxyzine HCl	●	…	…
Idarubicin HCl	●	…	…
Ifosfamide	●	…	…
Imipenem–cilastatin sodium	…	…	●
Leucovorin calcium	●	…	…
Lorazepam	●	…	…
Mannitol	…	●	…
Mechlorethamine HCl	●	…	…
Melphalan HCl	●	…	…
Meperidine HCl	●	…	…
Mesna	●	…	…
Methotrexate sodium	●	…	…
Methylprednisolone sod. succ.	…	●	…
Metoclopramide HCl	●	…	…
Metronidazole	…	●	…
Mitomycin	…	●	…
Mitoxantrone HCl	●	…	…
Morphine sulfate	●	…	…
Nalbuphine HCl	●	…	…
Ondansetron HCl	●	…	…
Piperacillin sodium	…	●	…
Potassium chloride	●	…	…
Prochlorperazine edisylate	…	●	…
Promethazine HCl	●	…	…
Ranitidine HCl	●	…	…
Sodium bicarbonate	●	…	…
Streptozocin	●	…	…
Thiotepa	…	●	…
Ticarcillin disod.–clavulanate pot. . . .	●	…	…
Tobramycin sulfate	●	…	…
Trimethoprim–sulfamethoxazole	●	…	…
Vancomycin HCl	●	…	…
Vinblastine sulfate	●	…	…
Vincristine sulfate	●	…	…
Vinorelbine tartrate	●	…	…
Zidovudine	●	…	…

Fluconazole

Handbook on Injectable Drugs pp. 722–729.

Description: A synthetic triazole-derived antifungal agent.

Products: Diflucan; 2 mg/mL in 100- and 200-mL bottles and bags. *pH:* From 4 to 8 in sodium chloride diluent and 3.5 to 6.5 in dextrose diluent.

Administration: Administer by IV infusion at a rate not exceeding 200 mg/hr.

Stability: Store fluconazole at room temperature or under refrigeration with protection from freezing. Do not use a cloudy or precipitated solution.

Compatibility Table

Drugs	Compatible	Incompatible	Variable
Acyclovir sodium	●	…	…
Aldesleukin	●	…	…
Allopurinol sodium	●	…	…
Amifostine	●	…	…
Amikacin sulfate	●	…	…
Aminophylline	●	…	…
Amiodarone HCl	●	…	…
Amphotericin B	…	…	●
Amphotericin B cholesteryl sulfate complex	…	●	…
Ampicillin sodium	…	●	…
Ampicillin sod.–sulbactam sod.	●	…	…
Anakinra	…	…	●
Aztreonam	●	…	…
Bivalirudin	●	…	…
Calcium gluconate	…	●	…
Cefazolin sodium	●	…	…
Cefepime HCl	●	…	…
Cefotaxime sodium	…	●	…
Cefotetan disodium	●	…	…
Cefoxitin sodium	●	…	…
Ceftazidime	…	…	●
Ceftriaxone sodium	…	●	…
Cefuroxime sodium	…	●	…
Chloramphenicol sodium succinate	…	●	…

Drugs	Compatible	Incompatible	Variable
Chlorpromazine HCl	●	...	...
Cimetidine HCl	●	...	...
Ciprofloxacin	●	...	...
Cisatracurium besylate	●	...	...
Clindamycin phosphate	...	...	●
Daptomycin	●	...	...
Dexamethasone sodium phosphate ...	●	...	...
Dexmedetomidine HCl	●	...	...
Diazepam	...	●	...
Digoxin	...	●	...
Diltiazem HCl	●	...	...
Dimenhydrinate	●	...	...
Diphenhydramine HCl	●	...	...
Dobutamine HCl	●	...	...
Docetaxel	●	...	...
Dopamine HCl	●	...	...
Doxorubicin HCl liposome injection	●	...	...
Droperidol	●	...	...
Drotrecogin alfa (activated)	●	...	...
Etoposide phosphate	●	...	...
Famotidine	●	...	...
Fenoldopam mesylate	●	...	...
Filgrastim	●	...	...
Fludarabine phosphate	●	...	...
Foscarnet sodium	●	...	...
Furosemide	...	●	...
Gallium nitrate	●	...	...
Ganciclovir sodium	●	...	...
Gemcitabine HCl	●	...	...
Gentamicin sulfate	●	...	...
Granisetron HCl	●	...	...
Haloperidol lactate	...	●	...
Heparin sodium	●	...	...
Hextend	●	...	...
Hydrocortisone sodium succinate	●	...	...
Hydroxyzine HCl	...	●	...
Imipenem–cilastatin sodium	...	●	...
Immune globulin intravenous	●	...	...
Lansoprazole	●	...	...
Leucovorin calcium	●	...	...

Drugs	Compatible	Incompatible	Variable
Linezolid	●	...	...
Lorazepam	●	...	...
Melphalan HCl	●	...	...
Meperidine HCl	●	...	...
Meropenem	●	...	...
Metoclopramide HCl	●	...	...
Metronidazole	●	...	...
Midazolam HCl	●	...	...
Morphine sulfate	●	...	...
Nafcillin sodium	●	...	...
Nitroglycerin	●	...	...
Ondansetron HCl	●	...	...
Oxacillin sodium	●	...	...
Paclitaxel	●	...	...
Pancuronium bromide	●	...	...
Pantoprazole sodium	...	●	...
Pemetrexed disodium	●	...	...
Penicillin G potassium	●	...	...
Pentamidine isethionate	...	●	...
Phenytoin sodium	●	...	...
Piperacillin sodium	...	...	●
Piperacillin sod.–tazobactam sod.	●	...	...
Potassium chloride	●	...	...
Prochlorperazine edisylate	●	...	...
Promethazine HCl	●	...	...
Propofol	●	...	...
Quinupristin–dalfopristin	●	...	...
Ranitidine HCl	●	...	...
Remifentanil HCl	●	...	...
Sargramostim	●	...	...
Tacrolimus	●	...	...
Teniposide	●	...	...
Theophylline	●	...	...
Thiotepa	●	...	...
Ticarcillin disod.–clavulanate pot.	●	...	...
Tobramycin sulfate	●	...	...
Trimethoprim–sulfamethoxazole	...	●	...
Vancomycin HCl	●	...	...
Vecuronium bromide	●	...	...
Vinorelbine tartrate	●	...	...
Zidovudine	●	...	...

Fludarabine Phosphate

Handbook on Injectable Drugs pp. 730–734.

Description: A synthetic nucleoside antineoplastic agent.

Products: Fludara; 50-mg vials. *pH:* From 7.2 to 8.2.

Preparation: Reconstitute with 2 mL of sterile water for injection to yield a 25-mg/mL solution. For IV infusion, dilute the dose in 100 or 125 mL of dextrose 5% or sodium chloride 0.9%.

Administration: Administer by IV infusion over 30 minutes.

Stability: Store fludarabine phosphate under refrigeration. The reconstituted solution exhibits less than a 2% loss in 16 days at room temperature. No sorption to PVC plastic bags has been noted.

Compatibility Table

Solutions	Compatible	Incompatible	Variable
Dextrose 5%	●	...	...
Sodium chloride 0.9%	●	...	...

Drugs			
Acyclovir sodium	...	●	...
Allopurinol sodium	●	...	...
Amifostine	●	...	...
Amikacin sulfate	●	...	...
Aminophylline	●	...	...
Amphotericin B	...	●	...
Ampicillin sodium	●	...	...
Ampicillin sod.–sulbactam sod.	●	...	...
Aztreonam	●	...	...
Bleomycin sulfate	●	...	...
Butorphanol tartrate	●	...	...
Carboplatin	●	...	...
Carmustine	●	...	...
Cefazolin sodium	●	...	...
Cefepime HCl	●	...	...
Cefotaxime sodium	●	...	...
Cefotetan disodium	●	...	...
Ceftazidime	●	...	...
Ceftizoxime sodium	●	...	...
Ceftriaxone sodium	●	...	...

Drugs	Compatible	Incompatible	Variable
Cefuroxime sodium	●	...	...
Chlorpromazine HCl	...	●	...
Cimetidine HCl	●	...	...
Cisplatin	●	...	...
Clindamycin phosphate	●	...	...
Cyclophosphamide	●	...	...
Cytarabine	●	...	...
Dacarbazine	●	...	...
Dactinomycin	●	...	...
Daunorubicin HCl	...	●	...
Dexamethasone sodium phosphate	●	...	...
Diphenhydramine HCl	●	...	...
Doxorubicin HCl	●	...	...
Doxycycline hyclate	●	...	...
Droperidol	●	...	...
Etoposide	●	...	...
Etoposide phosphate	●	...	...
Famotidine	●	...	...
Filgrastim	●	...	...
Fluconazole	●	...	...
Fluorouracil	●	...	...
Furosemide	●	...	...
Ganciclovir sodium	...	●	...
Gemcitabine HCl	●	...	...
Gentamicin sulfate	●	...	...
Granisetron HCl	●	...	...
Haloperidol lactate	●	...	...
Heparin sodium	●	...	...
Hydrocortisone sodium phosphate	●	...	...
Hydrocortisone sodium succinate	●	...	...
Hydromorphone HCl	●	...	...
Hydroxyzine HCl	...	●	...
Ifosfamide	●	...	...
Imipenem–cilastatin sodium	●	...	...
Lorazepam	●	...	...
Magnesium sulfate	●	...	...
Mannitol	●	...	...
Mechlorethamine HCl	●	...	...
Melphalan HCl	●	...	...
Meperidine HCl	●	...	...

Drugs	Compatible	Incompatible	Variable
Mesna	●	...	...
Methotrexate sodium	●	...	...
Methylprednisolone sod. succ.	●	...	...
Metoclopramide HCl	●	...	...
Mitoxantrone HCl	●	...	...
Morphine sulfate	●	...	...
Multivitamins	●	...	...
Nalbuphine HCl	●	...	...
Ondansetron HCl	●	...	...
Pentostatin	●	...	...
Piperacillin sodium	●	...	...
Piperacillin sod.–tazobactam sod.	●	...	...
Potassium chloride	●	...	...
Prochlorperazine edisylate	...	●	...
Promethazine HCl	●	...	...
Ranitidine HCl	●	...	...
Sodium bicarbonate	●	...	...
Teniposide	●	...	...
Thiotepa	●	...	...
Ticarcillin disod.–clavulanate pot.	●	...	...
Tobramycin sulfate	●	...	...
Trimethoprim–sulfamethoxazole	●	...	...
Vancomycin HCl	●	...	...
Vinblastine sulfate	●	...	...
Vincristine sulfate	●	...	...
Vinorelbine tartrate	●	...	...
Zidovudine	●	...	...

Fluorouracil

Handbook on Injectable Drugs pp. 736–745.

Description: An antineoplastic agent which acts as a pyrimidine antagonist.

Products: 50 mg/mL in 10- and 20-mL vials and ampuls and 100-mL bulk packages. *pH:* Approximately 9.2.

Administration: Administer IV, carefully avoiding extravasation. Fluorouracil may be given by infusion or direct IV injection. Dilution is not required.

Stability: Potency is not affected by slight discoloration during storage. The solution is normally colorless to faint yellow. However, a dark yellow, amber, or brown solution should be discarded. Store at room temperature. Exposure to low temperatures may result in a precipitate, which may be resolubilized by heating to 60 °C with vigorous shaking.

No significant sorption to plastic IV bags, sets, tubing, or syringes has been noted.

Compatibility Table

Solutions	Compatible	Incompatible	Variable
Dextrose 5%	●	...	...
Dextrose 5% in Ringer's injection, lactated	●	...	...
Sodium chloride 0.9%	●	...	...

Drugs	Compatible	Incompatible	Variable
Aldesleukin	...	●	...
Allopurinol sodium	●	...	...
Amifostine	●	...	...
Amphotericin B cholesteryl sulfate complex	...	●	...
Aztreonam	●	...	...
Bleomycin sulfate	●	...	...
Carboplatin	...	●	...
Cefepime HCl	●	...	...
Cisplatin	...	...	●

Drugs	Compatible	Incompatible	Variable
Cyclophosphamide	●	...	...
Cytarabine	...	●	...
Diazepam	...	●	...
Doxorubicin HCl	...	●	...
Doxorubicin HCl liposome injection	●	...	...
Droperidol	...	●	...
Epirubicin HCl	...	●	...
Etoposide	●	...	...
Etoposide phosphate	●	...	...
Fentanyl citrate	...	●	...
Filgrastim	...	●	...
Fludarabine phosphate	●	...	...
Furosemide	●	...	...
Gallium nitrate	...	●	...
Gemcitabine HCl	●	...	...
Granisetron HCl	●	...	...
Heparin sodium	●	...	...
Hydrocortisone sodium succinate	●	...	...
Hydromorphone HCl	●	...	...
Ifosfamide	●	...	...
Lansoprazole	...	●	...
Leucovorin calcium	...	...	●
Linezolid	●	...	...
Mannitol	●	...	...
Melphalan HCl	●	...	...
Methotrexate sodium	...	...	●
Metoclopramide HCl	...	...	●
Mitomycin	●	...	...
Mitoxantrone HCl	●	...	...
Morphine sulfate	...	●	...
Ondansetron HCl	...	●	...
Paclitaxel	●	...	...
Pemetrexed disodium	●	...	...
Piperacillin sod.–tazobactam sod.	●	...	...
Potassium chloride	●	...	...
Propofol	●	...	...
Sargramostim	●	...	...
Teniposide	●	...	...
Thiotepa	●	...	...
Topotecan HCl	...	●	...
Vinblastine sulfate	●	...	...
Vincristine sulfate	●	...	...
Vinorelbine tartrate	...	●	...

Foscarnet Sodium

Handbook on Injectable Drugs pp. 748–753.

Description: An organic analog of pyrophosphate that acts as an antiviral agent.

Products: Foscavir; 24 mg/mL in 250- and 500-mL bottles. *pH:* 7.4.

Preparation: For peripheral administration, dilute to 12 mg/mL with dextrose 5% or sodium chloride 0.9%.

Administration: Administer by IV infusion, using a pump at a rate not exceeding 1 mg/kg/min, undiluted through a central line or diluted to 12 mg/mL for peripheral use.

Stability: Foscarnet sodium injection is a clear, colorless solution. Store it at room temperature and protect it from freezing and excessive heat. Use only if the container seal is intact and a vacuum is present. Diluted in a compatible diluent, the drug is stable for 24 hours at room or refrigeration temperature.

Compatibility Table

Solutions	Compatible	Incompatible	Variable
Dextrose 5%	●	...	...
Sodium chloride 0.9%	●	...	...

Drugs	Compatible	Incompatible	Variable
Acyclovir sodium	...	●	...
Aldesleukin	●	...	...
Amikacin sulfate	●	...	...
Aminophylline	●	...	...
Amphotericin B	...	●	...
Ampicillin sodium	●	...	...
Aztreonam	●	...	...
Cefazolin sodium	●	...	...
Cefoxitin sodium	●	...	...
Ceftazidime	●	...	...
Ceftizoxime sodium	●	...	...
Ceftriaxone sodium	●	...	...
Cefuroxime sodium	●	...	...
Chloramphenicol sodium succinate	●	...	...

Drugs	Compatible	Incompatible	Variable
Cimetidine HCl	●	...	...
Clindamycin phosphate	●	...	...
Dexamethasone sodium phosphate ...	●	...	...
Diazepam	...	●	...
Digoxin	...	●	...
Diphenhydramine HCl	...	●	...
Dobutamine HCl	...	●	...
Dopamine HCl	●	...	...
Droperidol	...	●	...
Erythromycin lactobionate	●	...	...
Fluconazole	●	...	...
Furosemide	●	...	...
Ganciclovir sodium	...	●	...
Gentamicin sulfate	●	...	...
Haloperidol lactate	...	●	...
Heparin sodium	●	...	...
Hydrocortisone sodium succinate	●	...	...
Hydromorphone HCl	●	...	...
Hydroxyzine HCl	●	...	...
Imipenem–cilastatin sodium	●	...	...
Leucovorin calcium	...	●	...
Lorazepam	...	...	●
Metoclopramide HCl	●	...	...
Metronidazole	●	...	...
Midazolam HCl	...	●	...
Morphine sulfate	●	...	...
Nafcillin sodium	●	...	...
Oxacillin sodium	●	...	...
Penicillin G potassium	●	...	...
Pentamidine isethionate	...	●	...
Phenytoin sodium	●	...	...
Piperacillin sodium	●	...	...
Potassium chloride	●	...	...
Prochlorperazine edisylate	...	●	...
Promethazine HCl	...	●	...
Ranitidine HCl	●	...	...
Ticarcillin disod.–clavulanate pot.	●	...	...
Tobramycin sulfate	●	...	...
Trimethoprim–sulfamethoxazole	...	...	●
Trimetrexate glucuronate	...	●	...
Vancomycin HCl	...	...	●

Furosemide

Handbook on Injectable Drugs pp. 757–768.

Description: A potent diuretic.

Products: **Lasix;** 10-mg/mL solution in 2-, 4-, and 10-mL amber ampuls, prefilled syringes, and single-use vials. *pH:* From 8 to 9.3.

Administration: Administer by IM or direct IV (slowly over one or two minutes) injection or by IV infusion at a rate not exceeding 4 mg/min.

Stability: Exposure to light may cause discoloration. Do not use furosemide solutions if they have a yellow color.

Store furosemide at room temperature; refrigeration may result in precipitation. Furosemide may precipitate in solutions having a pH below 5.5. No loss due to binding to filters has been found.

Compatibility Table

Solutions	Compatible	Incompatible	Variable
Dextrose 5%	●	...	...
Dextrose 5% in Ringer's injection, lactated	●	...	...
Dextrose 5% in sodium chloride 0.9%	●	...	...
Mannitol 20%	●	...	...
Ringer's injection, lactated	●	...	...
Sodium chloride 0.9%	●	...	...

Drugs			
Allopurinol sodium	●	...	...
Amifostine	●	...	...
Amikacin sulfate	●	...	...
Aminophylline	●	...	...
Amiodarone HCl	...	...	●
Amphotericin B cholesteryl sulfate complex	●	...	...
Ampicillin sodium	●	...	...
Argatroban	●	...	...
Atropine sulfate	●	...	...

Drugs	Compatible	Incompatible	Variable
Azithromycin	...	●	...
Aztreonam	●	...	...
Bivalirudin	●	...	...
Bleomycin sulfate	●	...	...
Bumetanide	●	...	...
Buprenorphine HCl	...	●	...
Caffeine citrate	...	●	...
Calcium gluconate	●	...	...
Cefamandole nafate	●	...	...
Cefepime HCl	●	...	...
Ceftazidime	●	...	...
Cefuroxime sodium	●	...	...
Chlorpromazine HCl	...	●	...
Cimetidine HCl	●	...	...
Ciprofloxacin	...	●	...
Cisatracurium besylate	...	...	●
Cisplatin	●	...	...
Cladribine	●	...	...
Cloxacillin sodium	●	...	...
Cyclophosphamide	●	...	...
Cytarabine	●	...	...
Dexamethasone sodium phosphate	●	...	...
Dexmedetomidine HCl	●	...	...
Diazepam	...	●	...
Digoxin	●	...	...
Diltiazem HCl	...	●	...
Dimenhydrinate	...	●	...
Dobutamine HCl	...	...	●
Docetaxel	●	...	...
Dopamine HCl	...	...	●
Doxapram HCl	...	●	...
Doxorubicin HCl	...	...	●
Doxorubicin HCl liposome injection	●	...	...
Droperidol	...	●	...
Drotrecogin alfa (activated)	...	...	●
Epinephrine HCl	...	...	●
Erythromycin lactobionate	...	●	...
Esmolol HCl	...	●	...
Etoposide phosphate	●	...	...

Drugs	Compatible	Incompatible	Variable
Famotidine	...	...	●
Fenoldopam mesylate	...	●	...
Fentanyl citrate	●	...	...
Filgrastim	...	●	...
Fluconazole	...	●	...
Fludarabine phosphate	●	...	...
Fluorouracil	●	...	...
Foscarnet sodium	●	...	...
Gallium nitrate	●	...	...
Gemcitabine HCl	...	●	...
Gentamicin sulfate	...	...	●
Granisetron HCl	●	...	...
Heparin sodium	●	...	...
Hextend	●	...	...
Hydralazine HCl	...	●	...
Hydrocortisone sodium succinate	...	...	●
Hydromorphone HCl	●	...	...
Idarubicin HCl	...	●	...
Indomethacin sodium trihydrate	●	...	...
Isoproterenol HCl	...	●	...
Kanamycin sulfate	●	...	...
Labetalol HCl	...	...	●
Lansoprazole	...	●	...
Leucovorin calcium	●	...	...
Levofloxacin	...	●	...
Lidocaine HCl	●	...	...
Linezolid	●	...	...
Lorazepam	●	...	...
Melphalan HCl	●	...	...
Meperidine HCl	...	...	●
Meropenem	●	...	...
Methotrexate sodium	●	...	...
Metoclopramide HCl	...	●	...
Midazolam HCl	...	●	...
Milrinone lactate	...	●	...
Mitomycin	●	...	...
Morphine sulfate	...	...	●
Nicardipine HCl	...	●	...
Nitroglycerin	●	...	...
Norepinephrine bitartrate	...	...	●

Drugs	Compatible	Incompatible	Variable
Ondansetron HCl	...	●	...
Oxaliplatin	●	...	...
Paclitaxel	●	...	...
Pantoprazole sodium	...	...	●
Piperacillin sod.–tazobactam sod.	●	...	...
Potassium chloride	●	...	...
Prochlorperazine edisylate	...	●	...
Promethazine HCl	...	●	...
Propofol	●	...	...
Quinidine gluconate	...	●	...
Ranitidine HCl	●	...	...
Remifentanil HCl	●	...	...
Sargramostim	●	...	...
Sodium bicarbonate	●	...	...
Sodium nitroprusside	●	...	...
Tacrolimus	●	...	...
Teniposide	●	...	...
Theophylline	●	...	...
Thiopental sodium	●	...	...
Thiotepa	●	...	...
Tirofiban HCl	●	...	...
Tobramycin sulfate	●	...	...
Vecuronium bromide	...	●	...
Verapamil HCl	...	...	●
Vinblastine sulfate	...	●	...
Vincristine sulfate	...	●	...
Vinorelbine tartrate	...	●	...

Ganciclovir Sodium

Handbook on Injectable Drugs pp. 773–777.

Description: A nucleoside analog of guanine that acts as an antiviral agent.

Products: **Cytovene-IV;** 500-mg vials. *pH:* Approximately 11.

Preparation: Reconstitute with 10 mL of sterile water for injection and shake to obtain a 50-mg/mL solution. Do not use paraben-containing diluents. Dilute further in 50 to 250 mL (usually 100 mL) of compatible infusion solution to a concentration not greater than 10 mg/mL.

Administration: Administer by IV infusion using an inline filter. Do not administer rapidly or by other routes.

Stability: Store at room temperature protected from heat. The reconstituted solution is stable for 12 hours at room temperature and should not be refrigerated due to possible precipitation. According to the manufacturer, admixtures of ganciclovir in infusion solutions may be refrigerated but should not be frozen. Sorption to PVC containers has not been found.

Compatibility Table

Solutions	Compatible	Incompatible	Variable
Dextrose 5%	●	...	...
Sodium chloride 0.9%	●	...	...

Drugs			
Aldesleukin	...	●	...
Allopurinol sodium	●	...	...
Amifostine	...	●	...
Amphotericin B cholesteryl sulfate complex	●	...	...
Aztreonam	...	●	...
Cefepime HCl	...	●	...
Cisatracurium besylate	...	...	●
Cisplatin	●	...	...
Cyclophosphamide	●	...	...

Drugs	Compatible	Incompatible	Variable
Cytarabine	...	●	...
Docetaxel	●	...	...
Doxorubicin HCl	...	●	...
Doxorubicin HCl liposome injection	●	...	...
Enalaprilat	●	...	...
Etoposide phosphate	●	...	...
Filgrastim	●	...	...
Fluconazole	●	...	...
Fludarabine phosphate	...	●	...
Foscarnet sodium	...	●	...
Gemcitabine HCl	...	●	...
Granisetron HCl	●	...	...
Lansoprazole	●	...	...
Linezolid	●	...	...
Melphalan HCl	●	...	...
Methotrexate sodium	●	...	...
Ondansetron HCl	...	●	...
Paclitaxel	●	...	...
Pemetrexed disodium	●	...	...
Piperacillin sod.–tazobactam sod.	...	●	...
Propofol	●	...	...
Remifentanil HCl	●	...	...
Sargramostim	...	●	...
Tacrolimus	...	...	●
Teniposide	●	...	...
Thiotepa	●	...	...
Vinorelbine tartrate	...	●	...

Gemcitabine Hydrochloride

Handbook on Injectable Drugs pp. 785–792.

Description: A synthetic pyrimidine nucleoside antineoplastic agent.

Products: **Gemzar;** 200-mg and 1-g vials. *pH:* 2.7 to 3.3.

Preparation: Reconstitute the 200-mg vials with 5 mL and the 1-g vials with 25 mL of sodium chloride 0.9% (without preservatives) and shake to obtain a 38-mg/mL solution. The reconstituted drug may be diluted with additional sodium chloride 0.9% for infusion to concentrations as low as 0.1 mg/mL.

Administration: Administer weekly by IV infusion over 30 minutes. Gemcitabine hydrochloride may be administered as the reconstituted solution or may be further diluted for infusion.

Stability: The reconstituted solution is stable for at least 24 hours at room temperature according to the manufacturer. Other research indicates the reconstituted solution is stable for at least 35 days at room temperature as are dilutions in sodium chloride 0.9% and dextrose 5%. However, the solutions should not be refrigerated because of the potential to develop colorless crystals that do not redissolve upon warming. No sorption to containers or sets has been found.

Compatibility Table

Solutions	Compatible	Incompatible	Variable
Dextrose 5%	●	...	...
Sodium chloride 0.9%	●	...	...

Drugs			
Acyclovir sodium	...	●	...
Amifostine	●	...	...
Amikacin sulfate	●	...	...
Aminophylline	●	...	...
Amphotericin B	...	●	...

Drugs	Compatible	Incompatible	Variable
Ampicillin sodium	●	...	...
Ampicillin sod.–sulbactam sod.	●	...	...
Aztreonam	●	...	...
Bleomycin sulfate	●	...	...
Bumetanide	●	...	...
Buprenorphine HCl	●	...	...
Butorphanol tartrate	●	...	...
Calcium gluconate	●	...	...
Carboplatin	●	...	...
Carmustine	●	...	...
Cefazolin sodium	●	...	...
Cefotaxime sodium	...	●	...
Cefotetan disodium	●	...	...
Cefoxitin sodium	●	...	...
Ceftazidime	●	...	...
Ceftizoxime sodium	●	...	...
Ceftriaxone sodium	●	...	...
Cefuroxime sodium	●	...	...
Chlorpromazine HCl	●	...	...
Cimetidine HCl	●	...	...
Ciprofloxacin	●	...	...
Cisplatin	●	...	...
Clindamycin phosphate	●	...	...
Cyclophosphamide	●	...	...
Cytarabine	●	...	...
Dactinomycin	●	...	...
Daunorubicin HCl	●	...	...
Dexamethasone sodium phosphate	●	...	...
Dexrazoxane	●	...	...
Diphenhydramine HCl	●	...	...
Dobutamine HCl	●	...	...
Docetaxel	●	...	...
Dopamine HCl	●	...	...
Doxorubicin HCl	●	...	...
Doxycycline hyclate	●	...	...
Droperidol	●	...	...
Enalaprilat	●	...	...
Etoposide	●	...	...
Etoposide phosphate	●	...	...
Famotidine	●	...	...

Drugs	Compatible	Incompatible	Variable
Fluconazole	●	...	...
Fludarabine phosphate	●	...	...
Fluorouracil	●	...	...
Furosemide	...	●	...
Ganciclovir sodium	...	●	...
Gentamicin sulfate	●	...	...
Granisetron HCl	●	...	...
Haloperidol lactate	●	...	...
Heparin sodium	●	...	...
Hydrocortisone sodium phosphate	●	...	...
Hydrocortisone sodium succinate	●	...	...
Hydromorphone HCl	●	...	...
Hydroxyzine HCl	●	...	...
Idarubicin HCl	●	...	...
Ifosfamide	●	...	...
Imipenem–cilastatin sodium	...	●	...
Irinotecan HCl	...	●	...
Lansoprazole	...	●	...
Leucovorin calcium	●	...	...
Linezolid	●	...	...
Lorazepam	●	...	...
Mannitol	●	...	...
Meperidine HCl	●	...	...
Mesna	●	...	...
Methotrexate sodium	...	●	...
Methylprednisolone sod. succ.	...	●	...
Metoclopramide HCl	●	...	...
Metronidazole	●	...	...
Mitomycin	...	●	...
Mitoxantrone HCl	●	...	...
Morphine sulfate	●	...	...
Nalbuphine HCl	●	...	...
Ondansetron HCl	●	...	...
Oxaliplatin	●	...	...
Paclitaxel	●	...	...
Pemetrexed disodium	...	●	...
Piperacillin sodium	...	●	...
Piperacillin sod.–tazobactam sod.	...	●	...
Potassium chloride	●	...	...
Prochlorperazine edisylate	...	●	...

Drugs	Compatible	Incompatible	Variable
Promethazine HCl	●	...	...
Ranitidine HCl	●	...	...
Sodium bicarbonate	●	...	...
Streptozocin	●	...	...
Teniposide	●	...	...
Thiotepa	●	...	...
Ticarcillin disod.–clavulanate pot.	●	...	...
Tobramycin sulfate	●	...	...
Topotecan HCl	●	...	...
Trimethoprim–sulfamethoxazole	●	...	...
Vancomycin HCl	●	...	...
Vinblastine sulfate	●	...	...
Vincristine sulfate	●	...	...
Vinorelbine tartrate	●	...	...
Zidovudine	●	...	...

Gentamicin Sulfate

Handbook on Injectable Drugs pp. 793–809.

Description: An aminoglycoside antibiotic.

Products: Garamycin; 40 and 10 (pediatric) mg/mL. It is also available in several concentrations as premixed infusions in sodium chloride 0.9%. *pH:* From 3 to 5.5.

Preparation: For intermittent IV infusion to adults, dilute the dose in 50 to 200 mL of sodium chloride 0.9% or dextrose 5%. For pediatric patients, use a reduced volume consistent with the patient's needs but sufficient to permit a 30- to 120-minute infusion.

Administration: Administer IM or by IV infusion over 30 to 120 minutes.

Stability: Intact vials should be stored between 2 and 30 °C. The injection is colorless to slightly yellow; potency loss is unrelated to color. Gentamicin sulfate diluted for infusion in dextrose 5% or sodium chloride 0.9% is stable for at least 24 hours at room temperature, up to 17 days refrigerated, and 30 days frozen at –20 °C. No loss of potency due to filtration or sorption has been reported.

Compatibility Table

Solutions	Compatible	Incompatible	Variable
Dextrose 5 & 10%	●	...	...
Dextrose 5% in sodium chloride 0.2%	●	...	...
Fat emulsion 10%, IV	...	●	...
Ringer's injection, lactated	●	...	...
Sodium chloride 0.9%	●	...	...

Drugs			
Acyclovir sodium	●	...	...
Aldesleukin	●	...	...
Allopurinol sodium	...	●	...
Amifostine	●	...	...
Amiodarone HCl	●	...	...

Drugs	Compatible	Incompatible	Variable
Amphotericin B	...	●	...
Amphotericin B cholesteryl sulfate complex	...	●	...
Ampicillin sodium	...	●	...
Atracurium besylate	●	...	...
Azithromycin	...	●	...
Aztreonam	●	...	...
Bivalirudin	●	...	...
Bleomycin sulfate	●	...	...
Caffeine citrate	●	...	...
Cefamandole nafate	...	●	...
Cefepime HCl	...	●	...
Cefotaxime sodium	...	...	●
Cefotetan disodium	...	●	...
Cefoxitin sodium	●	...	...
Ceftazidime	...	...	●
Ceftriaxone sodium	...	...	●
Cefuroxime sodium	...	...	●
Cimetidine HCl	●	...	...
Ciprofloxacin	●	...	...
Cisatracurium besylate	●	...	...
Clindamycin phosphate	●	...	...
Cloxacillin sodium	...	●	...
Cyclophosphamide	●	...	...
Cytarabine	...	...	●
Daptomycin	●	...	...
Dexmedetomidine HCl	●	...	...
Diatrizoate sodium	●	...	...
Diltiazem HCl	●	...	...
Dimenhydrinate	●	...	...
Docetaxel	●	...	...
Dopamine HCl	...	...	●
Doxapram HCl	●	...	...
Doxorubicin HCl liposome injection	●	...	...
Drotrecogin alfa (activated)	...	●	...
Enalaprilat	●	...	...
Esmolol HCl	●	...	...
Etoposide phosphate	●	...	...
Famotidine HCl	●	...	...

Drugs	Compatible	Incompatible	Variable
Fenoldopam mesylate	●	...	...
Filgrastim	...	...	●
Fluconazole	●	...	...
Fludarabine phosphate	●	...	...
Foscarnet sodium	●	...	...
Furosemide	...	...	●
Gemcitabine HCl	●	...	...
Granisetron HCl	●	...	...
Heparin sodium	...	●	...
Hetastarch in sodium chloride 0.9%	...	●	...
Hextend	●	...	...
Hydromorphone HCl	●	...	...
Idarubicin HCl	...	●	...
IL-2	●	...	...
Indomethacin sodium trihydrate	...	●	...
Insulin, regular	●	...	...
Iodipamide meglumine	...	●	...
Iothalamate meglumine	●	...	...
Ioxaglate meglumine & sodium	...	...	●
Labetalol HCl	●	...	...
Lansoprazole	●	...	...
Levofloxacin	●	...	...
Lidocaine HCl	●	...	...
Linezolid	●	...	...
Lorazepam	●	...	...
Magnesium sulfate	●	...	...
Melphalan HCl	●	...	...
Meperidine HCl	●	...	...
Meropenem	●	...	...
Metronidazole	●	...	...
Midazolam HCl	●	...	...
Milrinone lactate	●	...	...
Morphine sulfate	●	...	...
Multivitamins	●	...	...
Nafcillin sodium	...	●	...
Nicardipine HCl	●	...	...
Ondansetron HCl	●	...	...
Paclitaxel	●	...	...
Pancuronium bromide	●	...	...
Pantoprazole sodium	...	●	...

Drugs	Compatible	Incompatible	Variable
Pemetrexed disodium	...	●	...
Penicillin G sodium	●	...	...
Propofol	...	●	...
Ranitidine HCl	●	...	...
Remifentanil HCl	●	...	...
Sargramostim	●	...	...
Tacrolimus	●	...	...
Teniposide	●	...	...
Theophylline	●	...	...
Thiotepa	●	...	...
Vancomycin HCl	...	...	●
Vecuronium bromide	●	...	...
Verapamil HCl	●	...	...
Vinorelbine tartrate	●	...	...
Warfarin sodium	...	●	...
Zidovudine	●	...	...

Granisetron Hydrochloride

Handbook on Injectable Drugs pp. 816–825.

Description: A serotonin antagonist antiemetic.

Products: **Kytril;** 1-mg/mL. *pH:* Single-dose containers from 4.7 to 7.3; multiple-dose containers from 4 to 6.

Preparation: For infusion, dilute the dose in 20 or 50 mL of dextrose 5% or sodium chloride 0.9%.

Administration: Granisetron hydrochloride may be administered undiluted IV over 30 seconds or administered by IV infusion over 5 minutes after dilution in 20 to 50 mL of dextrose 5% or sodium chloride 0.9%.

Stability: Store intact vials at less than 30 °C protected from freezing and light. The injection is clear and colorless. Admixtures in dextrose 5% or sodium chloride 0.9% are stable for at least 24 hours.

Compatibility Table

Solutions	Compatible	Incompatible	Variable
Dextrose 5%	●	...	...
Dextrose 5% in sodium chloride 0.45 & 0.9%	●	...	...
Sodium chloride 0.9%	●	...	...

Drugs	Compatible	Incompatible	Variable
Acyclovir sodium	●	...	...
Allopurinol sodium	●	...	...
Amifostine	●	...	...
Amikacin sulfate	●	...	...
Aminophylline	●	...	...
Amphotericin B	...	●	...
Amphotericin B cholesteryl sulfate complex	●	...	...
Ampicillin sodium	●	...	...
Ampicillin sod.–sulbactam sod.	●	...	...

Drugs	Compatible	Incompatible	Variable
Aztreonam	●	...	...
Bleomycin sulfate	●	...	...
Bumetanide	●	...	...
Buprenorphine HCl	●	...	...
Butorphanol tartrate	●	...	...
Calcium gluconate	●	...	...
Carboplatin	●	...	...
Carmustine	●	...	...
Cefazolin sodium	●	...	...
Cefepime HCl	●	...	...
Cefotaxime sodium	●	...	...
Cefotetan disodium	●	...	...
Cefoxitin sodium	●	...	...
Ceftazidime	●	...	...
Ceftizoxime sodium	●	...	...
Ceftriaxone sodium	●	...	...
Cefuroxime sodium	●	...	...
Chlorpromazine HCl	●	...	...
Cimetidine HCl	●	...	...
Ciprofloxacin	●	...	...
Cisplatin	●	...	...
Cladribine	●	...	...
Clindamycin phosphate	●	...	...
Cyclophosphamide	●	...	...
Cytarabine	●	...	...
Dacarbazine	●	...	...
Dactinomycin	●	...	...
Daunorubicin HCl	●	...	...
Dexamethasone sodium phosphate	●	...	...
Dexmedetomidine HCl	●	...	...
Diphenhydramine HCl	●	...	...
Dobutamine HCl	●	...	...
Docetaxel	●	...	...
Dopamine HCl	●	...	...
Doxorubicin HCl	●	...	...
Doxorubicin HCl liposome injection	●	...	...
Doxycycline hyclate	●	...	...
Droperidol	●	...	...
Enalaprilat	●	...	...

Drugs	Compatible	Incompatible	Variable
Etoposide	●	...	...
Etoposide phosphate	●	...	...
Famotidine	●	...	...
Fenoldopam mesylate	●	...	...
Filgrastim	●	...	...
Fluconazole	●	...	...
Fludarabine phosphate	●	...	...
Fluorouracil	●	...	...
Furosemide	●	...	...
Gallium nitrate	●	...	...
Ganciclovir sodium	●	...	...
Gemcitabine HCl	●	...	...
Gentamicin sulfate	●	...	...
Haloperidol lactate	●	...	...
Heparin sodium	●	...	...
Hextend	●	...	...
Hydrocortisone sodium phosphate	●	...	...
Hydrocortisone sodium succinate	●	...	...
Hydromorphone HCl	●	...	...
Hydroxyzine HCl	●	...	...
Idarubicin HCl	●	...	...
Ifosfamide	●	...	...
Imipenem–cilastatin sodium	●	...	...
Lansoprazole	...	●	...
Leucovorin calcium	●	...	...
Linezolid	●	...	...
Lorazepam	●	...	...
Magnesium sulfate	●	...	...
Mechlorethamine HCl	●	...	...
Melphalan HCl	●	...	...
Meperidine HCl	●	...	...
Mesna	●	...	...
Methotrexate sodium	●	...	...
Methylprednisolone sod. succ.	●	...	...
Metoclopramide HCl	●	...	...
Metronidazole	●	...	...
Mitomycin	●	...	...
Mitoxantrone HCl	●	...	...
Morphine sulfate	●	...	...
Nalbuphine HCl	●	...	...

Drugs	Compatible	Incompatible	Variable
Oxaliplatin	●	...	...
Paclitaxel	●	...	...
Pemetrexed disodium	●	...	...
Piperacillin sodium	●	...	...
Piperacillin sod.–tazobactam sod.	●	...	...
Potassium chloride	●	...	...
Prochlorperazine edisylate	●	...	...
Promethazine HCl	●	...	...
Propofol	●	...	...
Ranitidine HCl	●	...	...
Sargramostim	●	...	...
Sodium bicarbonate	●	...	...
Streptozocin	●	...	...
Teniposide	●	...	...
Thiotepa	●	...	...
Ticarcillin disod.–clavulanate pot.	●	...	...
Tobramycin sulfate	●	...	...
Topotecan HCl	●	...	...
Trimethoprim–sulfamethoxazole	●	...	...
Vancomycin HCl	●	...	...
Vinblastine sulfate	●	...	...
Vincristine sulfate	●	...	...
Vinorelbine tartrate	●	...	...
Zidovudine	●	...	...

Heparin Sodium

Handbook on Injectable Drugs pp. 833–867.

Description: A mixture of natural substances which prolongs clotting time.

Products: 1000 to 20,000 units/mL packaged in sizes from 0.5 to 30 mL. Available as dilute solutions of 10 and 100 units/mL in disposable units for flushing heparin locks. *pH:* From 5 to 8.

Preparation: For intermittent IV injection, the dose may be diluted in 50 to 100 mL of dextrose 5% or sodium chloride 0.9% or given undiluted. For continuous IV infusion to adults, appropriate doses are added to a liter of compatible solution.

Administration: Administer by deep SC injection, by intermittent IV injection, or by continuous IV infusion diluted in a compatible diluent, preferably using an electronic rate control device.

Stability: Store intact containers at room temperature. The drug is colorless to slightly yellow. Minor color variations do not affect efficacy. No loss due to sorption to glass containers, plastic syringes, or filters has been noted.

Compatibility Table

Solutions	Compatible	Incompatible	Variable
NOTE: Although conflicting results exist, most studies showed that heparin sodium can be administered in dextrose-containing solutions.			
Dextrose 5%	...	...	●
Dextrose 5% in sodium chloride 0.2, 0.45, & 0.9%	...	...	●
Ringer's injection, lactated	...	...	●
Sodium chloride 0.9%	...	...	●

Drugs	Compatible	Incompatible	Variable
Acyclovir sodium	●	...	...
Aldesleukin	...	...	●
Allopurinol sodium	●	...	...
Alteplase	...	●	...
Amifostine	●	...	...

Drugs	Compatible	Incompatible	Variable
Amikacin sulfate	...	●	...
Aminophylline	●	...	...
Amiodarone HCl	...	●	...
Amphotericin B	●	...	...
Amphotericin B cholesteryl sulfate complex	...	●	...
Ampicillin sodium	...	...	●
Ampicillin sod.–sulbactam sod.	●	...	...
Antithymocyte globulin (rabbit)	...	...	●
Atracurium besylate	...	...	●
Atropine sulfate	●	...	...
Aztreonam	●	...	...
Betamethasone sodium phosphate	●	...	...
Bivalirudin	●	...	...
Bleomycin sulfate	●	...	...
Buprenorphine HCl	●	...	...
Caffeine citrate	●	...	...
Calcium gluconate	●	...	...
Cefamandole nafate	●	...	...
Cefazolin sodium	●	...	...
Cefepime HCl	●	...	...
Cefotaxime sodium	●	...	...
Cefotetan disodium	●	...	...
Cefoxitin sodium	●	...	...
Ceftazidime	●	...	...
Ceftriaxone sodium	●	...	...
Chloramphenicol sod. succ.	●	...	...
Chlorpromazine HCl	...	...	●
Cimetidine HCl	●	...	...
Ciprofloxacin	...	●	...
Cisatracurium besylate	...	...	●
Cisplatin	●	...	...
Cladribine	●	...	...
Clindamycin phosphate	●	...	...
Clonidine HCl	●	...	...
Cloxacillin sodium	●	...	...
Colistimethate sodium	●	...	...
Corticotropin	●	...	...
Cyclophosphamide	●	...	...
Cytarabine	...	...	●
Dacarbazine	...	...	●

Drugs	Compatible	Incompatible	Variable
Daptomycin	●	…	…
Daunorubicin HCl	…	●	…
Dexamethasone sodium phosphate	●	…	…
Dexmedetomidine HCl	●	…	…
Diazepam	…	●	…
Diazoxide	●	…	…
Digoxin	●	…	…
Diltiazem HCl	…	…	●
Dimenhydrinate	…	…	●
Diphenhydramine HCl	●	…	…
Dobutamine HCl	…	…	●
Docetaxel	●	…	…
Dopamine HCl	…	…	●
Doxapram HCl	●	…	…
Doxorubicin HCl	…	…	●
Doxycycline hyclate	…	●	…
Droperidol	…	…	●
Drotrecogin alfa (activated)	…	…	●
Enalaprilat	●	…	…
Epinephrine HCl	●	…	…
Ergotamine tartrate	…	●	…
Ertapenem	●	…	…
Erythromycin lactobionate	…	●	…
Esmolol HCl	●	…	…
Etomidate	●	…	…
Etoposide phosphate	●	…	…
Famotidine	●	…	…
Fenoldopam mesylate	●	…	…
Fentanyl citrate	●	…	…
Filgrastim	…	●	…
Fluconazole	●	…	…
Fludarabine phosphate	●	…	…
Flumazenil	●	…	…
Fluorouracil	●	…	…
Foscarnet sodium	●	…	…
Furosemide	●	…	…
Gallium nitrate	●	…	…
Gemcitabine HCl	●	…	…
Gentamicin sulfate	…	●	…
Granisetron HCl	●	…	…

211

Drugs	Compatible	Incompatible	Variable
Haloperidol lactate	...	●	...
Hextend	●	...	...
Hyaluronidase	...	●	...
Hydralazine HCl	●	...	...
Hydrocortisone sodium succinate	...	...	●
Hydromorphone HCl	...	...	●
Idarubicin HCl	...	●	...
Insulin, regular	●	...	...
Isoproterenol HCl	●	...	...
Kanamycin sulfate	...	...	●
Labetalol HCl	...	...	●
Lansoprazole	●	...	...
Leucovorin calcium	●	...	...
Levofloxacin	...	●	...
Lidocaine HCl	●	...	...
Lincomycin HCl	●	...	...
Linezolid	●	...	...
Lorazepam	●	...	...
Magnesium sulfate	●	...	...
Melphalan HCl	●	...	...
Meperidine HCl	...	...	●
Meropenem	●	...	...
Methotrexate sodium	●	...	...
Methyldopate HCl	●	...	...
Methylprednisolone sod. succ.	...	...	●
Metoclopramide HCl	●	...	...
Metronidazole	●	...	...
Midazolam HCl	●	...	...
Milrinone lactate	●	...	...
Mitomycin	...	...	●
Morphine sulfate	...	...	●
Nafcillin sodium	●	...	...
Naloxone HCl	●	...	...
Neostigmine methylsulfate	●	...	...
Nicardipine HCl	...	...	●
Nitroglycerin	●	...	...
Norepinephrine HCl	●	...	...
Octreotide acetate	●	...	...
Ondansetron HCl	●	...	...
Oxacillin sodium	●	...	...

Drugs	Compatible	Incompatible	Variable
Oxaliplatin	●	...	...
Oxytocin	●	...	...
Paclitaxel	●	...	...
Pancuronium bromide	●	...	...
Pantoprazole sodium	...	●	...
Pemetrexed disodium	●	...	...
Penicillin G potassium & sodium	...	...	●
Pentazocine lactate	...	...	●
Phenobarbital sodium	●	...	...
Phenytoin sodium	...	●	...
Phytonadione	●	...	...
Piperacillin sodium	●	...	...
Piperacillin sod.–tazobactam sod.	●	...	...
Polymyxin B sulfate	...	●	...
Potassium chloride	●	...	...
Procainamide HCl	●	...	...
Prochlorperazine edisylate	...	...	●
Promethazine HCl	...	...	●
Propofol	●	...	...
Propranolol HCl	●	...	...
Quinidine gluconate	...	...	●
Ranitidine HCl	●	...	...
Remifentanil HCl	●	...	...
Sargramostim	●	...	...
Scopolamine HBr	●	...	...
Sodium bicarbonate	●	...	...
Sodium nitroprusside	●	...	...
Streptokinase	●	...	...
Streptomycin sulfate	...	●	...
Succinylcholine chloride	●	...	...
Tacrolimus	●	...	...
Theophylline	●	...	...
Thiopental sodium	●	...	...
Thiotepa	●	...	...
Ticarcillin disod.–clavulanate pot.	●	...	...
Tirofiban HCl	●	...	...
Tobramycin sulfate	...	●	...
Triflupromazine HCl	...	●	...
Trimethoprim–sulfamethoxazole	●	...	...
Vancomycin HCl	...	...	●

Drugs	Compatible	Incompatible	Variable
Vasopressin	●	...	...
Vecuronium bromide	●	...	...
Verapamil HCl	●	...	...
Vinblastine sulfate	...	...	●
Vincristine sulfate	●	...	...
Vinorelbine tartrate	...	...	●
Warfarin sodium	●	...	...
Zidovudine	●	...	...

Hetastarch in Lactated Electrolyte Injection

Handbook on Injectable Drugs pp. 867–874.

Description: A synthetic polymer derived from starch used as a plasma volume expander.

Products: **Hextend;** 6% in a lactated multielectrolyte ready-to-use solution packaged in single-use plastic containers of 500- and 1000-mL. *pH:* Approximately 5.9.

Administration: The ready-to-use solution is administered only by IV infusion. The amount administered and rate depend on the patient's clinical condition. This product contains calcium and should not be administered simultaneously with blood through the same set because of possible coagulation.

Stability: The clear pale yellow to amber solution should be stored at room temperature and protected from freezing and excessive heat. Brief exposure to temperatures up to 40 °C does not adversely affect the product. However, prolonged exposure may result in the formation of a turbid deep brown appearance or crystalline precipitate and should not be used.

Compatibility Table

Drugs	Compatible	Incompatible	Variable
Alfentanil HCl	●	...	...
Amikacin sulfate	●	...	...
Aminophylline	●	...	...
Amiodarone HCl	●	...	...
Amphotericin B	...	●	...
Ampicillin sodium	●	...	...
Ampicillin sod.–sulbactam sod.	●	...	...
Atracurium besylate	●	...	...
Azithromycin	●	...	...
Aztreonam	●	...	...
Bumetanide	●	...	...
Butorphanol tartrate	●	...	...
Calcium gluconate	●	...	...
Cefazolin sodium	●	...	...
Cefepime HCl	●	...	...

Drugs	Compatible	Incompatible	Variable
Cefotaxime sodium	●	. . .	. . .
Cefotetan disodium	●	. . .	. . .
Cefoxitin sodium	●	. . .	. . .
Ceftazidime	●	. . .	. . .
Ceftizoxime sodium	●	. . .	. . .
Ceftriaxone sodium	●	. . .	. . .
Cefuroxime sodium	●	. . .	. . .
Chlorpromazine HCl	●	. . .	. . .
Cimetidine HCl	●	. . .	. . .
Ciprofloxacin	●	. . .	. . .
Cisatracurium besylate	●	. . .	. . .
Clindamycin phosphate	●	. . .	. . .
Dexamethasone sodium phosphate . . .	●	. . .	. . .
Diazepam	. . .	●	. . .
Digoxin	●	. . .	. . .
Diltiazem HCl	●	. . .	. . .
Diphenhydramine HCl	●	. . .	. . .
Dobutamine HCl	●	. . .	. . .
Dolasetron mesylate	●	. . .	. . .
Dopamine HCl	●	. . .	. . .
Doxycycline hyclate	●	. . .	. . .
Droperidol	●	. . .	. . .
Enalaprilat	●	. . .	. . .
Ephedrine sulfate	●	. . .	. . .
Epinephrine HCl	●	. . .	. . .
Erythromycin lactobionate	●	. . .	. . .
Esmolol HCl	●	. . .	. . .
Famotidine	●	. . .	. . .
Fenoldopam mesylate	●	. . .	. . .
Fentanyl citrate	●	. . .	. . .
Fluconazole	●	. . .	. . .
Furosemide	●	. . .	. . .
Gentamicin sulfate	●	. . .	. . .
Granisetron HCl	●	. . .	. . .
Haloperidol lactate	●	. . .	. . .
Heparin sodium	●	. . .	. . .
Hydrocortisone sodium succinate	●	. . .	. . .
Hydromorphone HCl	●	. . .	. . .
Hydroxyzine HCl	●	. . .	. . .
Isoproterenol HCl	●	. . .	. . .

Drugs	Compatible	Incompatible	Variable
Ketorolac tromethamine	●	...	...
Labetalol HCl	●	...	...
Levofloxacin	●	...	...
Lidocaine HCl	●	...	...
Lorazepam	●	...	...
Magnesium sulfate	●	...	...
Mannitol	●	...	...
Meperidine HCl	●	...	...
Methylprednisolone sod. succ.	●	...	...
Metoclopramide HCl	●	...	...
Metronidazole	●	...	...
Midazolam HCl	●	...	...
Milrinone lactate	●	...	...
Mivacurium chloride	●	...	...
Morphine sulfate	●	...	...
Nalbuphine HCl	●	...	...
Nitroglycerin	●	...	...
Norepinephrine bitartrate	●	...	...
Ondansetron HCl	●	...	...
Pancuronium bromide	●	...	...
Phenylephrine HCl	●	...	...
Piperacillin sodium	●	...	...
Piperacillin sod.–tazobactam sod.	●	...	...
Potassium chloride	●	...	...
Procainamide HCl	●	...	...
Prochlorperazine edisylate	●	...	...
Promethazine HCl	●	...	...
Ranitidine HCl	●	...	...
Rocuronium bromide	●	...	...
Sodium bicarbonate	...	●	...
Sodium nitroprusside	●	...	...
Succinylcholine chloride	●	...	...
Sufentanil citrate	●	...	...
Theophylline	●	...	...
Thiopental sodium	●	...	...
Ticarcillin disod.–clavulanate pot.	●	...	...
Tobramycin sulfate	●	...	...
Trimethoprim–sulfamethoxazole	●	...	...
Vancomycin HCl	●	...	...
Vecuronium bromide	●	...	...
Verapamil HCl	●	...	...

Hetastarch in Lactated Electrolyte Injection

Hydrocortisone Sodium Succinate

Handbook on Injectable Drugs pp. 885–900.

Description: An anti-inflammatory adrenocortical steroid.

Products: Solu-Cortef; A variety of sizes and containers ranging from 100 to 1000 mg. *pH:* From 7 to 8 when reconstituted.

Preparation: Reconstitute with not more than 2 mL of bacteriostatic (preserved) diluent for IM or IV use or unpreserved diluent for intrathecal use.

Administration: Administer IM, by direct IV injection over 30 seconds to several minutes, or by IV infusion of a 0.1- to 1-mg/mL solution. For intrathecal injection, use only unpreserved diluent.

Stability: Reconstituted solutions are stable at room temperature or below if protected from light. Unused solutions should be discarded after three days. The drug is heat labile and should not be autoclaved. No sorption to plastic IV bags, tubing, syringes, or filters has been noted.

Compatibility Table

Solutions	Compatible	Incompatible	Variable
Dextrose 5%	●	...	...
Dextrose 5% in Ringer's injection, lactated	●	...	...
Dextrose 5% in sodium chloride 0.2, 0.45, & 0.9%	●	...	...
Ringer's injection, lactated	●	...	...
Sodium chloride 0.45 & 0.9%	●	...	...

Drugs			
Acyclovir sodium	●	...	...
Allopurinol sodium	●	...	...
Amifostine	●	...	...
Amikacin sulfate	●	...	...
Aminophylline	●	...	...

Drugs	Compatible	Incompatible	Variable
Amobarbital sodium	...	...	●
Amphotericin B	●	...	...
Amphotericin B cholesteryl sulfate complex	●	...	...
Ampicillin sodium	...	...	●
Antithymocyte globulin (rabbit)	●	...	...
Argatroban	●	...	...
Atracurium besylate	●	...	...
Atropine sulfate	●	...	...
Aztreonam	●	...	...
Betamethasone sodium phosphate	●	...	...
Bivalirudin	●	...	...
Bleomycin sulfate	...	●	...
Calcium chloride & gluconate	●	...	...
Cefepime HCl	●	...	...
Chloramphenicol sodium succinate	●	...	...
Chlordiazepoxide HCl	●	...	...
Chlorpromazine HCl	●	...	...
Ciprofloxacin	...	●	...
Cisatracurium besylate	●	...	...
Cladribine	●	...	...
Clindamycin phosphate	●	...	...
Cloxacillin sodium	●	...	...
Colistimethate sodium	...	●	...
Corticotropin	●	...	...
Cyanocobalamin	●	...	...
Cytarabine	...	...	●
Dacarbazine	...	●	...
Daunorubicin HCl	●	...	...
Dexamethasone sodium phosphate ...	●	...	...
Diatrizoate meglumine & sodium	●	...	...
Diazepam	...	●	...
Digoxin	●	...	...
Diltiazem HCl	...	...	●
Dimenhydrinate	...	...	●
Diphenhydramine HCl	●	...	...
Docetaxel	●	...	...
Dopamine HCl	●	...	...
Doxapram HCl	...	●	...
Doxorubicin HCl	...	●	...

Hydrocortisone Sodium Succinate

Drugs	Compatible	Incompatible	Variable
Doxorubicin HCl liposome injection	●	...	...
Droperidol	●	...	...
Edrophonium chloride	●	...	...
Enalaprilat	●	...	...
Ephedrine sulfate	...	...	●
Epinephrine HCl	●	...	...
Erythromycin lactobionate	●	...	...
Esmolol HCl	●	...	...
Estrogens, conjugated	●	...	...
Ethacrynate sodium	●	...	...
Etoposide phosphate	●	...	...
Famotidine	●	...	...
Fenoldopam mesylate	●	...	...
Fentanyl citrate	●	...	...
Filgrastim	●	...	...
Fludarabine phosphate	●	...	...
Fluorouracil	●	...	...
Foscarnet sodium	●	...	...
Furosemide	...	...	●
Gallium nitrate	●	...	...
Gemcitabine HCl	●	...	...
Granisetron HCl	●	...	...
Heparin sodium	...	...	●
Hextend	●	...	...
Hydralazine HCl	...	...	●
Idarubicin HCl......................	...	●	...
Insulin, regular	●	...	...
Iothalamate sodium	●	...	...
Ioxaglate meglumine & sodium	●	...	...
Isoproterenol HCl...................	●	...	...
Kanamycin sulfate	...	...	●
Lansoprazole	...	●	...
Lidocaine HCl	●	...	...
Linezolid	●	...	...
Lorazepam	●	...	...
Magnesium sulfate	...	...	●
Melphalan HCl......................	●	...	...
Meperidine HCl.....................	●	...	...
Mephentermine sulfate	●	...	...

Drugs	Compatible	Incompatible	Variable
Methylergonovine maleate	●	...	...
Methylprednisolone sod. succ.	...	...	●
Metoclopramide HCl	●	...	...
Metronidazole	...	...	●
Midazolam HCl	...	●	...
Mitomycin	●	...	...
Mitoxantrone HCl	●	...	...
Morphine sulfate	●	...	...
Nafcillin sodium	...	●	...
Neostigmine methylsulfate	●	...	...
Nicardipine HCl	●	...	...
Norepinephrine bitartrate	●	...	...
Ondansetron HCl	●	...	...
Oxacillin sodium	●	...	...
Oxaliplatin	●	...	...
Oxytocin	●	...	...
Paclitaxel	●	...	...
Pancuronium bromide	●	...	...
Pantoprazole sodium	...	●	...
Penicillin G potassium	...	...	●
Penicillin G sodium	●	...	...
Pentazocine lactate	●	...	...
Pentobarbital sodium	...	...	●
Phenobarbital sodium	...	●	...
Phenytoin sodium	...	●	...
Phytonadione	●	...	...
Piperacillin sodium	●	...	...
Piperacillin sod.–tazobactam sod.	●	...	...
Polymyxin B sulfate	●	...	...
Potassium chloride	●	...	...
Procainamide HCl	●	...	...
Procaine HCl	●	...	...
Prochlorperazine edisylate	...	...	●
Promethazine HCl	...	...	●
Propofol	●	...	...
Propranolol HCl	●	...	...
Remifentanil HCl	●	...	...
Sargramostim	...	●	...
Scopolamine HBr	●	...	...
Sodium bicarbonate	●	...	...

Hydrocortisone Sodium Succinate

Drugs	Compatible	Incompatible	Variable
Succinylcholine chloride	●	...	...
Tacrolimus	●	...	...
Teniposide	●	...	...
Theophylline	●	...	...
Thiopental sodium	●	...	...
Thiotepa	●	...	...
Trimethobenzamide HCl	●	...	...
Vancomycin HCl	...	...	●
Vecuronium bromide	●	...	...
Verapamil HCl	●	...	...
Vinorelbine tartrate	●	...	...

Hydromorphone Hydrochloride

Handbook on Injectable Drugs pp. 900–912.

Description: A semisynthetic opiate analgesic.

Products: Dilaudid HCl; 1-, 2-, and 4-mg/mL in 1-mL ampuls and 2-mg/mL in 20-mL multiple-dose vials. Also high potency **Dilaudid-HP**; 10 mg/mL. *pH:* From 4 to 5.5.

Administration: Administer SC, IM, or by slow direct IV injection over at least two to three minutes.

Stability: Store at room temperature protected from light; do not refrigerate. Refrigeration may result in precipitation or crystallization, but the drug may be resolubilized at room temperature without affecting stability. A slight yellow discoloration may develop but is not associated with a loss of potency.

Compatibility Table

Solutions	Compatible	Incompatible	Variable
Dextrose 5%	●	...	...
Dextrose 5% in Ringer's injection	●	...	...
Dextrose 5% in Ringer's injection, lactated	●	...	...
Dextrose 5% in sodium chloride 0.45 & 0.9%	●	...	...
Ringer's injection	●	...	...
Ringer's injection, lactated	●	...	...
Sodium chloride 0.45 & 0.9%	●	...	...

Drugs	Compatible	Incompatible	Variable
Acyclovir sodium	●	...	...
Allopurinol sodium	●	...	...
Amifostine	●	...	...
Amikacin sulfate	●	...	...
Amphotericin B cholesteryl sulfate complex	...	●	...

Drugs	Compatible	Incompatible	Variable
Ampicillin sodium	...	...	●
Atropine sulfate	●	...	...
Aztreonam	●	...	...
Bivalirudin	●	...	...
Bupivacaine HCl	●	...	...
Cefamandole nafate	●	...	...
Cefazolin sodium	...	...	●
Cefepime HCl	●	...	...
Cefotaxime sodium	●	...	...
Cefoxitin sodium	●	...	...
Ceftazidime	●	...	...
Ceftizoxime sodium	●	...	...
Cefuroxime sodium	●	...	...
Chloramphenicol sodium succinate	●	...	...
Chlorpromazine HCl	●	...	...
Cimetidine HCl	●	...	...
Cisatracurium besylate	●	...	...
Cisplatin	●	...	...
Cladribine	●	...	...
Clindamycin phosphate	●	...	...
Clonidine HCl	●	...	...
Cloxacillin sodium	...	...	●
Cyclophosphamide	●	...	...
Cytarabine	●	...	...
Dexamethasone sodium phosphate ...	...	...	●
Dexmedetomidine HCl	●	...	...
Diazepam	...	●	...
Diltiazem HCl	●	...	...
Dimenhydrinate	...	...	●
Diphenhydramine HCl	●	...	...
Dobutamine HCl	●	...	...
Docetaxel	●	...	...
Dopamine HCl	●	...	...
Doxorubicin HCl	●	...	...
Doxorubicin HCl liposome injection	●	...	...
Doxycycline hyclate	●	...	...
Epinephrine HCl	●	...	...
Erythromycin lactobionate	●	...	...

Drugs	Compatible	Incompatible	Variable
Etoposide phosphate	•	...	...
Famotidine	•	...	...
Fenoldopam mesylate	•	...	...
Fentanyl citrate	•	...	...
Filgrastim	•	...	...
Fludarabine phosphate	•	...	...
Fluorouracil	•	...	...
Foscarnet sodium	•	...	...
Furosemide	•	...	...
Gallium nitrate	...	•	...
Gemcitabine HCl	•	...	...
Gentamicin sulfate	•	...	...
Glycopyrrolate	•	...	...
Granisetron HCl	•	...	...
Haloperidol lactate	...	...	•
Heparin sodium	...	...	•
Hextend	•	...	...
Hyaluronidase	...	•	...
Hydroxyzine HCl	•	...	...
Kanamycin sulfate	•	...	...
Ketorolac tromethamine	...	...	•
Labetalol HCl	•	...	...
Lansoprazole	...	•	...
Linezolid	•	...	...
Lorazepam	•	...	...
Magnesium sulfate	•	...	...
Melphalan HCl	•	...	...
Methotrexate sodium	•	...	...
Metoclopramide HCl	•	...	...
Metronidazole	•	...	...
Midazolam HCl	•	...	...
Milrinone lactate	•	...	...
Morphine sulfate	•	...	...
Nafcillin sodium	•	...	...
Nicardipine HCl	•	...	...
Nitroglycerin	•	...	...
Norepinephrine bitartrate	•	...	...
Ondansetron HCl	•	...	...
Oxacillin sodium	•	...	...
Oxaliplatin	•	...	...

Drugs	Compatible	Incompatible	Variable
Paclitaxel	●	...	...
Pantoprazole sodium	...	●	...
Pemetrexed disodium	●	...	...
Penicillin G potassium	●	...	...
Pentazocine lactate	●	...	...
Pentobarbital sodium	●	...	...
Phenobarbital sodium	...	...	●
Phenytoin sodium	...	●	...
Piperacillin sodium	●	...	...
Piperacillin sod.–tazobactam sod.	●	...	...
Potassium chloride	●	...	...
Prochlorperazine edisylate	...	...	●
Promethazine HCl	●	...	...
Propofol	●	...	...
Ranitidine HCl	●	...	...
Remifentanil HCl	●	...	...
Sargramostim	...	●	...
Scopolamine HBr	●	...	...
Sodium bicarbonate	...	●	...
Tacrolimus	●	...	...
Teniposide	●	...	...
Thiethylperazine malate	●	...	...
Thiopental sodium	...	●	...
Thiotepa	●	...	...
Tobramycin sulfate	●	...	...
Trimethobenzamide HCl	●	...	...
Trimethoprim–sulfamethoxazole	●	...	...
Vancomycin HCl	●	...	...
Vecuronium bromide	●	...	...
Verapamil HCl	●	...	...
Vinorelbine tartrate	●	...	...

Hydroxyzine Hydrochloride

Handbook on Injectable Drugs pp. 913–919.

Description: An antihistamine used in the management of anxiety and tension as well as for its antipruritic effect.

Products: Vistaril; 25 mg/mL in 10-mL vials; 50 mg/mL in 1-, 2-, and 10-mL sizes. *pH:* From 3.5 to 6.

Administration: Administer undiluted by deep IM injection into a large muscle mass.

Stability: Store intact containers at room temperature and protect from excessive heat and freezing.

Compatibility Table

Drugs	Compatible	Incompatible	Variable
Allopurinol sodium	...	●	...
Amifostine	...	●	...
Aminophylline	...	●	...
Amobarbital sodium	...	●	...
Amphotericin B cholesteryl sulfate complex	...	●	...
Atropine sulfate	●	...	...
Aztreonam	●	...	...
Buprenorphine HCl	●	...	...
Butorphanol tartrate	●	...	...
Cefepime HCl	...	●	...
Chloramphenicol sodium succinate	...	●	...
Chlorpromazine HCl	●	...	...
Cimetidine HCl	●	...	...
Ciprofloxacin	●	...	...
Cisatracurium besylate	●	...	...
Cisplatin	●	...	...
Cladribine	●	...	...
Codeine phosphate	●	...	...
Cyclophosphamide	●	...	...

Drugs	Compatible	Incompatible	Variable
Cytarabine	•	...	...
Dexmedetomidine HCl	•	...	...
Dimenhydrinate	...	...	•
Diphenhydramine HCl	•	...	...
Docetaxel	•	...	...
Doxapram HCl	•	...	...
Doxorubicin HCl liposome injection	...	•	...
Droperidol	•	...	...
Etoposide	•	...	...
Etoposide phosphate	•	...	...
Famotidine	•	...	...
Fenoldopam mesylate	•	...	...
Fentanyl citrate	•	...	...
Filgrastim	•	...	...
Fluconazole	...	•	...
Fludarabine phosphate	...	•	...
Fluphenazine HCl	•	...	...
Foscarnet sodium	•	...	...
Gemcitabine HCl	•	...	...
Glycopyrrolate	•	...	...
Granisetron HCl	•	...	...
Haloperidol lactate	...	•	...
Heparin sodium	...	•	...
Hextend	•	...	...
Hydromorphone HCl	•	...	...
Ketorolac tromethamine	...	•	...
Lansoprazole	...	•	...
Lidocaine HCl	•	...	...
Linezolid	•	...	...
Melphalan HCl	•	...	...
Meperidine HCl	•	...	...
Mesna	•	...	...
Methadone HCl	•	...	...
Methotrexate sodium	•	...	...
Metoclopramide HCl	•	...	...
Midazolam HCl	•	...	...
Morphine sulfate	•	...	...
Nafcillin sodium	•	...	...
Nalbuphine HCl	•	...	...

Drugs	Compatible	Incompatible	Variable
Ondansetron HCl	●	...	...
Oxaliplatin	●	...	...
Oxymorphone HCl	●	...	...
Paclitaxel	...	●	...
Pemetrexed disodium	●	...	...
Penicillin G potassium & sodium	...	●	...
Pentazocine lactate	●	...	...
Pentobarbital sodium	...	●	...
Phenobarbital sodium	...	●	...
Phenytoin sodium	...	●	...
Piperacillin sod.–tazobactam sod.	...	●	...
Procaine HCl	●	...	...
Prochlorperazine edisylate	●	...	...
Promethazine HCl	●	...	...
Propofol	●	...	...
Ranitidine HCl	...	●	...
Remifentanil HCl	●	...	...
Sargramostim	...	●	...
Scopolamine HBr	●	...	...
Sufentanil citrate	●	...	...
Teniposide	●	...	...
Thiotepa	●	...	...
Vinorelbine tartrate	●	...	...

Ifosfamide

Handbook on Injectable Drugs pp. 923–927.

Description: An antineoplastic alkylating agent structurally similar to cyclophosphamide.

Products: Ifex; 1- and 3-g vials. *pH:* Approximately 6.

Preparation: Reconstitute the 1- and 3-g vials with 20 or 60 mL, respectively, of sterile water for injection or bacteriostatic water for injection to obtain a 50-mg/mL solution. Dilute further to a concentration of 0.6 to 20 mg/mL in a compatible infusion solution.

Administration: Administer by IV infusion over a minimum of 30 minutes. To prevent bladder toxicity, mesna and at least 2 L/day of fluid should also be given.

Stability: Vials should be stored at room temperature; the drug may liquefy at temperatures above 35 °C.

The reconstituted solution is stable for seven days at 30 °C and for at least three weeks under refrigeration.

Compatibility Table

Solutions	Compatible	Incompatible	Variable
Dextrose 5%	●	...	...
Dextrose 5% in Ringer's injection	●	...	...
Dextrose 5% in sodium chloride 0.9%	●	...	...
Ringer's injection, lactated	●	...	...
Sodium chloride 0.45 & 0.9%	●	...	...

Drugs	Compatible	Incompatible	Variable
Allopurinol sodium	●	...	...
Amifostine	●	...	...
Amphotericin B cholesteryl sulfate complex	●	...	...
Aztreonam	●	...	...
Carboplatin	●	...	...
Cefepime HCl	...	●	...
Cisplatin	●	...	...
Doxorubicin HCl liposome injection	●	...	...

Drugs	Compatible	Incompatible	Variable
Epirubicin HCl	●	...	...
Etoposide	●	...	...
Etoposide phosphate	●	...	...
Filgrastim	●	...	...
Fludarabine phosphate	●	...	...
Fluorouracil	●	...	...
Gallium nitrate	●	...	...
Gemcitabine HCl	●	...	...
Granisetron HCl	●	...	...
Lansoprazole	●	...	...
Linezolid	●	...	...
Melphalan HCl	●	...	...
Mesna	●	...	...
Methotrexate sodium	...	●	...
Ondansetron HCl	●	...	...
Oxaliplatin	●	...	...
Paclitaxel	●	...	...
Pemetrexed disodium	●	...	...
Piperacillin sod.–tazobactam sod.	●	...	...
Propofol	●	...	...
Sargramostim	●	...	...
Sodium bicarbonate	●	...	...
Teniposide	●	...	...
Thiotepa	●	...	...
Topotecan HCl	●	...	...
Vinorelbine tartrate	●	...	...

Imipenem–Cilastatin Sodium

Handbook on Injectable Drugs pp. 927–934.

Description: A combination of imipenem, a thienamycin antibiotic, and cilastatin sodium, an inhibitor of imipenem inactivation.

Products: Primaxin; Vials and piggyback infusion bottles for IV use containing 250 and 500 mg each of imipenem and cilastatin sodium; vials for IM use containing 500 and 750 mg of each component. *pH:* Buffered to 6.5 to 8.5 when reconstituted.

Preparation: Reconstitute the IV vials with 10 mL of diluent from a 100-mL container and shake well to form a suspension. Transfer the suspension to the remaining solution in the infusion container for dilution. Do *not* inject the suspension. Repeat the procedure. Agitate the admixture until it is clear to yield a 2.5- or 5-mg/mL concentration, depending on the vial content.

The piggyback bottles should be reconstituted with 100 mL of compatible diluent and shaken until clear.

Reconstitute the 500- and 750-mg IM vials with 2 and 3 mL, respectively, of lidocaine hydrochloride 1% (without epinephrine) and shake to form a suspension. Use within one hour.

Administration: Administer IV by intermittent infusion at a concentration not exceeding 5 mg/mL of each drug in 20 to 30 minutes for 250- or 500-mg doses or in 40 to 60 minutes for 1-g doses. Inject the IM suspension deeply into a large muscle mass.

Stability: Store at temperatures below 25 °C. Reconstituted solutions are colorless to yellow or tan; they should be discarded if they darken to brown. Reconstituted solutions are stable for four hours at room temperature or 24 hours under refrigeration. An exception is reconstitution with sodium chloride 0.9%, which is stable for 10 hours at room temperature or 48 hours under refrigeration.

Compatibility Table

Solutions	Compatible	Incompatible	Variable
Dextrose 5 & 10%*	...	...	•
Dextrose 5% in Ringer's injection, lactated	...	•	...
Dextrose 5% in sodium chloride 0.225, 0.45, & 0.9%*	...	...	•
Mannitol 2.5, 5, & 10% in water*	...	...	•
Ringer's injection, lactated*	...	...	•
Sodium bicarbonate 5%	...	•	...
Sodium chloride 0.9%*	...	...	•
Sodium lactate 1/6 M	...	•	...

*Stability in these solutions is insufficient to be considered truly compatible; the drug is sufficiently stable for use within a few hours.

Drugs	Compatible	Incompatible	Variable
Acyclovir sodium	•	...	...
Allopurinol sodium	...	•	...
Amifostine	•	...	...
Amiodarone HCl	...	•	...
Amphotericin B cholesteryl sulfate complex	...	•	...
Azithromycin	...	•	...
Aztreonam	•	...	...
Cefepime HCl	•	...	...
Cisatracurium besylate	•	...	...
Diltiazem HCl	•	...	...
Docetaxel	•	...	...
Drotrecogin alfa (activated)	...	•	...
Etoposide phosphate	...	•	...
Famotidine	•	...	...
Filgrastim	...	...	•
Fluconazole	...	•	...
Fludarabine phosphate	•	...	...
Foscarnet sodium	•	...	...
Gallium nitrate	...	•	...
Gemcitabine HCl	...	•	...

Drugs	Compatible	Incompatible	Variable
Granisetron HCl	●	...	...
Idarubicin HCl	●	...	...
Insulin, regular	●	...	...
Lansoprazole	...	●	...
Linezolid	●	...	...
Lorazepam	...	●	...
Melphalan HCl	●	...	...
Meperidine HCl	...	●	...
Methotrexate sodium	●	...	...
Midazolam HCl	...	●	...
Milrinone lactate	...	●	...
Ondansetron HCl	●	...	...
Propofol	●	...	...
Remifentanil HCl	●	...	...
Sargramostim	...	●	...
Sodium bicarbonate	...	●	...
Tacrolimus	●	...	...
Teniposide	●	...	...
Thiotepa	●	...	...
Vinorelbine tartrate	●	...	...
Zidovudine	●	...	...

Insulin

Handbook on Injectable Drugs pp. 941–948.

Description: The hormone secreted by the beta cells of the pancreatic islets of Langerhans.

Products: **Humulin R, Novolin R, Velosulin;** 100 units/mL in 10-mL vials and 500 units/mL in 20-mL vials. *pH:* From 7 to 7.8.

Administration: Administer SC, IM, or IV. Regular insulin is the only form that can be given IV.

Stability: The newer neutral formulation of insulin is stable at room temperature for 24 to 30 months, but refrigeration is still recommended. It should not be frozen.

Discoloration, turbidity, or unusual viscosity indicates deterioration or contamination. Regular insulin should not be used unless it is clear and colorless.

Compatibility Table

Solutions	Compatible	Incompatible	Variable
NOTE: The adsorption of insulin to the surfaces of IV infusion solution containers (both glass and plastic), tubing, and filters has been demonstrated. Estimates of the potency loss range up to about 80%, although varying results have been obtained. The percent adsorbed is inversely proportional to concentration. The container surface area and length of contact also may play a role. However, the clinical significance of this adsorption is uncertain.			
Parenteral nutrition solutions	...	...	●

Drugs			
Aminophylline	...	●	...
Amiodarone HCl	●	...	...
Amobarbital sodium	...	●	...
Ampicillin sodium	●	...	...
Ampicillin sod.–sulbactam sod.	●	...	...
Aztreonam	●	...	...
Cefazolin sodium	●	...	...
Cefepime HCl	●	...	...
Cefotetan disodium	●	...	...
Ceftazidime	●	...	...

Drugs	Compatible	Incompatible	Variable
Chlorothiazide sodium	...	●	...
Cimetidine HCl	●	...	...
Cytarabine.........................	...	●	...
Digoxin	...	...	●
Diltiazem HCl	...	...	●
Dobutamine HCl	...	...	●
Dopamine HCl	...	●	...
Doxapram HCl	●	...	...
Drotrecogin alfa (activated)	...	●	...
Esmolol HCl	●	...	...
Famotidine	●	...	...
Gentamicin sulfate	●	...	...
Heparin sodium	●	...	...
Imipenem–cilastatin sodium	●	...	...
Indomethacin sodium trihydrate	●	...	...
Labetalol HCl	...	...	●
Levofloxacin	...	...	●
Lidocaine HCl	●	...	...
Magnesium sulfate	●	...	...
Meperidine HCl	●	...	...
Meropenem	●	...	...
Methylprednisolone sod. succ.	...	●	...
Metoclopramide HCl	●	...	...
Midazolam HCl	●	...	...
Milrinone lactate	●	...	...
Morphine sulfate	●	...	...
Nafcillin sodium	...	●	...
Nitroglycerin	●	...	...
Norepinephrine bitartrate	...	●	...
Oxytocin	●	...	...
Pantoprazole sodium	...	...	●
Pentobarbital sodium	...	...	●
Phenobarbital sodium	...	●	...
Phenytoin sodium	...	●	...
Potassium chloride	●	...	...

Drugs	Compatible	Incompatible	Variable
Propofol	●	...	...
Ranitidine HCl	...	...	●
Sodium bicarbonate	●	...	...
Sodium nitroprusside	●	...	...
Tacrolimus	●	...	...
Terbutaline sulfate	●	...	...
Thiopental sodium	...	●	...
Ticarcillin disod.–clavulanate pot.	●	...	...
Tobramycin sulfate	●	...	...
Vancomycin HCl	●	...	...
Verapamil HCl	●	...	...

Isoproterenol Hydrochloride

Handbook on Injectable Drugs pp. 962–967.

Description: A synthetic sympathomimetic amine.

Products: **Isuprel HCl;** 0.02 mg/mL (1:50,000) in syringes and 0.2 mg/mL (1:5000) in ampuls and syringes. *pH:* From 2.5 to 4.5.

Administration: Administer by IV infusion or direct IV, IM, or SC injection. In extreme emergencies, administer by intracardiac injection. For direct IV injection, 1 mL of the 0.2-mg/mL injection should be diluted to 10 mL with sodium chloride 0.9% or dextrose 5% to provide a 20-mcg/mL solution. IV infusions are prepared by adding 1 to 10 mL of the 0.2-mg/mL injection to 500 mL of compatible diluent.

Stability: Store intact containers at controlled room temperature protected from light. Exposure to air, light, or heat may cause a pink to brownish pink color to develop. Do not use if a color or precipitate is present. In solutions with a pH greater than 6, significant decomposition occurs.

Compatibility Table

Solutions	Compatible	Incompatible	Variable
Dextrose 5%	●	…	…
Dextrose 5% in Ringer's injection, lactated	●	…	…
Dextrose 5% in sodium chloride 0.9%	●	…	…
Ringer's injection, lactated	●	…	…
Sodium bicarbonate 5%	…	●	…
Sodium chloride 0.9%	●	…	…

Drugs	Compatible	Incompatible	Variable
Aminophylline	…	●	…
Amiodarone HCl	●	…	…
Atracurium besylate	●	…	…
Barbiturates	…	●	…
Bivalirudin	●	…	…

Drugs	Compatible	Incompatible	Variable
Caffeine citrate	●	...	...
Calcium chloride	●	...	...
Cimetidine HCl	●	...	...
Cisatracurium besylate	●	...	...
Dexmedetomidine HCl	●	...	...
Dobutamine HCl	●	...	...
Famotidine	●	...	...
Fenoldopam mesylate	●	...	...
Furosemide	...	●	...
Heparin sodium	●	...	...
Hextend	●	...	...
Hydrocortisone sodium succinate	●	...	...
Levofloxacin	●	...	...
Lidocaine HCl	...	●	...
Magnesium sulfate	●	...	...
Milrinone lactate	●	...	...
Multivitamins	●	...	...
Pancuronium bromide	●	...	...
Pantoprazole sodium	...	●	...
Potassium chloride	●	...	...
Propofol	●	...	...
Ranitidine HCl	●	...	...
Remifentanil HCl	●	...	...
Sodium bicarbonate	...	●	...
Sodium nitroprusside	●	...	...
Succinylcholine chloride	●	...	...
Tacrolimus	●	...	...
Vecuronium bromide	●	...	...
Verapamil HCl	●	...	...

Itraconazole

Handbook on Injectable Drugs pp. 970.

Description: A synthetic azole derivative antifungal.

Products: Sporanox; Available as a kit containing a 25-mL ampul of a 10-mg/mL concentrate along with a special 50-mL sodium chloride 0.9% diluent in a plastic bag and a filter-bearing infusion set. *pH:* 4.5 after preparation.

Preparation: The manufacturer's preparation instructions must be followed completely. The special 50-mL bag of sodium chloride 0.9% must be used to prepare itraconazole; no other solution or container may be used. Transfer the full contents of the 25-mL ampul of itraconazole concentrate into the special 50-mL bag of sodium chloride 0.9% and mix gently to yield a total of 75 mL of itraconazole 3.33 mg/mL.

Administration: Itraconazole must be prepared only according to the manufacturer's instructions to avoid inadvertent precipitation. After dilution of the concentrate using the bag of sodium chloride provided in the kit, 60 mL (200 mg) of the itraconazole 3.33-mg/mL solution should be infused IV over 60 minutes using a flow-control device through a dedicated infusion line; do not give by bolus injection. Administration should be performed using an extension set and the filter-bearing infusion set provided in the kit. No other drugs or solutions should be administered through this dedicated line or added to the bag of itraconazole. After the itraconazole infusion has been completed, the infusion set should be flushed with 15 to 20 mL of sodium chloride 0.9% over 30 seconds to 15 minutes using the two-way stopcock. The entire infusion set should then be discarded. Administration of other drugs through the lumen used to administer itraconazole may only be done after performing the described flush process with sodium chloride 0.9%.

Stability: The colorless to slightly yellow solution should be stored at room temperature and protected from light and freezing. It should be inspected for particulates and discoloration prior to use. After preparation for use, the diluted solution can be stored for up to 48 hours at room temperature or under refrigeration protected from light. Exposure to normal room light during adminstration is acceptable.

Compatibility Table

Solutions	Compatible	Incompatible	Variable
Dextrose 5%	...	●	...
Dextrose 5% in Ringer's injection, lactated*	...	●	...
Dextrose 5% in sodium chloride 0.2, 0.45, & 0.9%	...	●	...
Ringer's injection, lactated	...	●	...
Sodium chloride 0.9%	...	...	●

*Itraconazole was found to be physically incompatible with aqueous solutions at most concentrations. It is essential for the physical stability of itraconazole injection that the preparation instructions be followed accurately to yield the required 3.33-mg/mL concentration in sodium chloride 0.9%. Any variation from this critical concentration, higher or lower, appears to result in rapid gross precipitation, even when no other drug is present and only a simple aqueous diluent is utilized. Consequently, itraconazole should be considered incompatible with all other medications and diluents in admixtures and by Y-site administration.

Labetalol Hydrochloride

Handbook on Injectable Drugs pp. 980–984.

Description: An α- and β-adrenergic blocking antihypertensive.

Products: Normodyne, Trandate; 5 mg/mL in 20- and 40-mL multiple-dose vials and 4- and 8-mL disposable syringes. *pH:* From 3 to 4.

Preparation: For continuous infusion, add 40 mL (200 mg) to 160 mL of compatible diluent to form a 1-mg/mL solution. For a 2-mg/3 mL solution, add 40 mL to 250 mL.

Administration: Administer by direct IV injection slowly over two minutes or continuous IV infusion using a controlled infusion device at an initial rate of 2 mg/min, with the rate adjusted according to the blood pressure response.

Stability: The solution is colorless to slightly yellow. Optimum stability is at pH 3 to 4. Precipitation may occur from alkaline solutions.

Compatibility Table

Solutions	Compatible	Incompatible	Variable
Dextrose 5%	●	...	...
Dextrose 5% in Ringer's injection, lactated	●	...	...
Dextrose 5% in sodium chloride 0.2, 0.33, & 0.9%	●	...	...
Ringer's injection	●	...	...
Ringer's injection, lactated	●	...	...
Sodium bicarbonate 5%	...	●	...
Sodium chloride 0.9%	●	...	...

Drugs			
Amikacin sulfate	●	...	...
Aminophylline	●	...	...
Amiodarone HCl	●	...	...
Amphotericin B cholesteryl sulfate complex	...	●	...

Drugs	Compatible	Incompatible	Variable
Ampicillin sodium	●	...	...
Bivalirudin	●	...	...
Butorphanol tartrate	●	...	...
Calcium gluconate	●	...	...
Cefazolin sodium	●	...	...
Ceftazidime	●	...	...
Ceftizoxime sodium	●	...	...
Ceftriaxone sodium	...	●	...
Chloramphenicol sod. succ.	●	...	...
Cimetidine HCl	●	...	...
Clindamycin phosphate	●	...	...
Dexmedetomidine HCl	●	...	...
Diltiazem HCl	●	...	...
Dobutamine HCl	●	...	...
Dopamine HCl	●	...	...
Enalaprilat	●	...	...
Epinephrine HCl	●	...	...
Erythromycin lactobionate	●	...	...
Esmolol HCl	●	...	...
Famotidine	●	...	...
Fenoldopam mesylate	●	...	...
Fentanyl citrate	●	...	...
Furosemide	...	...	●
Gentamicin sulfate	●	...	...
Heparin sodium	...	...	●
Hextend	●	...	...
Hydromorphone HCl	●	...	...
Insulin, regular	...	...	●
Lansoprazole	...	●	...
Lidocaine HCl	●	...	...
Linezolid	●	...	...
Lorazepam	●	...	...
Magnesium sulfate	●	...	...
Meperidine HCl	●	...	...
Metronidazole	●	...	...
Midazolam HCl	●	...	...
Milrinone lactate	●	...	...
Morphine sulfate	●	...	...
Nafcillin sodium	...	●	...
Nicardipine HCl	●	...	...

Drugs	Compatible	Incompatible	Variable
Nitroglycerin	●	...	...
Norepinephrine bitartrate	●	...	...
Oxacillin sodium	●	...	...
Pantoprazole sodium	...	●	...
Penicillin G potassium	●	...	...
Piperacillin sodium	●	...	...
Potassium chloride	●	...	...
Potassium phosphates	●	...	...
Propofol	●	...	...
Ranitidine HCl	●	...	...
Sodium acetate	●	...	...
Sodium nitroprusside	●	...	...
Thiopental sodium	...	●	...
Tobramycin sulfate	●	...	...
Trimethoprim–sulfamethoxazole	●	...	...
Vancomycin HCl	●	...	...
Vecuronium bromide	●	...	...
Warfarin sodium	...	●	...

Lansoprazole

Handbook on Injectable Drugs pp. 984–989.

Description: A proton-pump inhibitor used as a gastric antisecretory agent.

Products: **Prevacid I.V.;** 30-mg vials. *pH:* 11.

Preparation: Reconstitute with 5 mL of sterile water for injection and mix gently resulting in a 6-mg/mL solution. Other diluents should not be used. The reconstituted concentrated injection must be diluted for administration.

Administration: Administer by IV infusion after dilution in 50 mL of dextrose 5%, sodium chloride 0.9%, or Ringer's injection, lactated. The manufacturer provides an inline filter for administration of lansoprazole that must be used because of the potential for precipitation to occur upon dilution. The inline filter should be changed after 24 hours.

Stability: Store vials at room temperature and protect from light. The reconstituted solution may be stored for up to one hour at room temperature prior to dilution in an infusion solution. After dilution in dextrose 5%, sodium chloride 0.9%, or lactated Ringer's injection, the drug is stable for up to 12 hours, 24 hours, and 24 hours, respectively, at room temperature. The manufacturer states that refrigeration of the diluted solution is not required.

Compatibility Table

Solutions	Compatible	Incompatible	Variable
Dextrose 5%	●	...	...
Ringer's injection, lactated	●	...	...
Sodium chloride 0.9%	●	...	...

Drugs	Compatible	Incompatible	Variable
Acyclovir sodium	●	...	...
Alfentanil HCl	...	●	...
Amikacin sulfate	●	...	...
Aminophylline	...	●	...
Amphotericin B	...	●	...

Drugs	Compatible	Incompatible	Variable
Ampicillin sodium	...	●	...
Ampicillin sod.–sulbactam sod.	...	●	...
Aztreonam	...	●	...
Buprenorphine HCl	...	●	...
Butorphanol tartrate	...	●	...
Calcium chloride	...	●	...
Calcium gluconate	...	●	...
Carboplatin	...	●	...
Cefazolin sodium	...	●	...
Cefepime HCl	...	●	...
Cefotetan disodium	...	●	...
Cefoxitin sodium	...	●	...
Ceftazidime	...	●	...
Ceftizoxime sodium	...	●	...
Ceftriaxone sodium	●	...	...
Chlorpromazine HCl	...	●	...
Cimetidine HCl	...	●	...
Ciprofloxacin	...	●	...
Cisplatin	...	●	...
Clindamycin phosphate	...	●	...
Cyclophosphamide	...	●	...
Cyclosporine	●	...	...
Cytarabine	...	●	...
Daunorubicin HCl	...	●	...
Dexamethasone sodium phosphate ...	●	...	...
Diazepam	...	●	...
Digoxin	...	●	...
Diltiazem HCl	...	●	...
Diphenhydramine HCl	...	●	...
Dobutamine HCl	...	●	...
Dopamine HCl	...	●	...
Doxorubicin HCl	...	●	...
Droperidol	...	●	...
Enalaprilat	...	●	...
Esmolol HCl	...	●	...
Famotidine	...	●	...
Fentanyl citrate	●	...	...
Fluconazole	●	...	...
Fluorouracil	...	●	...
Furosemide	...	●	...

Drugs	Compatible	Incompatible	Variable
Ganciclovir sodium	●	...	...
Gemcitabine HCl	...	●	...
Gentamicin sulfate	●	...	...
Granisetron HCl	...	●	...
Haloperidol lactate	...	●	...
Heparin sodium	●	...	...
Hydrocortisone sodium succinate	...	●	...
Hydromorphone HCl	...	●	...
Hydroxyzine HCl	...	●	...
Ifosfamide	●	...	...
Imipenem–cilastatin sodium	...	●	...
Labetalol HCl	...	●	...
Leucovorin calcium	...	●	...
Levofloxacin	...	●	...
Lidocaine HCl	...	●	...
Lorazepam	...	●	...
Magnesium sulfate	...	●	...
Mannitol	●	...	...
Meperidine HCl	...	●	...
Mesna	...	●	...
Methotrexate sodium	●	...	...
Methylprednisolone sod. succ.	...	●	...
Metoclopramide HCl	...	●	...
Metronidazole	...	●	...
Midazolam HCl	...	●	...
Milrinone lactate	...	●	...
Mitoxantrone HCl	...	●	...
Morphine sulfate	...	●	...
Nalbuphine HCl	●	...	...
Naloxone HCl	...	●	...
Nicardipine HCl	...	●	...
Nitroglycerin	...	●	...
Ondansetron HCl	...	●	...
Paclitaxel	●	...	...
Pentamidine isethionate	...	●	...
Pentobarbital sodium	...	●	...
Phenobarbital sodium	...	●	...
Phenylephrine HCl	...	●	...
Phenytoin sodium	...	●	...
Piperacillin sodium	●	...	...

Drugs	Compatible	Incompatible	Variable
Piperacillin sod.–tazobactam sod.	●	...	...
Potassium chloride	...	●	...
Potassium phosphates	...	●	...
Procainamide HCl	...	●	...
Prochlorperazine edisylate	...	●	...
Promethazine HCl	...	●	...
Propranolol HCl	...	●	...
Ranitidine HCl	...	●	...
Sodium bicarbonate	...	●	...
Sodium phosphates	...	●	...
Sufentanil citrate	●	...	...
Theophylline	...	●	...
Ticarcillin disod.–clavulanate pot.	...	●	...
Tobramycin sulfate	...	●	...
Trimethoprim–sulfamethoxazole	●	...	...
Vancomycin HCl	...	●	...
Verapamil HCl	...	●	...
Vinblastine sulfate	...	●	...
Vincristine sulfate	...	●	...
Vinorelbine tartrate	...	●	...
Zidovudine	...	●	...

Leucovorin Calcium

Handbook on Injectable Drugs pp. 991–996.

Description: A water-soluble vitamin, similar to folic acid, useful as an antidote to inhibitors of the enzyme dihydrofolate reductase.

Products: Available in sizes ranging from 50 to 500 mg in both dry form and as a liquid injection of 10 mg/mL. *pH:* From 6.5 to 8.5.

Preparation: Reconstitute the dry forms with bacteriostatic water for injection containing benzyl alcohol (for doses less than 10 mg/m^2) or sterile water for injection. To yield a 10-mg/mL solution, reconstitute the dry 50-, 100-, 200-, or 500-mg vial with 5, 10, 20, or 50 mL, respectively. To yield a 20-mg/mL solution, reconstitute the 350-mg vial with 17.5 mL.

Administration: Administer by IM or IV injection or IV infusion at a rate not exceeding 160 mg/min.

Stability: Store at room temperature and protect from light. Reconstituted solutions are chemically stable for seven days but should be used immediately if reconstituted with a diluent containing no preservatives. Aqueous solutions are stable at pH 6.5 to 10. An increased rate of decomposition occurs below pH 6.

Compatibility Table

Solutions	Compatible	Incompatible	Variable
Dextrose 5 & 10%	●	...	...
Dextrose 10% in sodium chloride 0.9%	●	...	...
Ringer's injection	●	...	...
Ringer's injection, lactated	●	...	...
Sodium chloride 0.9%	...	...	●

Drugs	Compatible	Incompatible	Variable
Amifostine	●	...	...
Amphotericin B cholesteryl sulfate complex	...	●	...
Aztreonam	●	...	...
Bleomycin sulfate	●	...	...

Drugs	Compatible	Incompatible	Variable
Cefepime HCl	•	...	...
Cisplatin	•	...	...
Cladribine	•	...	...
Cyclophosphamide	•	...	...
Docetaxel	•	...	...
Doxorubicin HCl	•	...	...
Doxorubicin HCl liposome injection	•	...	...
Droperidol	...	•	...
Etoposide phosphate	•	...	...
Filgrastim	•	...	...
Floxuridine	•	...	...
Fluconazole	•	...	...
Fluorouracil	...	...	•
Foscarnet sodium	...	•	...
Furosemide	•	...	...
Gemcitabine HCl	•	...	...
Granisetron HCl	•	...	...
Heparin sodium	•	...	...
Lansoprazole	...	•	...
Linezolid	•	...	...
Methotrexate sodium	•	...	...
Metoclopramide HCl	•	...	...
Mitomycin	•	...	...
Oxaliplatin	•	...	...
Pemetrexed disodium	•	...	...
Piperacillin sod.–tazobactam sod.	•	...	...
Sodium bicarbonate	...	•	...
Tacrolimus	•	...	...
Teniposide	•	...	...
Thiotepa	•	...	...
Vinblastine sulfate	•	...	...
Vincristine sulfate	•	...	...

Levofloxacin

Handbook on Injectable Drugs pp. 997–1001.

Description: A synthetic fluoroquinolone anti-infective.

Products: Levaquin; 25-mg/mL concentrate in 20- and 30-mL single-use vials and a 5-mg/mL ready-to-use infusion solution in 50-, 100-, and 200-mL plastic bags. *pH:* From 3.8 to 5.8.

Preparation: The concentrate must be diluted to a final concentration of 5 mg/mL with a compatible infusion solution.

Administration: Administer a 5-mg/mL concentration by slow IV infusion only. The drug should not be given by any other route of administration or administered rapidly or as a bolus. Levofloxacin is infused over at least 60 minutes. Doses of 750 mg should be infused over 90 minutes.

Stability: The clear light yellow to greenish-yellow solution should be stored at room temperature and protected from light. The ready-to-use solution also should be protected from freezing and excessive heat. Dilution of the concentrate to 5 mg/mL in a compatible infusion solution results in a solution that is stable for 72 hours at room temperature, 14 days under refrigeration, and six months frozen. Frozen solutions should be thawed at room temperature or in the refrigerator.

Compatibility Table

Solutions	Compatible	Incompatible	Variable
Dextrose 5%	●	...	...
Dextrose 5% in Ringer's injection, lactated	●	...	...
Dextrose 5% in sodium chloride 0.45 & 0.9%	●	...	...
Mannitol 20%	...	...	●
Sodium chloride 0.9%	●	...	...

Drugs			
Acyclovir sodium	...	●	...
Alprostadil	...	●	...
Amikacin sulfate	●	...	...
Aminophylline	●	...	...
Ampicillin sodium	●	...	...

Drugs	Compatible	Incompatible	Variable
Azithromycin	...	●	...
Bivalirudin	●	...	...
Caffeine citrate	●	...	...
Cefotaxime sodium	●	...	...
Cimetidine HCl	●	...	...
Clindamycin phosphate	●	...	...
Daptomycin	●	...	...
Dexamethasone sodium phosphate	●	...	...
Dexmedetomidine HCl	●	...	...
Dobutamine HCl	●	...	...
Dopamine HCl	●	...	...
Drotrecogin alfa (activated)	...	●	...
Epinephrine HCl	●	...	...
Fenoldopam mesylate	●	...	...
Fentanyl citrate	●	...	...
Furosemide	...	●	...
Gentamicin sulfate	●	...	...
Heparin sodium	...	●	...
Hextend	●	...	...
Indomethacin sodium trihydrate	...	●	...
Insulin, regular	...	...	●
Isoproterenol HCl	●	...	...
Lansoprazole	...	●	...
Lidocaine HCl	●	...	...
Linezolid	●	...	...
Lorazepam	●	...	...
Metoclopramide HCl	●	...	...
Morphine sulfate	●	...	...
Nitroglycerin	●	...	...
Oxacillin sodium	●	...	...
Pancuronium bromide	●	...	...
Penicillin G sodium	●	...	...
Phenobarbital sodium	●	...	...
Phenylephrine HCl	●	...	...
Potassium chloride	●	...	...
Propofol	...	●	...
Sodium bicarbonate	...	...	●
Sodium nitroprusside	...	●	...
Vancomycin HCl	●	...	...

Lidocaine Hydrochloride

Handbook on Injectable Drugs pp. 1001–1012.

Description: An amide-type local anesthetic which is also used as an antiarrhythmic agent.

Products: Xylocaine; For IV use, 10 and 20 mg/mL in sizes ranging from 5 to 50 mL. For preparing IV infusions, 40-, 100-, and 200-mg/mL concentrates are available. Also available premixed in dextrose 5% in concentrations of 0.2, 0.4, and 0.8% (2, 4, and 8 mg/mL, respectively). *pH:* Vials from 5 to 7; premixed from 3 to 7.

Preparation: For IV infusion, 1 or 2 g of drug is usually added to a liter of dextrose 5% to form a 1- or 2-mg/mL (0.1 or 0.2%) solution, respectively. When fluid restriction is desired, more concentrated solutions (up to 8 mg/mL) have been recommended.

Administration: Usually administered by direct IV injection and continuous IV infusion. The concentrates must be diluted for IV use. The drug may also be administered by IM injection. Products containing epinephrine should not be used intravenously to treat arrhythmias.

Stability: Intact containers should be stored at controlled room temperature protected from heat and freezing. Lidocaine hydrochloride exhibits maximum stability at pH 3 to 6.

Compatibility Table

Solutions	Compatible	Incompatible	Variable
Dextrose 5%	●	...	...
Dextrose 5% in Ringer's injection, lactated	●	...	...
Dextrose 5% in sodium chloride 0.45 & 0.9%	●	...	...
Ringer's injection, lactated	●	...	...
Sodium chloride 0.45 & 0.9%	●	...	...

Drugs	Compatible	Incompatible	Variable
Alteplase	●	...	...
Aminophylline	●	...	...
Amiodarone HCl	●	...	...
Amphotericin B	...	●	...
Amphotericin B cholesteryl sulfate complex	...	●	...

Drugs	Compatible	Incompatible	Variable
Ampicillin sodium	...	...	●
Argatroban	●	...	...
Atracurium besylate	●	...	...
Bivalirudin	●	...	...
Caffeine citrate	●	...	...
Calcium chloride	●	...	...
Calcium gluconate	●	...	...
Cefazolin sodium	...	...	●
Ceftriaxone sodium	...	...	●
Chloramphenicol sodium succinate	●	...	...
Chlorothiazide sodium	●	...	...
Cimetidine HCl	●	...	...
Ciprofloxacin	●	...	...
Cisatracurium besylate	●	...	...
Cloxacillin sodium	●	...	...
Daptomycin	●	...	...
Dexamethasone sodium phosphate ...	●	...	...
Dexmedetomidine HCl	●	...	...
Digoxin	●	...	...
Diltiazem HCl	●	...	...
Diphenhydramine HCl	●	...	...
Dobutamine HCl	●	...	...
Dopamine HCl	●	...	...
Enalaprilat	●	...	...
Ephedrine sulfate	●	...	...
Epinephrine HCl	...	●	...
Erythromycin lactobionate	●	...	...
Etomidate	●	...	...
Famotidine	●	...	...
Fenoldopam mesylate	●	...	...
Fentanyl citrate	...	...	●
Flumazenil	●	...	...
Furosemide	●	...	...
Glycopyrrolate	●	...	...
Haloperidol lactate	●	...	...
Heparin sodium	●	...	...
Hextend	●	...	...
Hydrocortisone sodium succinate	●	...	...
Hydroxyzine HCl	●	...	...
Insulin, regular	●	...	...

Drugs	Compatible	Incompatible	Variable
Isoproterenol HCl	...	●	...
Labetalol HCl	●	...	...
Lansoprazole	...	●	...
Levofloxacin	●	...	...
Linezolid	●	...	...
Meperidine HCl	●	...	...
Mephentermine sulfate	●	...	...
Methohexital sodium	...	●	...
Metoclopramide HCl	●	...	...
Milrinone lactate	●	...	...
Morphine sulfate	●	...	...
Nafcillin sodium	●	...	...
Nalbuphine HCl	●	...	...
Nicardipine HCl	●	...	...
Nitroglycerin	●	...	...
Norepinephrine bitartrate	...	●	...
Pantoprazole sodium	...	●	...
Penicillin G potassium	●	...	...
Pentobarbital sodium	●	...	...
Phenylephrine HCl	●	...	...
Phenytoin sodium	...	●	...
Potassium chloride	●	...	...
Procainamide HCl	●	...	...
Prochlorperazine edisylate	●	...	...
Propofol	...	...	●
Ranitidine HCl	●	...	...
Remifentanil HCl	●	...	...
Sodium bicarbonate	...	...	●
Sodium lactate	●	...	...
Sodium nitroprusside	●	...	...
Streptokinase	●	...	...
Theophylline	●	...	...
Thiopental sodium	...	●	...
Tirofiban HCl	●	...	...
Vasopressin	●	...	...
Verapamil HCl	●	...	...
Warfarin sodium	●	...	...

Linezolid

Handbook on Injectable Drugs pp. 1014–1023.

Description: A synthetic fluoroquinolone anti-infective.

Products: Zyvox; 2-mg/mL as a ready-to-use infusion solution in single-use plastic containers of 100, 200, and 300 mL. *pH:* Adjusted to 4.8.

Administration: The ready-to-use solution is administered only by IV infusion over 30 to 120 minutes.

Stability: The clear colorless to yellow solution should be stored at room temperature and protected from light and freezing. The containers should be kept in the protective overwrap until use.

Compatibility Table

Solutions	Compatible	Incompatible	Variable
Dextrose 5%	●	...	...
Dextrose 5% in Ringer's injection, lactated	●	...	...
Dextrose 5% in sodium chloride 0.2, 0.45, & 0.9%	●	...	...
Ringer's injection, lactated	●	...	...
Sodium chloride 0.9%	●	...	...

Drugs			
Acyclovir sodium	●	...	...
Alfentanil HCl	●	...	...
Amikacin sulfate	●	...	...
Aminophylline	●	...	...
Amphotericin B	...	●	...
Ampicillin sodium	●	...	...
Ampicillin sod.–sulbactam sod.	●	...	...
Aztreonam	●	...	...
Buprenorphine HCl	●	...	...
Butorphanol tartrate	●	...	...
Calcium gluconate	●	...	...
Carboplatin	●	...	...
Cefazolin sodium	●	...	...
Cefotetan disodium	●	...	...
Cefoxitin sodium	●	...	...

Drugs	Compatible	Incompatible	Variable
Ceftazidime	●	...	...
Ceftizoxime sodium	●	...	...
Ceftriaxone sodium	●	...	...
Cefuroxime sodium	●	...	...
Chlorpromazine HCl	...	●	...
Cimetidine HCl	●	...	...
Ciprofloxacin	●	...	...
Cisatracurium besylate	●	...	...
Cisplatin	●	...	...
Clindamycin phosphate	●	...	...
Cyclophosphamide	●	...	...
Cyclosporine	●	...	...
Cytarabine	●	...	...
Dexamethasone sodium phosphate	●	...	...
Dexmedetomidine HCl	●	...	...
Diazepam	...	●	...
Digoxin	●	...	...
Diphenhydramine HCl	●	...	...
Dobutamine HCl	●	...	...
Dopamine HCl	●	...	...
Doxorubicin HCl	●	...	...
Doxycycline hyclate	●	...	...
Droperidol	●	...	...
Enalaprilat	●	...	...
Erythromycin lactobionate	...	●	...
Esmolol HCl	●	...	...
Etoposide phosphate	●	...	...
Famotidine	●	...	...
Fenoldopam mesylate	●	...	...
Fentanyl citrate	●	...	...
Fluconazole	●	...	...
Fluorouracil	●	...	...
Furosemide	●	...	...
Ganciclovir sodium	●	...	...
Gemcitabine HCl	●	...	...
Gentamicin sulfate	●	...	...
Granisetron HCl	●	...	...
Haloperidol lactate	●	...	...
Heparin sodium	●	...	...
Hydrocortisone sodium succinate	●	...	...

Drugs	Compatible	Incompatible	Variable
Hydromorphone HCl	●	...	...
Hydroxyzine HCl	●	...	...
Ifosfamide	●	...	...
Imipenem–cilastatin sodium	●	...	...
Labetalol HCl	●	...	...
Leucovorin calcium	●	...	...
Levofloxacin	●	...	...
Lidocaine HCl	●	...	...
Lorazepam	●	...	...
Magnesium sulfate	●	...	...
Mannitol	●	...	...
Meperidine HCl	●	...	...
Meropenem	●	...	...
Mesna	●	...	...
Methotrexate sodium	●	...	...
Methylprednisolone sod. succ.	●	...	...
Metoclopramide HCl	●	...	...
Metronidazole	●	...	...
Midazolam HCl	●	...	...
Mitoxantrone HCl	●	...	...
Morphine sulfate	●	...	...
Nalbuphine HCl	●	...	...
Naloxone HCl	●	...	...
Nicardipine HCl	●	...	...
Nitroglycerin	●	...	...
Ondansetron HCl	●	...	...
Paclitaxel	●	...	...
Pentamidine isethionate	...	●	...
Pentobarbital sodium	●	...	...
Phenobarbital sodium	●	...	...
Phenytoin sodium	...	●	...
Piperacillin sodium	●	...	...
Piperacillin sod.–tazobactam sod.	●	...	...
Potassium chloride	●	...	...
Prochlorperazine edisylate	●	...	...
Promethazine HCl	●	...	...
Propranolol HCl	●	...	...
Ranitidine HCl	●	...	...
Remifentanil HCl	●	...	...
Sodium bicarbonate	●	...	...

Drugs	Compatible	Incompatible	Variable
Sufentanil citrate	●	...	...
Theophylline	●	...	...
Tobramycin sulfate	●	...	...
Trimethoprim–sulfamethoxazole	●	...	...
Vancomycin HCl	●	...	...
Vecuronium bromide	●	...	...
Verapamil HCl	●	...	...
Vincristine sulfate	●	...	...
Zidovudine	●	...	...

Lorazepam

Handbook on Injectable Drugs pp. 1023–1031.

Description: A benzodiazepine sedative.

Products: Ativan; 2 and 4 mg/mL in 1- and 10-mL vials, 2 mg/mL in 0.5- and 1-mL syringe cartridges, and 4 mg/mL in 1-mL syringe units.

Preparation: For IV use, dilute immediately prior to injection with an equal volume of compatible diluent. To dilute in a syringe, first eliminate all air and then aspirate the diluent. Pull the plunger back slightly to provide some mixing space and gently invert the syringe repeatedly to mix the contents. Do not shake.

Administration: Administer by IM injection deep into the muscle mass or by IV injection at a rate not exceeding 2 mg/min.

Stability: Store under refrigeration and protect from light and freezing. The drug is stable for up to 60 days at room temperature. Lorazepam undergoes significant sorption into PVC fluid bags and administration sets. Losses of over 10% in two hours have been observed.

The physical stability of dilutions is dependent on the concentration of lorazepam and the commercial lorazepam injection used. Concentrations of 1 and 2 mg/mL and those below 0.08 mg/mL have been reported to be physically stable. Concentrations in the middle range of 0.08 to 1 mg/mL may be problematic. Use of the 2-mg/mL commercial product is more likely to result in physically stable admixtures than the 4-mg/mL concentration because of the larger amounts of solubilizing solvents per milligram of drug.

Compatibility Table

Solutions	Compatible	Incompatible	Variable
Dextrose 5%	...	...	●
Ringer's injection, lactated	...	...	●
Sodium chloride 0.9%	...	...	●

Drugs			
Acyclovir sodium	●	...	...
Albumin	●	...	...
Aldesleukin	...	●	...
Allopurinol sodium	●	...	...
Amifostine	●	...	...

Drugs	Compatible	Incompatible	Variable
Amikacin sulfate	●	...	...
Amiodarone HCl	●	...	...
Amphotericin B cholesteryl sulfate complex	●	...	...
Anakinra	●	...	...
Atracurium besylate	●	...	...
Aztreonam	...	●	...
Bivalirudin	●	...	...
Bumetanide	●	...	...
Buprenorphine HCl	...	●	...
Caffeine citrate	...	●	...
Cefepime HCl	●	...	...
Cefotaxime sodium	●	...	...
Cimetidine HCl	●	...	...
Ciprofloxacin	●	...	...
Cisatracurium besylate	●	...	...
Cisplatin	●	...	...
Cladribine	●	...	...
Clonidine HCl	●	...	...
Cyclophosphamide	●	...	...
Cytarabine	●	...	...
Dexamethasone sodium phosphate ...	●	...	...
Dexmedetomidine HCl	●	...	...
Diltiazem HCl	●	...	...
Dimenhydrinate	●	...	...
Dobutamine HCl	●	...	...
Docetaxel	●	...	...
Dopamine HCl	●	...	...
Doxorubicin HCl	●	...	...
Doxorubicin HCl liposome injection	●	...	...
Epinephrine HCl	●	...	...
Erythromycin lactobionate	●	...	...
Etomidate	●	...	...
Etoposide phosphate	●	...	...
Famotidine	●	...	...
Fenoldopam mesylate	●	...	...
Fentanyl citrate	●	...	...
Filgrastim	●	...	...
Fluconazole	●	...	...
Fludarabine phosphate	●	...	...

Drugs	Compatible	Incompatible	Variable
Foscarnet sodium	...	...	●
Fosphenytoin sodium	●	...	...
Furosemide	●	...	...
Gallium nitrate	...	●	...
Gemcitabine HCl	●	...	...
Gentamicin sulfate	●	...	...
Granisetron HCl	●	...	...
Haloperidol lactate	●	...	...
Heparin sodium	●	...	...
Hextend	●	...	...
Hydrocortisone sodium succinate	●	...	...
Hydromorphone HCl	●	...	...
Idarubicin HCl	...	●	...
Imipenem–cilastatin sodium	...	●	...
Labetalol HCl	●	...	...
Lansoprazole	...	●	...
Levofloxacin	●	...	...
Linezolid	●	...	...
Melphalan HCl	●	...	...
Methadone HCl	●	...	...
Methotrexate sodium	●	...	...
Metronidazole	●	...	...
Midazolam HCl	●	...	...
Milrinone lactate	●	...	...
Morphine sulfate	●	...	...
Nicardipine HCl	●	...	...
Nitroglycerin	●	...	...
Norepinephrine bitartrate	●	...	...
Ondansetron HCl	...	●	...
Oxaliplatin	●	...	...
Paclitaxel	●	...	...
Palonosetron HCl	●	...	...
Pancuronium bromide	●	...	...
Pantoprazole sodium	...	●	...
Pemetrexed disodium	●	...	...
Piperacillin sodium	●	...	...
Piperacillin sod.–tazobactam sod.	●	...	...
Potassium chloride	●	...	...
Propofol	●	...	...
Ranitidine HCl	...	...	●

Drugs	Compatible	Incompatible	Variable
Remifentanil HCl	●	...	...
Sargramostim	...	●	...
Sufentanil citrate	...	●	...
Tacrolimus	●	...	...
Teniposide	●	...	...
Thiopental sodium	...	...	●
Thiotepa	●	...	...
Trimethoprim–sulfamethoxazole	●	...	...
Vancomycin HCl	●	...	...
Vecuronium bromide	●	...	...
Vinorelbine tartrate	●	...	...
Zidovudine	●	...	...

Magnesium Sulfate

Handbook on Injectable Drugs pp. 1032–1038.

Description: A magnesium salt with anticonvulsant properties used to treat or prevent magnesium deficiency.

Products: Available in concentrations of 1 to 50% in a variety of container sizes. Each milliliter of the 50% solution contains 500 mg of magnesium sulfate, providing 4 mEq of magnesium. Each milliliter of the 12.5% solution contains 125 mg of magnesium sulfate, providing 1 mEq of magnesium. *pH:* From 5.5 to 7.

Preparation: For IV injection, a concentration of 20% or less should be used. For IM injection, a 25 or 50% concentration is satisfactory for adults, but dilution to 20% is recommended for children.

Administration: Administer by direct IV injection, IV infusion, and IM injection. By IV injection, concentrations of 20% or less should be used; the rate of injection should not exceed 1.5 mL of a 10% solution (or the equivalent) per minute.

Stability: Intact containers should be stored at room temperature and protected from temperatures above 40 °C and from freezing. Refrigeration of the concentrated solution may result in precipitation.

Compatibility Table

Solutions	Compatible	Incompatible	Variable
Dextrose 5%	●	...	...
Fat emulsion 10%, IV	...	●	...
Ringer's injection, lactated	●	...	...
Sodium chloride 0.9%	●	...	...

Magnesium sulfate is compatible in most common IV infusion solutions.

Drugs	Compatible	Incompatible	Variable
Acyclovir sodium	●	...	...
Aldesleukin	●	...	...
Amifostine	●	...	...
Amikacin sulfate	●	...	...
Amiodarone HCl	...	...	●

Drugs	Compatible	Incompatible	Variable
Amphotericin B	…	●	…
Amphotericin B cholesteryl sulfate complex	…	●	…
Ampicillin sodium	●	…	…
Aztreonam	●	…	…
Bivalirudin	●	…	…
Calcium chloride	…	…	●
Calcium gluconate	…	…	●
Cefamandole nafate	●	…	…
Cefazolin sodium	●	…	…
Cefepime HCl	…	●	…
Cefotaxime sodium	●	…	…
Cefoxitin sodium	●	…	…
Chloramphenicol sodium succinate	●	…	…
Ciprofloxacin	…	…	●
Cisatracurium besylate	●	…	…
Cisplatin	●	…	…
Clindamycin phosphate	…	…	●
Cyclosporine	…	●	…
Dexmedetomidine HCl	●	…	…
Dimenhydrinate	●	…	…
Dobutamine HCl	…	…	●
Docetaxel	●	…	…
Doxorubicin HCl liposome injection	●	…	…
Doxycycline hyclate	●	…	…
Drotrecogin alfa (activated)	…	●	…
Enalaprilat	●	…	…
Erythromycin lactobionate	●	…	…
Esmolol HCl	●	…	…
Etoposide phosphate	●	…	…
Famotidine HCl	●	…	…
Fenoldopam mesylate	●	…	…
Fludarabine phosphate	●	…	…
Gallium nitrate	●	…	…
Gentamicin sulfate	●	…	…
Granisetron HCl	●	…	…
Heparin sodium	●	…	…
Hextend	●	…	…
Hydrocortisone sodium succinate	…	…	●

Magnesium Sulfate

Drugs	Compatible	Incompatible	Variable
Hydromorphone HCl	●	...	...
Idarubicin HCl	●	...	...
Insulin, regular	●	...	...
Isoproterenol HCl	●	...	...
Kanamycin sulfate	●	...	...
Labetalol HCl	●	...	...
Lansoprazole	...	●	...
Linezolid	●	...	...
Meperidine HCl	●	...	...
Meropenem	●	...	...
Methyldopa HCl	●	...	...
Metoclopramide HCl	●	...	...
Metronidazole	●	...	...
Milrinone lactate	●	...	...
Morphine sulfate	●	...	...
Nafcillin sodium	●	...	...
Nicardipine HCl	●	...	...
Norepinephrine bitartrate	●	...	...
Ondansetron HCl	●	...	...
Oxacillin sodium	●	...	...
Oxaliplatin	●	...	...
Paclitaxel	●	...	...
Pantoprazole sodium	...	●	...
Penicillin G potassium	●	...	...
Piperacillin sodium	●	...	...
Piperacillin sod.–tazobactam sod.	●	...	...
Polymyxin B sulfate	...	●	...
Potassium chloride	●	...	...
Potassium phosphates	●	...	...
Procaine HCl	...	●	...
Propofol	●	...	...
Remifentanil HCl	●	...	...
Sargramostim	●	...	...
Sodium bicarbonate	...	●	...
Sodium nitroprusside	●	...	...
Sodium phosphates	...	...	●
Thiotepa	●	...	...
Tobramycin sulfate	...	...	●
Trimethoprim–sulfamethoxazole	●	...	...
Vancomycin HCl	●	...	...
Verapamil HCl	●	...	...

Meperidine Hydrochloride

Handbook on Injectable Drugs pp. 1053–1063.

Description: A synthetic narcotic analgesic.

Products: **Demerol Hydrochloride;** available in concentrations ranging from 10 to 100 mg/mL in ampuls, vials, and disposable syringe cartridges. *pH:* 3.5 to 6.

Preparation: As a supplement to anesthesia, dilution to 10 mg/mL for repeated slow IV injections or 1 mg/mL for continuous IV infusion has been recommended.

Administration: Administer as an IM injection into a large muscle mass. It also may be given SC or by slow IV injection in a diluted solution.

Stability: Store intact containers at room temperature protected from light and freezing. No sorption to plastic IV bags, sets, or syringes has been noted.

Compatibility Table

Solutions	Compatible	Incompatible	Variable
Dextrose 5%	●	…	…
Dextrose 5% in Ringer's injection	●	…	…
Dextrose 5% in Ringer's injection, lactated	●	…	…
Dextrose 5% in sodium chloride 0.2, 0.45, & 0.9%	●	…	…
Ringer's injection	●	…	…
Ringer's injection, lactated	●	…	…
Sodium chloride 0.45 & 0.9%	●	…	…

Drugs	Compatible	Incompatible	Variable
Acyclovir sodium	…	…	●
Allopurinol sodium	…	●	…
Amifostine	●	…	…
Amikacin sulfate	●	…	…
Aminophylline	…	●	…

Drugs	Compatible	Incompatible	Variable
Amobarbital sodium	...	●	...
Amphotericin B cholesteryl sulfate complex	...	●	...
Ampicillin sodium	●	...	...
Ampicillin sod.–sulbactam sod.	●	...	...
Atenolol	●	...	...
Atropine sulfate	●	...	...
Aztreonam	●	...	...
Bivalirudin	●	...	...
Bumetanide	●	...	...
Butorphanol tartrate	●	...	...
Cefamandole nafate	●	...	...
Cefazolin sodium	●	...	...
Cefepime HCl	...	●	...
Cefotaxime sodium	●	...	...
Cefotetan disodium	●	...	...
Cefoxitin sodium	●	...	...
Ceftazidime	●	...	...
Ceftizoxime sodium	●	...	...
Ceftriaxone sodium	●	...	...
Cefuroxime sodium	●	...	...
Chloramphenicol sodium succinate	●	...	...
Chlorpromazine HCl	●	...	...
Cimetidine HCl	●	...	...
Cisatracurium besylate	●	...	...
Cladribine	●	...	...
Clindamycin phosphate	●	...	...
Dexamethasone sodium phosphate ...	●	...	...
Dexmedetomidine HCl	●	...	...
Digoxin	●	...	...
Diltiazem HCl	●	...	...
Dimenhydrinate	●	...	...
Diphenhydramine HCl	●	...	...
Dobutamine HCl	●	...	...
Docetaxel	●	...	...
Dopamine HCl	●	...	...
Doxorubicin HCl liposome injection	...	●	...
Doxycycline hyclate	●	...	...

Drugs	Compatible	Incompatible	Variable
Droperidol	●	...	...
Erythromycin lactobionate	●	...	...
Etoposide phosphate	●	...	...
Famotidine	●	...	...
Fenoldopam mesylate	●	...	...
Fentanyl citrate	●	...	...
Filgrastim	●	...	...
Fluconazole	●	...	...
Fludarabine phosphate	●	...	...
Furosemide	...	...	●
Gallium nitrate	●	...	...
Gemcitabine HCl	●	...	...
Gentamicin sulfate	●	...	...
Glycopyrrolate	●	...	...
Granisetron HCl	●	...	...
Heparin sodium	...	...	●
Hextend	●	...	...
Hydrocortisone sodium succinate	●	...	...
Hydroxyzine HCl	●	...	...
Idarubicin HCl	...	●	...
Imipenem–cilastatin sodium	...	●	...
Insulin, regular	●	...	...
Kanamycin sulfate	●	...	...
Ketamine HCl	●	...	...
Labetalol HCl	●	...	...
Lansoprazole	...	●	...
Lidocaine HCl	●	...	...
Linezolid	●	...	...
Magnesium sulfate	●	...	...
Melphalan HCl	●	...	...
Methyldopate HCl	●	...	...
Methylprednisolone sod. succ.	●	...	...
Metoclopramide HCl	●	...	...
Metoprolol tartrate	●	...	...
Metronidazole	●	...	...
Midazolam HCl	●	...	...
Morphine sulfate	...	●	...
Nafcillin sodium	...	...	●
Ondansetron HCl	●	...	...
Oxacillin sodium	●	...	...

Drugs	Compatible	Incompatible	Variable
Oxaliplatin	●	…	…
Oxytocin	●	…	…
Paclitaxel	●	…	…
Pantoprazole sodium	…	●	…
Pemetrexed disodium	●	…	…
Penicillin G potassium	●	…	…
Pentazocine lactate	●	…	…
Pentobarbital sodium	…	●	…
Phenobarbital sodium	…	●	…
Phenytoin sodium	…	●	…
Piperacillin sodium	●	…	…
Piperacillin sod.–tazobactam sod.	●	…	…
Potassium chloride	●	…	…
Prochlorperazine edisylate	●	…	…
Promethazine HCl	●	…	…
Propofol	●	…	…
Propranolol HCl	●	…	…
Ranitidine HCl	●	…	…
Remifentanil HCl	●	…	…
Sargramostim	●	…	…
Scopolamine HBr	●	…	…
Sodium bicarbonate	…	…	●
Succinylcholine chloride	●	…	…
Teniposide	●	…	…
Thiopental sodium	…	●	…
Thiotepa	●	…	…
Ticarcillin disod.–clavulanate pot.	●	…	…
Tobramycin sulfate	●	…	…
Triflupromazine HCl	●	…	…
Trimethoprim–sulfamethoxazole	●	…	…
Vancomycin HCl	●	…	…
Verapamil HCl	●	…	…
Vinorelbine tartrate	●	…	…

Meropenem

Handbook on Injectable Drugs pp. 1064–1071.

Description: A synthetic carbapenem antibiotic.

Products: Merrem; 500-mg and 1-g vials, ADD-Vantage vials, and infusion vials. *pH:* From 7.3 to 8.3 when reconstituted.

Preparation: Reconstitute the 500-mg vials with 10 mL and the 1-g vials with 20 mL of sterile water for injection, shake, and allow to stand until clear. The solution will contain meropenem 50 mg/mL.

The 500-mg and 1-g ADD-Vantage vials should be reconstituted with sodium chloride 0.45%, sodium chloride 0.9%, or dextrose 5% in 50-, 100-, or 250-mL ADD-Vantage containers. The 500-mg and 1-g infusion vials should be reconstituted directly with 100 mL of a compatible diluent.

Administration: Administer by direct IV injection over three to five minutes or by IV infusion diluted in a compatible infusion solution over 15 to 30 minutes.

Stability: Store intact vials at room temperature. The reconstituted solution in vials up to 50 mg/mL is stable for two hours at room temperature and up to 12 hours under refrigeration. Meropenem 2.5 to 50 mg/mL in sodium chloride 0.9% in infusion vials is stable for two hours at room temperature and 18 hours under refrigeration; in dextrose 5% at these concentrations, stability is only one hour at room temperature and eight hours under refrigeration. In ADD-Vantage vials at 5 to 20 mg/mL in sodium chloride 0.45% or 1 to 20 mg/mL in sodium chloride 0.9%, the drug is stable for six or four hours, respectively, at room temperature and up to 24 hours under refrigeration. However, a 1 to 20 mg/mL concentration in dextrose 5% is stable for only one hour at room temperature and up to eight hours under refrigeration. Solutions should not be frozen.

Compatibility Table

Drugs	Compatible	Incompatible	Variable

NOTE: Unstable in infusion solutions. Unacceptable drug decomposition occurs in one to four hours in some solutions at room temperature. See **Stability.**

Drugs	Compatible	Incompatible	Variable
Acyclovir sodium	...	...	●
Aminophylline	●	...	...
Amphotericin B	...	●	...
Atenolol	●	...	...
Atropine sulfate	●	...	...
Calcium gluconate	...	...	●
Cimetidine HCl	●	...	...
Dexamethasone sodium phosphate	●	...	...
Diazepam	...	●	...
Digoxin	●	...	...
Diphenhydramine HCl	●	...	...
Dobutamine HCl	●	...	...
Docetaxel	●	...	...
Dopamine HCl	●	...	...
Doxycycline hyclate	...	...	●
Enalaprilat	●	...	...
Fluconazole	●	...	...
Furosemide	●	...	...
Gentamicin sulfate	●	...	...
Heparin sodium	●	...	...
Insulin, regular	●	...	...
Linezolid	●	...	...
Magnesium sulfate	●	...	...
Metoclopramide HCl	●	...	...
Metronidazole HCl	...	●	...
Milrinone lactate	●	...	...
Morphine sulfate	●	...	...
Multivitamins	...	●	...
Norepinephrine bitartrate	●	...	...
Ondansetron HCl	...	...	●
Pantoprazole sodium	...	●	...
Phenobarbital sodium	●	...	...
Potassium chloride	●	...	...
Ranitidine HCl	●	...	...
Vancomycin HCl	●	...	...
Zidovudine	...	...	●

Methotrexate Sodium

Description: A folic acid antagonist antineoplastic agent.

Products: Available in a 25-mg/mL liquid form and in lyophilized form in 1-g vials. *pH:* Approximately 8.5.

Preparation: Reconstitute the 1-g size with 19.4 mL to yield a 50-mg/mL solution. Reconstitute with a sterile, preservative-free diluent.

For high-dose IV therapy, use only the preservative-free forms of methotrexate.

For intrathecal injection, dilute preservative-free methotrexate to 1 mg/mL with a preservative-free diluent such as sodium chloride 0.9% or Elliott's B Solution.

Administration: Administer by IM or direct IV injection, continuous or intermittent IV infusion, and intra-arterial or intrathecal injection.

Stability: Store intact containers at room temperature protected from light. The commercial manufacturers recommend reconstitution immediately prior to use. In dilute solutions, methotrexate may undergo unacceptable photodegradation within days if exposed to light and within hours if exposed to direct sunlight. No sorption to plastic administration sets has been noted.

Compatibility Table

Solutions	Compatible	Incompatible	Variable
Dextrose 5%	●	...	...
Dextrose 5% in sodium chloride 0.9%	●	...	...
Sodium bicarbonate 0.05 M	●	...	...
Sodium chloride 0.9%	●	...	...

Drugs			
Allopurinol sodium	●	...	...
Amifostine	●	...	...
Amphotericin B cholesteryl sulfate complex	●	...	...
Asparaginase	●	...	...

Drugs	Compatible	Incompatible	Variable
Aztreonam	●	...	...
Bleomycin sulfate	...	...	●
Cefepime HCl	●	...	...
Ceftriaxone sodium	●	...	...
Chlorpromazine HCl	...	●	...
Cimetidine HCl	●	...	...
Cisplatin	●	...	...
Cyclophosphamide	●	...	...
Cytarabine	●	...	...
Daunorubicin HCl	●	...	...
Dexamethasone sodium phosphate ...	...	...	●
Diphenhydramine HCl	●	...	...
Doxapram HCl	●	...	...
Doxorubicin HCl	●	...	...
Doxorubicin HCl liposome injection	●	...	...
Droperidol	...	...	●
Etoposide	●	...	...
Etoposide phosphate	●	...	...
Famotidine	●	...	...
Filgrastim	●	...	...
Fludarabine phosphate	●	...	...
Fluorouracil	...	...	●
Furosemide	●	...	...
Gallium nitrate	●	...	...
Ganciclovir sodium	●	...	...
Gemcitabine HCl	...	●	...
Granisetron HCl	●	...	...
Heparin sodium	●	...	...
Hydromorphone HCl	●	...	...
Hydroxyzine HCl	●	...	...
Idarubicin HCl	...	●	...
Ifosfamide	...	●	...
Imipenem–cilastatin sodium	●	...	...
Lansoprazole	●	...	...
Leucovorin calcium	●	...	...
Linezolid	●	...	...
Lorazepam	●	...	...
Melphalan HCl	●	...	...
Mesna	●	...	...
Methylprednisolone sod. succ.	●	...	...

Drugs	Compatible	Incompatible	Variable
Metoclopramide HCl	...	...	●
Midazolam HCl	...	●	...
Mitomycin	●	...	...
Morphine sulfate	●	...	...
Nalbuphine HCl	...	●	...
Ondansetron HCl	●	...	...
Oxacillin sodium	●	...	...
Oxaliplatin	●	...	...
Paclitaxel	●	...	...
Piperacillin sod.–tazobactam sod.	●	...	...
Prochlorperazine edisylate	●	...	...
Promethazine HCl	...	●	...
Propofol	...	●	...
Ranitidine HCl	●	...	...
Sargramostim	●	...	...
Sodium bicarbonate	●	...	...
Teniposide	●	...	...
Thiotepa	●	...	...
Vancomycin HCl	...	...	●
Vinblastine sulfate	●	...	...
Vincristine sulfate	●	...	...
Vindesine sulfate	●	...	...
Vinorelbine tartrate	●	...	...

Methylprednisolone Sodium Succinate

Handbook on Injectable Drugs pp. 1097–1106.

Description: A synthetic glucocorticoid used primarily for its anti-inflammatory effect.

Products: A-Methapred, Solu-Medrol; 40-, 125-, and 500-mg and 1- and 2-g sizes. *pH:* From 7 to 8 when reconstituted.

Preparation: When reconstituted with the supplied diluent or bacteriostatic water for injection with benzyl alcohol if a diluent is not supplied, the solutions have the following concentrations:

Vial Size	Diluent Volume	Methylprednisolone Concentration
40 mg	1 mL	40 mg/mL
125 mg	2 mL	62.5 mg/mL
500 mg	8 mL	62.5 mg/mL
1000 mg	16 mL	62.5 mg/mL
2000 mg	30.6 mL	62.5 mg/mL

Administration: Administer by IV infusion, IM injection, or direct IV injection over one to several minutes. High-dose therapy is given IV over at least 30 minutes.

Stability: Store intact vials at room temperature. Reconstituted vials should be stored at room temperature and used within 48 hours.

Compatibility Table

Solutions	Compatible	Incompatible	Variable

NOTE: Haze formation in infusion fluids may be caused by hydrolysis of the ester to free methylprednisolone. Haze forms in variable time periods, even among solutions with the same concentration.

Solutions	Compatible	Incompatible	Variable
Dextrose 5%	...	...	•
Dextrose 5% in sodium chloride 0.45 & 0.9%	...	...	•
Ringer's injection, lactated	...	...	•
Sodium chloride 0.9%	...	...	•

Drugs	Compatible	Incompatible	Variable
Acyclovir sodium	●	…	…
Allopurinol sodium	…	●	…
Amifostine	●	…	…
Aminophylline	…	…	●
Amiodarone HCl	●	…	…
Amphotericin B cholesteryl sulfate complex	●	…	…
Aztreonam	●	…	…
Bivalirudin	●	…	…
Calcium gluconate	…	●	…
Cefepime HCl	●	…	…
Ceftazidime	●	…	…
Chloramphenicol sodium succinate	●	…	…
Cimetidine HCl	●	…	…
Ciprofloxacin	…	●	…
Cisatracurium besylate	…	…	●
Cisplatin	●	…	…
Cladribine	●	…	…
Clindamycin phosphate	●	…	…
Cyclophosphamide	●	…	…
Cytarabine	…	…	●
Dexmedetomidine HCl	●	…	…
Diatrizoate meglumine & sodium	●	…	…
Diltiazem HCl	…	…	●
Docetaxel	…	●	…
Dopamine HCl	●	…	…
Doxapram HCl	…	●	…
Doxorubicin HCl	●	…	…
Doxorubicin HCl liposome injection	●	…	…
Enalaprilat	●	…	…
Etoposide phosphate	…	●	…
Famotidine	●	…	…
Fenoldopam mesylate	…	●	…
Filgrastim	…	●	…
Fludarabine phosphate	●	…	…
Gemcitabine HCl	…	●	…
Glycopyrrolate	…	●	…
Granisetron HCl	●	…	…
Heparin sodium	…	…	●

Drugs	Compatible	Incompatible	Variable
Hextend	●	...	...
Insulin, regular	...	●	...
Iohexol	●	...	...
Iopamidol	●	...	...
Iothalamate sodium	●	...	...
Ioxaglate meglumine & sodium	●	...	...
Lansoprazole	...	●	...
Linezolid	●	...	...
Melphalan HCl	●	...	...
Meperidine HCl	●	...	...
Methotrexate sodium	●	...	...
Metoclopramide HCl	●	...	...
Metronidazole	●	...	...
Midazolam HCl	●	...	...
Milrinone lactate	●	...	...
Morphine sulfate	●	...	...
Nafcillin sodium	...	●	...
Nicardipine HCl	●	...	...
Norepinephrine bitartrate	●	...	...
Ondansetron HCl	...	●	...
Oxaliplatin	●	...	...
Paclitaxel	...	●	...
Pantoprazole sodium	...	●	...
Pemetrexed disodium	●	...	...
Penicillin G potassium	●	...	...
Penicillin G sodium	...	●	...
Piperacillin sod.–tazobactam sod.	●	...	...
Potassium chloride	...	...	●
Propofol	...	●	...
Ranitidine HCl	●	...	...
Remifentanil HCl	●	...	...
Sargramostim	...	●	...
Sodium bicarbonate	...	...	●
Tacrolimus	●	...	...
Teniposide	●	...	...
Theophylline	●	...	...
Thiotepa	●	...	...
Topotecan HCl	●	...	...
Verapamil HCl	●	...	...
Vinorelbine tartrate	...	●	...

Metoclopramide Hydrochloride

Handbook on Injectable Drugs pp. 1106–1120.

Description: A synthetic substituted benzamide that is a dopamine receptor antagonist, an antiemetic, and a stimulant of upper gastrointestinal motility.

Products: Reglan; 5 mg/mL in 2-mL ampuls and syringe cartridges and 2-, 10-, 20-, and 30-mL vials. *pH:* From 2.5 to 6.5.

Administration: Administer by IM injection, direct IV injection without dilution slowly over one to two minutes for 10-mg doses, or intermittent IV infusion in 50 mL of compatible diluent over at least 15 minutes.

Stability: Metoclopramide hydrochloride, a colorless solution, is light sensitive, but dilutions do not require light protection for storage up to 24 hours. Store intact containers at controlled room temperature and protected from freezing and light.

Compatibility Table

Solutions	Compatible	Incompatible	Variable
Dextrose 5%	●	…	…
Dextrose 5% in sodium chloride 0.45%	●	…	…
Ringer's injection	●	…	…
Ringer's injection, lactated	●	…	…
Sodium chloride 0.9%	●	…	…

Drugs	Compatible	Incompatible	Variable
Acyclovir sodium	●	…	…
Aldesleukin	●	…	…
Allopurinol sodium	…	●	…
Amifostine	●	…	…
Aminophylline	●	…	…
Amphotericin B cholesteryl sulfate complex	…	●	…
Ampicillin sodium	…	●	…
Atropine sulfate	●	…	…
Aztreonam	●	…	…

Drugs	Compatible	Incompatible	Variable
Bivalirudin	●	...	...
Bleomycin sulfate	●	...	...
Butorphanol tartrate	●	...	...
Caffeine citrate	●	...	...
Calcium gluconate	...	●	...
Cefepime HCl	...	●	...
Chloramphenicol sodium succinate	...	●	...
Chlorpromazine HCl	●	...	...
Cimetidine HCl	...	...	●
Ciprofloxacin	●	...	...
Cisatracurium besylate	●	...	...
Cisplatin	●	...	...
Cladribine	●	...	...
Clindamycin phosphate	●	...	...
Cyclophosphamide	●	...	...
Cytarabine	●	...	...
Dexamethasone sodium phosphate	●	...	...
Dexmedetomidine HCl	●	...	...
Diltiazem HCl	●	...	...
Dimenhydrinate	●	...	...
Diphenhydramine HCl	●	...	...
Docetaxel	●	...	...
Doxapram HCl	●	...	...
Doxorubicin HCl	●	...	...
Doxorubicin HCl liposome injection	...	●	...
Droperidol	●	...	...
Erythromycin lactobionate	...	●	...
Etoposide phosphate	●	...	...
Famotidine	●	...	...
Fenoldopam mesylate	●	...	...
Fentanyl citrate	●	...	...
Filgrastim	●	...	...
Fluconazole	●	...	...
Fludarabine phosphate	●	...	...
Fluorouracil	...	...	●
Foscarnet sodium	●	...	...
Furosemide	...	●	...
Gallium nitrate	●	...	...

Drugs	Compatible	Incompatible	Variable
Gemcitabine HCl	●	…	…
Granisetron HCl	●	…	…
Heparin sodium	●	…	…
Hextend	●	…	…
Hydrocortisone sodium phosphate	●	…	…
Hydrocortisone sodium succinate	●	…	…
Hydromorphone HCl	●	…	…
Hydroxyzine HCl	●	…	…
Idarubicin HCl	●	…	…
Insulin, regular	●	…	…
Lansoprazole	…	●	…
Leucovorin calcium	●	…	…
Levofloxacin	●	…	…
Lidocaine HCl	●	…	…
Linezolid	●	…	…
Magnesium sulfate	●	…	…
Melphalan HCl	●	…	…
Meperidine HCl	●	…	…
Meropenem	●	…	…
Methadone HCl	●	…	…
Methotrexate sodium	…	…	●
Methylprednisolone sod. succ.	●	…	…
Midazolam HCl	●	…	…
Mitomycin	●	…	…
Morphine sulfate	●	…	…
Multivitamins	●	…	…
Ondansetron HCl	●	…	…
Oxaliplatin	●	…	…
Paclitaxel	●	…	…
Pantoprazole sodium	…	●	…
Pemetrexed disodium	●	…	…
Penicillin G potassium	…	●	…
Pentazocine lactate	●	…	…
Piperacillin sod.–tazobactam sod.	●	…	…
Potassium acetate & chloride	●	…	…
Potassium phosphates	●	…	…
Prochlorperazine edisylate	●	…	…
Promethazine HCl	●	…	…
Propofol	…	●	…
Quinupristin–dalfopristin	●	…	…

Drugs	Compatible	Incompatible	Variable
Ranitidine HCl	●	...	...
Remifentanil HCl	●	...	...
Sargramostim	●	...	...
Scopolamine HBr	●	...	...
Sodium bicarbonate	...	●	...
Sufentanil citrate	●	...	...
Tacrolimus	●	...	...
Teniposide	●	...	...
Thiotepa	●	...	...
Topotecan HCl	●	...	...
Verapamil HCl	●	...	...
Vinblastine sulfate	●	...	...
Vincristine sulfate	●	...	...
Vinorelbine tartrate	●	...	...
Zidovudine	●	...	...

Metronidazole

Handbook on Injectable Drugs pp. 1121–1128.

Description: A synthetic nitroimidazole antibacterial and antiprotozoal agent.

Products: Flagyl I.V. RTU; 500 mg/100-mL bags. *pH:* From 4.5 to 7.

Preparation: Metronidazole (Flagyl I.V. RTU) is ready to use, requiring no dilution or buffer.

Administration: Administer by continuous IV infusion or intermittent IV infusion over one hour. If administration is to be through the tubing of an ongoing infusion, that infusion should be stopped during metronidazole administration.

Stability: Metronidazole should be stored at room temperature and protected from light. Refrigeration may result in crystal formation. Exposure to light causes darkening.

Compatibility Table

Drugs	Compatible	Incompatible	Variable
Acyclovir sodium	●	…	…
Allopurinol sodium	●	…	…
Amifostine	●	…	…
Amikacin sulfate	●	…	…
Amphotericin B cholesteryl sulfate complex	…	●	…
Ampicillin sodium	…	…	●
Aztreonam	…	●	…
Bivalirudin	●	…	…
Cefamandole nafate	…	…	●
Cefazolin sodium	●	…	…
Cefepime HCl	●	…	…
Cefotaxime sodium	●	…	…
Cefoxitin sodium	…	…	●
Ceftazidime	●	…	…
Ceftizoxime sodium	●	…	…
Ceftriaxone sodium	●	…	…
Cefuroxime sodium	●	…	…
Chloramphenicol sodium succinate	●	…	…
Ciprofloxacin	●	…	…

Drugs	Compatible	Incompatible	Variable
Cisatracurium besylate	●	...	...
Clindamycin phosphate	●	...	...
Cyclophosphamide	●	...	...
Dexmedetomidine HCl	●	...	...
Diltiazem HCl	●	...	...
Dimenhydrinate	●	...	...
Docetaxel	●	...	...
Dopamine HCl	...	...	●
Doxapram HCl	●	...	...
Doxorubicin HCl liposome injection	●	...	...
Drotrecogin alfa (activated)	...	●	...
Enalaprilat	●	...	...
Esmolol HCl	●	...	...
Etoposide phosphate	●	...	...
Fenoldopam mesylate	●	...	...
Filgrastim	...	●	...
Fluconazole	●	...	...
Foscarnet sodium	●	...	...
Gemcitabine HCl	●	...	...
Gentamicin sulfate	●	...	...
Granisetron HCl	●	...	...
Heparin sodium	●	...	...
Hextend	●	...	...
Hydrocortisone sodium succinate	...	...	●
Hydromorphone HCl	●	...	...
Labetalol HCl	●	...	...
Lansoprazole	...	●	...
Linezolid	●	...	...
Lorazepam	●	...	...
Magnesium sulfate	●	...	...
Melphalan HCl	●	...	...
Meperidine HCl	●	...	...
Methylprednisolone sod. succ.	●	...	...
Midazolam HCl	●	...	...
Milrinone lactate	●	...	...
Morphine sulfate	●	...	...
Nicardipine HCl	●	...	...
Pantoprazole sodium	...	●	...
Pemetrexed disodium	...	●	...
Penicillin G potassium	...	...	●

Drugs	Compatible	Incompatible	Variable
Piperacillin sod.–tazobactam sod.	●	...	...
Remifentanil HCl	●	...	...
Sargramostim	●	...	...
Tacrolimus	●	...	...
Teniposide	●	...	...
Theophylline	●	...	...
Thiotepa	●	...	...
Tobramycin sulfate	●	...	...
Vinorelbine tartrate	●	...	...

Metronidazole

Midazolam Hydrochloride

Handbook on Injectable Drugs pp. 1133–1144.

Description: A benzodiazepine sedative.

Products: **Versed;** 1 and 5 mg/mL in vials containing 1 to 10 mL and in 2-mL prefilled syringes. *pH:* From 2.9 to 3.7.

Administration: Administer by IM injection deep into a large muscle mass, by slow IV injection over at least two minutes, or by IV infusion diluted in sodium chloride 0.9% or dextrose 5%.

Stability: Store at room temperature and protect from light. Admixtures in compatible solutions do not require light protection for short-term storage and administration. Midazolam hydrochloride is highly water soluble at pH 4 or below; at higher pH values, increased lipid solubility occurs.

Compatibility Table

Solutions	Compatible	Incompatible	Variable
Dextrose 5%	●	…	…
Dextrose 5% in sodium chloride 0.9%	●	…	…
Ringer's injection, lactated*	…	●	…
Sodium chloride 0.9%	●	…	…

*Stable for only four hours.

Drugs	Compatible	Incompatible	Variable
Abciximab	●	…	…
Albumin	…	●	…
Alfentanil HCl	●	…	…
Amikacin sulfate	●	…	…
Aminophylline	…	…	●
Amiodarone HCl	●	…	…
Amphotericin B cholesteryl sulfate complex	…	●	…
Ampicillin sodium	…	●	…
Argatroban	●	…	…

Drugs	Compatible	Incompatible	Variable
Atracurium besylate	●	. . .	. . .
Atropine sulfate	●	. . .	. . .
Bivalirudin	●	. . .	. . .
Bumetanide	. . .	●	. . .
Buprenorphine HCl	●	. . .	. . .
Butorphanol tartrate	. . .	. . .	●
Calcium gluconate	●	. . .	. . .
Cefazolin sodium	●	. . .	. . .
Cefepime HCl	. . .	●	. . .
Cefotaxime sodium	●	. . .	. . .
Ceftazidime	. . .	●	. . .
Cefuroxime sodium	. . .	. . .	●
Chlorpromazine HCl	●	. . .	. . .
Cimetidine HCl	●	. . .	. . .
Ciprofloxacin	●	. . .	. . .
Cisatracurium besylate	●	. . .	. . .
Clindamycin phosphate	●	. . .	. . .
Clonidine HCl	. . .	●	. . .
Dexamethasone sodium phosphate . . .	. . .	. . .	●
Digoxin	●	. . .	. . .
Diltiazem HCl	●	. . .	. . .
Dimenhydrinate	. . .	●	. . .
Diphenhydramine HCl	●	. . .	. . .
Dobutamine HCl	. . .	. . .	●
Dopamine HCl	●	. . .	. . .
Droperidol	●	. . .	. . .
Drotrecogin alfa (activated)	. . .	●	. . .
Epinephrine HCl	●	. . .	. . .
Erythromycin lactobionate	●	. . .	. . .
Esmolol HCl	●	. . .	. . .
Etomidate	●	. . .	. . .
Famotidine	●	. . .	. . .
Fenoldopam mesylate	●	. . .	. . .
Fentanyl citrate	●	. . .	. . .
Fluconazole	●	. . .	. . .
Foscarnet sodium	. . .	●	. . .
Fosphenytoin sodium	. . .	●	. . .
Furosemide	. . .	. . .	●
Gentamicin sulfate	●	. . .	. . .
Glycopyrrolate	●	. . .	. . .

Drugs	Compatible	Incompatible	Variable
Haloperidol lactate	●	. . .	. . .
Heparin sodium	. . .	. . .	●
Hextend	●	. . .	. . .
Hydrocortisone sodium succinate	. . .	●	. . .
Hydromorphone HCl	●	. . .	. . .
Hydroxyzine HCl	●	. . .	. . .
Imipenem–cilastatin sodium	. . .	●	. . .
Insulin, regular	●	. . .	. . .
Labetalol HCl	●	. . .	. . .
Lansoprazole	. . .	●	. . .
Linezolid	●	. . .	. . .
Lorazepam	●	. . .	. . .
Meperidine HCl	●	. . .	. . .
Methadone HCl	●	. . .	. . .
Methotrexate sodium	. . .	●	. . .
Methylprednisolone sod. succ.	●	. . .	. . .
Metoclopramide HCl	●	. . .	. . .
Metronidazole	●	. . .	. . .
Milrinone lactate	●	. . .	. . .
Morphine sulfate	●	. . .	. . .
Nafcillin sodium	. . .	●	. . .
Nalbuphine HCl	●	. . .	. . .
Nicardipine HCl	●	. . .	. . .
Nitroglycerin	●	. . .	. . .
Norepinephrine bitartrate	●	. . .	. . .
Ondansetron HCl	●	. . .	. . .
Palonosetron HCl	●	. . .	. . .
Pancuronium bromide	●	. . .	. . .
Pantoprazole sodium	. . .	●	. . .
Pentobarbital sodium	. . .	●	. . .
Piperacillin sodium	●	. . .	. . .
Potassium chloride	●	. . .	. . .
Prochlorperazine edisylate	. . .	●	. . .
Promethazine HCl	●	. . .	. . .
Propofol	. . .	. . .	●
Ranitidine HCl	. . .	. . .	●
Remifentanil HCl	●	. . .	. . .
Scopolamine HBr	●	. . .	. . .
Sodium bicarbonate	. . .	●	. . .
Sodium nitroprusside	●	. . .	. . .

Drugs	Compatible	Incompatible	Variable
Sufentanil citrate	●	...	...
Theophylline	●	...	...
Thiethylperazine malate	●	...	...
Thiopental sodium	...	●	...
Tirofiban HCl	●	...	...
Tobramycin sulfate	●	...	...
Trimethobenzamide HCl	●	...	...
Trimethoprim–sulfamethoxazole	...	●	...
Vancomycin HCl	●	...	...
Vecuronium bromide	●	...	...

Midazolam Hydrochloride

Milrinone Lactate

Handbook on Injectable Drugs pp. 1144–1149.

Description: A cardiac inotropic agent.

Products: Primacor; 1 mg/mL in vials and syringe cartridges and 200 mcg/mL ready-to-use solution in flexible plastic containers. *pH:* From 3.2 to 4.

Administration: Administer IV. For continuous IV infusion, the drug is usually diluted to 200 mcg/mL and administered using a calibrated electronic infusion device.

Stability: Store intact vials at controlled room temperature protected from freezing. At a concentration of 200 mcg/mL in sodium chloride 0.45 or 0.9% and dextrose 5%, milrinone lactate is stable for 72 hours at room temperature in normal light. Milrinone lactate has not shown sorption to glass or plastic containers.

Compatibility Table

Solutions	Compatible	Incompatible	Variable
Dextrose 5%	●	...	...
Ringer's injection, lactated	●	...	...
Sodium chloride 0.45 & 0.9%	●	...	...

Drugs	Compatible	Incompatible	Variable
Acyclovir sodium	●	...	...
Amikacin sulfate	●	...	...
Amiodarone HCl	●	...	...
Ampicillin sodium	●	...	...
Argatroban	●	...	...
Atracurium besylate	●	...	...
Atropine sulfate	●	...	...
Bivalirudin	●	...	...
Bumetanide	...	...	●
Calcium chloride	●	...	...
Calcium gluconate	●	...	...
Cefazolin sodium	●	...	...
Cefepime HCl	●	...	...
Cefotaxime sodium	●	...	...
Ceftazidime	●	...	...

Drugs	Compatible	Incompatible	Variable
Cefuroxime sodium	●	...	...
Cimetidine HCl	●	...	...
Ciprofloxacin	●	...	...
Clindamycin phosphate	●	...	...
Dexamethasone sodium phosphate ...	●	...	...
Dexmedetomidine HCl	●	...	...
Digoxin	●	...	...
Diltiazem HCl	●	...	...
Dobutamine HCl	●	...	...
Dopamine HCl	●	...	...
Epinephrine HCl	●	...	...
Fenoldopam mesylate	●	...	...
Fentanyl citrate	●	...	...
Furosemide	...	●	...
Gentamicin sulfate	●	...	...
Heparin sodium	●	...	...
Hextend	●	...	...
Hydromorphone HCl	●	...	...
Imipenem–cilastatin sodium	...	●	...
Insulin, regular human	●	...	...
Isoproterenol HCl	●	...	...
Labetalol HCl	●	...	...
Lansoprazole	...	●	...
Lidocaine HCl	●	...	...
Lorazepam	●	...	...
Magnesium sulfate	●	...	...
Meropenem	●	...	...
Methylprednisolone sodium succinate	●	...	...
Metronidazole	●	...	...
Midazolam HCl	●	...	...
Morphine sulfate	●	...	...
Nicardipine HCl	●	...	...
Nitroglycerin	●	...	...
Norepinephrine bitartrate	●	...	...
Oxacillin sodium	●	...	...
Pancuronium bromide	●	...	...
Piperacillin sodium	●	...	...
Piperacillin sodium–tazobactam sodium	●	...	...

Drugs	Compatible	Incompatible	Variable
Potassium chloride	●	...	...
Procainamide HCl	...	●	...
Propofol	●	...	...
Propranolol HCl	●	...	...
Quinidine gluconate	●	...	...
Ranitidine HCl	●	...	...
Rocuronium bromide	●	...	...
Sodium bicarbonate	●	...	...
Sodium nitroprusside	●	...	...
Theophylline	●	...	...
Thiopental sodium	●	...	...
Ticarcillin disodium–clavulanate potassium	●	...	...
Tobramycin sulfate	●	...	...
Torsemide	●	...	...
Vancomycin HCl	●	...	...
Vasopressin	●	...	...
Vecuronium bromide	●	...	...
Verapamil HCl	●	...	...

Morphine Sulfate

Handbook on Injectable Drugs pp. 1159–1181.

Description: A narcotic analgesic.

Products: Available in concentrations of 0.5 to 50 mg/mL. *pH:* From 2.5 to 6.

Administration: Administer by SC, IM, or slow IV injection or by slow continuous SC or IV infusion. Preservative-free dosage forms may be administered epidurally or intrathecally.

Stability: The clear, colorless injection in intact containers should be stored at controlled room temperature and protected from freezing and light. Degradation is often accompanied by a yellow or brown discoloration. No sorption to plastic IV bags, sets, or syringes has been noted.

Compatibility Table

Solutions	Compatible	Incompatible	Variable
Dextrose 5%	●	…	…
Dextrose 5% in Ringer's injection	●	…	…
Dextrose 5% in Ringer's injection, lactated	●	…	…
Dextrose 5% in sodium chloride 0.2, 0.45, & 0.9%	●	…	…
Ringer's injection	●	…	…
Ringer's injection, lactated	●	…	…
Sodium chloride 0.45 & 0.9%	●	…	…

Drugs	Compatible	Incompatible	Variable
Acyclovir sodium	…	…	●
Aldesleukin	●	…	…
Alfentanil HCl	●	…	…
Allopurinol sodium	●	…	…
Alteplase	●	…	…
Amifostine	●	…	…
Amikacin sulfate	●	…	…
Aminophylline	…	…	●
Amiodarone HCl	●	…	…
Amobarbital sodium	…	●	…

Drugs	Compatible	Incompatible	Variable
Amphotericin B cholesteryl sulfate complex	...	●	...
Ampicillin sodium	●	...	...
Ampicillin sod.–sulbactam sod.	●	...	...
Argatroban	●	...	...
Atenolol	●	...	...
Atracurium besylate	●	...	...
Atropine sulfate	●	...	...
Azithromycin	...	●	...
Aztreonam	●	...	...
Baclofen	●	...	...
Bivalirudin	●	...	...
Bumetanide	●	...	...
Bupivacaine HCl	●	...	...
Butorphanol tartrate	●	...	...
Caffeine citrate	●	...	...
Calcium chloride	●	...	...
Cefamandole nafate	●	...	...
Cefazolin sodium	●	...	...
Cefepime HCl	...	...	●
Cefotaxime sodium	●	...	...
Cefotetan disodium	●	...	...
Cefoxitin sodium	●	...	...
Ceftazidime	●	...	...
Ceftizoxime sodium	●	...	...
Ceftriaxone sodium	●	...	...
Cefuroxime sodium	●	...	...
Chloramphenicol sodium succinate	●	...	...
Chlorothiazide sodium	...	●	...
Chlorpromazine HCl	...	...	●
Cimetidine HCl	●	...	...
Cisatracurium besylate	●	...	...
Cisplatin	●	...	...
Cladribine	●	...	...
Clindamycin phosphate	●	...	...
Clonidine HCl	●	...	...
Cyclophosphamide	●	...	...
Cytarabine	●	...	...
Dexamethasone sodium phosphate ...	●	...	...

Drugs	Compatible	Incompatible	Variable
Digoxin	●	…	…
Diltiazem HCl	●	…	…
Dimenhydrinate	●	…	…
Diphenhydramine HCl	●	…	…
Dobutamine HCl	●	…	…
Docetaxel	●	…	…
Dopamine HCl	●	…	…
Doxorubicin HCl	●	…	…
Doxorubicin HCl liposome injection	…	●	…
Doxycycline hyclate	●	…	…
Droperidol	●	…	…
Enalaprilat	●	…	…
Epinephrine HCl	●	…	…
Erythromycin lactobionate	●	…	…
Esmolol HCl	●	…	…
Etomidate	●	…	…
Etoposide phosphate	●	…	…
Famotidine	●	…	…
Fenoldopam mesylate	●	…	…
Fentanyl citrate	●	…	…
Filgrastim	●	…	…
Fluconazole	●	…	…
Fludarabine phosphate	●	…	…
Fluorouracil	…	●	…
Foscarnet sodium	●	…	…
Furosemide	…	…	●
Gallium nitrate	…	●	…
Gemcitabine HCl	●	…	…
Gentamicin sulfate	●	…	…
Glycopyrrolate	●	…	…
Granisetron HCl	●	…	…
Haloperidol lactate	…	…	●
Heparin sodium	…	…	●
Hextend	●	…	…
Hydrocortisone sodium succinate	●	…	…
Hydromorphone HCl	●	…	…
Hydroxyzine HCl	●	…	…
Insulin, regular	●	…	…
Kanamycin sulfate	●	…	…

Drugs	Compatible	Incompatible	Variable
Ketamine HCl	●	...	...
Ketorolac tromethamine	●	...	...
Labetalol HCl	●	...	...
Lansoprazole	...	●	...
Levofloxacin	●	...	...
Lidocaine HCl	●	...	...
Linezolid	●	...	...
Lorazepam	●	...	...
Magnesium sulfate	●	...	...
Melphalan HCl	●	...	...
Meperidine HCl	...	●	...
Meropenem	●	...	...
Methotrexate sodium	●	...	...
Methyldopate HCl	●	...	...
Methylprednisolone sod. succ.	●	...	...
Metoclopramide HCl	●	...	...
Metoprolol tartrate	●	...	...
Metronidazole	●	...	...
Midazolam HCl	...	...	●
Milrinone lactate	●	...	...
Nafcillin sodium	●	...	...
Nicardipine HCl	●	...	...
Nitroglycerin	●	...	...
Norepinephrine bitartrate	●	...	...
Ondansetron HCl	●	...	...
Oxacillin sodium	●	...	...
Oxaliplatin	●	...	...
Oxytocin	●	...	...
Paclitaxel	●	...	...
Pancuronium bromide	●	...	...
Pantoprazole sodium	...	...	●
Pemetrexed disodium	●	...	...
Penicillin G potassium	●	...	...
Pentazocine lactate	●	...	...
Pentobarbital sodium	...	...	●
Phenobarbital sodium	...	●	...
Phenytoin sodium	...	●	...
Piperacillin sodium	●	...	...
Piperacillin sod.–tazobactam sod.	●	...	...
Potassium chloride	●	...	...

Drugs	Compatible	Incompatible	Variable
Prochlorperazine edisylate	...	...	•
Promethazine HCl	...	...	•
Propofol	...	...	•
Propranolol HCl	•	...	...
Ranitidine HCl	•	...	...
Remifentanil HCl	•	...	...
Ropivacaine HCl	•	...	...
Sargramostim	...	•	...
Scopolamine HBr	•	...	...
Sodium bicarbonate	...	...	•
Sodium nitroprusside	•	...	...
Succinylcholine chloride	•	...	...
Tacrolimus	•	...	...
Teniposide	•	...	...
Thiopental sodium	...	...	•
Thiotepa	•	...	...
Ticarcillin disod.–clavulanate pot.	•	...	...
Tirofiban HCl	•	...	...
Tobramycin sulfate	•	...	...
Trimethoprim–sulfamethoxazole	•	...	...
Vancomycin HCl	•	...	...
Vecuronium bromide	•	...	...
Verapamil HCl	•	...	...
Vinorelbine tartrate	•	...	...
Warfarin sodium	•	...	...
Zidovudine	•	...	...

Nafcillin Sodium

Handbook on Injectable Drugs pp. 1188–1195.

Description: A semisynthetic, penicillinase-resistant penicillin.

Products: **Nallpen**; 1- and 2-g vials and frozen premixed solutions. *pH:* From 6 to 8.5 when reconstituted.

Preparation: To prepare a 250-mg/mL solution, reconstitute the 1- and 2-g sizes with 3.4 and 6.6 mL, respectively, of sterile or bacteriostatic water for injection or sodium chloride 0.9%. For direct IV injection, further dilute with 15 to 30 mL of sterile water for injection or sodium chloride 0.9%. For IV infusion, further dilute to a concentration of 2 to 40 mg/mL in a compatible IV solution.

Administration: Administer by deep IM or direct IV injection or by continuous or intermittent IV infusion at a concentration between 2 and 40 mg/mL.

Stability: Store intact vials at room temperature or lower. Nafcillin sodium 250 mg/mL is stable for three days at room temperature or seven days under refrigeration. At 10 to 40 mg/mL, the drug is stable for 24 hours at room temperature or 96 hours under refrigeration.

Compatibility Table

Solutions	Compatible	Incompatible	Variable
Dextrose 5%	●	...	...
Dextrose 5% in Ringer's injection	●	...	...
Dextrose 5% in Ringer's injection, lactated	●	...	...
Dextrose 5% in sodium chloride 0.2, 0.45, & 0.9%	●	...	...
Ringer's injection	●	...	...
Ringer's injection, lactated	●	...	...
Sodium chloride 0.9%	●	...	...

Drugs	Compatible	Incompatible	Variable
Acyclovir sodium	●	...	...
Aminophylline	...	...	●
Ascorbic acid injection	...	●	...
Atropine sulfate	●	...	...
Aztreonam	...	●	...

Drugs	Compatible	Incompatible	Variable
Bleomycin sulfate	...	●	...
Chloramphenicol sod. succ.	●	...	...
Chlorothiazide HCl	●	...	...
Cimetidine HCl	●	...	...
Cyclophosphamide	●	...	...
Cytarabine	...	●	...
Dexamethasone sodium phosphate ...	●	...	...
Diazepam	●	...	...
Diltiazem HCl	...	...	●
Diphenhydramine HCl	●	...	...
Droperidol	...	●	...
Enalaprilat	●	...	...
Ephedrine sulfate	●	...	...
Esmolol HCl	●	...	...
Famotidine	●	...	...
Fentanyl citrate	●	...	...
Fluconazole	●	...	...
Foscarnet sodium	●	...	...
Gentamicin sulfate	...	●	...
Heparin sodium	●	...	...
Hydrocortisone sodium succinate	...	●	...
Hydromorphone HCl	●	...	...
Hydroxyzine HCl	●	...	...
Insulin, regular	...	●	...
Labetalol HCl	...	●	...
Lidocaine HCl	●	...	...
Magnesium sulfate	●	...	...
Meperidine HCl	...	...	●
Methylprednisolone sod. succ.	...	●	...
Midazolam HCl	...	●	...
Morphine sulfate	●	...	...
Nalbuphine HCl	...	●	...
Nicardipine HCl	●	...	...
Pentazocine lactate	...	●	...
Potassium chloride	●	...	...
Prochlorperazine edisylate	●	...	...
Propofol	●	...	...
Sodium bicarbonate	●	...	...
Sodium lactate	●	...	...
Succinylcholine chloride	...	●	...
Theophylline	●	...	...
Vancomycin HCl	...	...	●
Verapamil HCl	...	...	●
Zidovudine	●	...	...

Nalbuphine Hydrochloride

Handbook on Injectable Drugs pp. 1195–1200.

Description: A synthetic opiate analgesic.

Products: **Nubain;** 10 mg/mL in 1-mL ampuls and 10-mL vials and 20 mg/mL in 1-mL ampuls and 10-mL vials. *pH:* From 3 to 4.5. The product in ampuls is provided without parabens, while the product in vials contains them.

Administration: Administer by IM, SC, or IV injection.

Stability: Store intact containers at room temperature, protected from excessive light.

Compatibility Table

Solutions	Compatible	Incompatible	Variable
Dextrose 5% in sodium chloride 0.9%	●	...	...
Dextrose 10%	●	...	...
Ringer's injection, lactated	●	...	...
Sodium chloride 0.9%	●	...	...

Drugs	Compatible	Incompatible	Variable
Allopurinol sodium	...	●	...
Amifostine	●	...	...
Amphotericin B cholesteryl sulfate complex	...	●	...
Atropine sulfate	●	...	...
Aztreonam	●	...	...
Bivalirudin	●	...	...
Cefepime HCl	...	●	...
Cimetidine HCl	●	...	...
Cisatracurium besylate	●	...	...
Cladribine	●	...	...
Dexmedetomidine HCl	●	...	...
Diazepam	...	●	...
Dimenhydrinate	...	●	...
Diphenhydramine HCl	●	...	...

Drugs	Compatible	Incompatible	Variable
Docetaxel	...	●	...
Droperidol	●	...	...
Etoposide phosphate	●	...	...
Fenoldopam mesylate	●	...	...
Filgrastim	●	...	...
Fludarabine phosphate	●	...	...
Gemcitabine HCl	●	...	...
Glycopyrrolate	●	...	...
Granisetron HCl	●	...	...
Hextend	●	...	...
Hydroxyzine HCl	●	...	...
Ketorolac tromethamine	...	●	...
Lansoprazole	●	...	...
Lidocaine HCl	●	...	...
Linezolid	●	...	...
Melphalan HCl	●	...	...
Methotrexate sodium	...	●	...
Midazolam HCl	●	...	...
Nafcillin sodium	...	●	...
Oxaliplatin	●	...	...
Paclitaxel	●	...	...
Pemetrexed disodium	...	●	...
Pentobarbital sodium	...	●	...
Piperacillin sod.–tazobactam sod.	...	●	...
Prochlorperazine edisylate	●	...	...
Promethazine HCl	...	...	●
Propofol	●	...	...
Ranitidine HCl	●	...	...
Remifentanil HCl	●	...	...
Sargramostim	...	●	...
Scopolamine HBr	●	...	...
Sodium bicarbonate	...	●	...
Teniposide	●	...	...
Thiethylperazine malate	...	...	●
Thiotepa	●	...	...
Trimethobenzamide HCl	●	...	...
Vinorelbine tartrate	●	...	...

Nicardipine Hydrochloride

Handbook on Injectable Drugs pp. 1211–1216.

Description: A calcium-channel-blocking antihypertensive agent.

Products: **Cardene;** I.V.; 2.5-mg/mL concentrate in 10-mL ampuls. *pH:* Buffered to pH 3.5.

Preparation: The concentrate must be diluted for use with a compatible infusion solution to a concentration of 0.1 mg/mL. To prepare a 0.1-mg/mL dilution of the drug for administration, the manufacturer recommends adding 10 mL of the injection to 240 mL of compatible infusion solution with mixing.

Administration: Administer by slow continuous intravenous infusion at a concentration of 0.1 mg/mL. For peripheral infusion, the site should be changed every 12 hours.

Stability: The clear, yellow injection should be stored at room temperature and protected from light. Exposure to daylight resulted in 21% loss in 14 hours. Freezing does not adversely affect the drug. Excessive heat should be avoided.

Nicardipine hydrochloride undergoes sorptive loss to PVC bags and tubing; losses ranging from about 12 to 42% have occurred. The use of non-PVC containers and sets should be considered.

Compatibility Table

Solutions	Compatible	Incompatible	Variable
Dextrose 5%*	●	...	...
Dextrose 5% in sodium chloride 0.45 & 0.9%*	●	...	...
Ringer's injection, lactated*	●	...	...
Sodium chloride 0.9%*	●	...	...

*In non-PVC containers.

Drugs	Compatible	Incompatible	Variable
Amikacin sulfate	●	...	...
Aminophylline	●	...	...
Ampicillin sodium	...	●	...
Ampicillin sodium–sulbactam sodium	...	●	...

Drugs	Compatible	Incompatible	Variable
Aztreonam	●	...	...
Butorphanol tartrate	●	...	...
Calcium gluconate	●	...	...
Cefazolin sodium	●	...	...
Cefepime HCl	...	●	...
Ceftazidime	...	...	●
Ceftizoxime sodium	●	...	...
Chloramphenicol sodium succinate	●	...	...
Cimetidine HCl	●	...	...
Clindamycin phosphate	●	...	...
Dextran 40	●	...	...
Diltiazem HCl	●	...	...
Dobutamine HCl	●	...	...
Dopamine HCl	●	...	...
Enalaprilat	●	...	...
Epinephrine HCl	●	...	...
Erythromycin lactobionate	●	...	...
Esmolol HCl	●	...	...
Famotidine	●	...	...
Fenoldopam mesylate	●	...	...
Fentanyl citrate	●	...	...
Furosemide	...	●	...
Gentamicin sulfate	●	...	...
Heparin sodium	...	...	●
Hetastarch in sodium chloride 0.9%	●	...	...
Hydrocortisone sodium succinate	●	...	...
Hydromorphone HCl	●	...	...
Labetalol HCl	●	...	...
Lansoprazole	...	●	...
Lidocaine HCl	●	...	...
Linezolid	●	...	...
Lorazepam	●	...	...
Magnesium sulfate	●	...	...
Methylprednisolone sodium succinate	●	...	...
Metronidazole	●	...	...
Midazolam HCl	●	...	...
Milrinone lactate	●	...	...

Drugs	Compatible	Incompatible	Variable
Morphine sulfate	●	...	...
Nafcillin sodium	●	...	...
Nitroglycerin	●	...	...
Norepinephrine bitartrate	●	...	...
Penicillin G potassium	●	...	...
Piperacillin sodium	●	...	...
Potassium chloride	●	...	...
Potassium phosphates	●	...	...
Ranitidine HCl	●	...	...
Sodium acetate	●	...	...
Sodium nitroprusside	●	...	...
Thiopental sodium	...	●	...
Tobramycin sulfate	●	...	...
Trimethoprim–sulfamethoxazole	●	...	...
Vancomycin HCl	●	...	...
Vecuronium bromide	●	...	...

Nitroglycerin

Handbook on Injectable Drugs pp. 1217–1229.

Description: An organic nitrate vasodilator.

Products: 5-mg/mL concentrate for dilution. Also available pre-mixed in dextrose 5% at concentrations of 100, 200, and 400 mcg/mL. *pH:* From 3 to 6.5.

Preparation: Dilute the concentrate in dextrose 5% or sodium chloride 0.9% in glass bottles before use. Infusion concentrations may range from 50 to 400 mcg/mL.

Administration: Administer by IV infusion, using an infusion control device, after proper dilution. Because of nitroglycerin loss due to sorption to PVC, dosing is higher with PVC sets and lower when nonabsorbing administration sets are used.

Stability: Store at room temperature; protect from freezing. Nitroglycerin diluted in dextrose 5% or sodium chloride 0.9% in glass containers is stable for at least 48 hours at room temperature or at least seven days under refrigeration.

Nitroglycerin readily undergoes extensive sorption to PVC plastic, including IV bags and tubing. The loss to PVC tubing may be 40 to 80%. Use only glass IV solution bottles and the special high-density polyethylene administration sets provided by the manufacturers.

Compatibility Table

Solutions	Compatible	Incompatible	Variable
Dextrose 5%	●	...	...
Dextrose 5% in Ringer's injection, lactated	●	...	...
Dextrose 5% in sodium chloride 0.45 & 0.9%	●	...	...
Ringer's injection, lactated	●	...	...
Sodium chloride 0.45 & 0.9%	●	...	...

Drugs			
Alteplase	...	...	●
Aminophylline	●	...	...
Amiodarone hydrochloride	●	...	...
Amphotericin B cholesteryl sulfate complex	●	...	...

Drugs	Compatible	Incompatible	Variable
Argatroban	●	...	...
Atracurium besylate	●	...	...
Bivalirudin	●	...	...
Caffeine citrate	...	●	...
Cisatracurium besylate	●	...	...
Dexmedetomidine HCl	●	...	...
Diltiazem HCl	●	...	...
Dobutamine HCl	●	...	...
Dopamine HCl	●	...	...
Drotrecogin alfa (activated)	●	...	...
Enalaprilat	●	...	...
Epinephrine HCl	●	...	...
Esmolol hydrochloride	●	...	...
Famotidine	●	...	...
Fenoldopam mesylate	●	...	...
Fentanyl citrate	●	...	...
Fluconazole	●	...	...
Furosemide	●	...	...
Haloperidol lactate	●	...	...
Heparin sodium	●	...	...
Hextend	●	...	...
Hydralazine HCl	...	...	●
Hydromorphone HCl	●	...	...
Insulin, regular	●	...	...
Labetalol HCl	●	...	...
Lansoprazole	...	●	...
Levofloxacin	...	●	...
Lidocaine HCl	●	...	...
Linezolid	●	...	...
Lorazepam	●	...	...
Midazolam HCl	●	...	...
Milrinone lactate	●	...	...
Morphine sulfate	●	...	...
Nicardipine HCl	●	...	...
Norepinephrine bitartrate	●	...	...
Pancuronium bromide	●	...	...
Pantoprazole sodium	...	...	●
Phenytoin sodium	...	●	...
Propofol	●	...	...
Ranitidine HCl	●	...	...

Drugs	Compatible	Incompatible	Variable
Remifentanil HCl	●	...	...
Sodium nitroprusside	●	...	...
Streptokinase	●	...	...
Tacrolimus	●	...	...
Theophylline	●	...	...
Thiopental sodium	●	...	...
Tirofiban HCl	●	...	...
Vasopressin	●	...	...
Vecuronium bromide	●	...	...
Verapamil HCl	●	...	...
Warfarin sodium	●	...	...

Norepinephrine Bitartrate

Handbook on Injectable Drugs pp. 1231–1237.

Description: An endogenous catecholamine whose main effects are vasoconstriction and cardiac stimulation.

Products: Levophed; 1 mg/mL in 4-mL ampuls. *pH:* From 3 to 4.5.

Preparation: To prepare an infusion, 4 mg (4 mL) is added to 1000 mL of dextrose 5% with or without sodium chloride to yield a 4-mcg/mL solution.

Administration: Administer by IV infusion into a large vein, using a pump or other apparatus to control the flow rate. Avoid extravasation.

Stability: Store intact containers at controlled room temperature protected from light. The solution gradually darkens with exposure to light or air. Do not use if it is discolored or contains a precipitate. In solutions with a pH greater than 6, significant decomposition occurs.

Compatibility Table

Solutions	Compatible	Incompatible	Variable
Dextrose 5%	●	...	...
Dextrose 5% in sodium chloride 0.9%	●	...	...
Ringer's injection, lactated	●	...	...
Sodium chloride 0.9%	●	...	...

Drugs	Compatible	Incompatible	Variable
Amikacin sulfate	●	...	...
Aminophylline	...	●	...
Amiodarone hydrochloride	●	...	...
Amobarbital sodium	...	●	...
Argatroban	●	...	...
Bivalirudin	●	...	...
Calcium chloride	●	...	...
Calcium gluconate	●	...	...
Chlorothiazide sodium	...	●	...
Cimetidine HCl	●	...	...

Drugs	Compatible	Incompatible	Variable
Ciprofloxacin	●	...	...
Cisatracurium besylate	●	...	...
Corticotropin	●	...	...
Dexmedetomidine HCl	●	...	...
Diltiazem HCl	●	...	...
Dimenhydrinate	●	...	...
Dobutamine HCl	●	...	...
Dopamine HCl	●	...	...
Drotrecogin alfa (activated)	...	●	...
Epinephrine HCl	●	...	...
Esmolol HCl	●	...	...
Famotidine	●	...	...
Fenoldopam mesylate	●	...	...
Fentanyl citrate	●	...	...
Furosemide	●	...	...
Haloperidol lactate	●	...	...
Heparin sodium	●	...	...
Hextend	●	...	...
Hydrocortisone sodium succinate	●	...	...
Hydromorphone HCl	●	...	...
Insulin, regular	...	●	...
Labetalol HCl	●	...	...
Lidocaine HCl	...	●	...
Lorazepam	●	...	...
Magnesium sulfate	●	...	...
Meropenem	●	...	...
Methylprednisolone sod. succ.	●	...	...
Midazolam HCl	●	...	...
Milrinone lactate	●	...	...
Morphine sulfate	●	...	...
Multivitamins	●	...	...
Nafcillin sodium	...	...	●
Nicardipine HCl	●	...	...
Nitroglycerin	●	...	...
Pantoprazole sodium	...	...	●
Pentobarbital sodium	...	●	...
Phenobarbital sodium	...	●	...
Phenytoin sodium	...	●	...
Potassium chloride	●	...	...
Propofol	●	...	...

Drugs	Compatible	Incompatible	Variable
Ranitidine HCl	...	...	●
Remifentanil HCl	●	...	...
Sodium bicarbonate	...	●	...
Sodium nitroprusside	●	...	...
Streptomycin sulfate	...	●	...
Succinylcholine chloride	●	...	...
Thiopental sodium	...	●	...
Vasopressin	●	...	...
Vecuronium bromide	●	...	...
Verapamil HCl	●	...	...

Ondansetron Hydrochloride

Handbook on Injectable Drugs pp. 1244–1255.

Description: A serotonin antagonist antiemetic.

Products: **Zofran;** 2 mg/mL in 20-mL multiple-dose vials and 2-mL single-dose vials and 0.64 mg/mL premixed infusion in dextrose 5%. *pH:* Injection from 3.3 to 4. Premixed infusion from 3 to 4.

Preparation: For IV infusion of the 2-mg/mL concentration, dilute the dose with 50 mL of sodium chloride 0.9% or dextrose 5%.

Administration: Administer by IV infusion over 15 minutes. By IV injection, it is administered undiluted over two to five minutes.

Stability: Store at room temperature or under refrigeration and protect from light. The drug is stable for about a month when exposed to mixed daylight and fluorescent light. In solutions with a pH greater than 5.7, precipitation of ondansetron occurs. Alkaline drugs have caused precipitation.

Compatibility Table

Solutions	Compatible	Incompatible	Variable
Dextrose 5%	●	...	...
Dextrose 5% in sodium chloride 0.45 & 0.9%	●	...	...
Mannitol 10%	●	...	...
Ringer's injection	●	...	...
Ringer's injection, lactated	●	...	...
Sodium chloride 0.9%	●	...	...

Drugs	Compatible	Incompatible	Variable
Acyclovir sodium	...	●	...
Aldesleukin	●	...	...
Alfentanil HCl	●	...	...
Allopurinol sodium	...	●	...
Amifostine	●	...	...

Drugs	Compatible	Incompatible	Variable
Amikacin sulfate	●	...	...
Aminophylline	...	●	...
Amphotericin B	...	●	...
Amphotericin B cholesteryl sulfate complex	...	●	...
Ampicillin sodium	...	●	...
Ampicillin sod.–sulbactam sod.	...	●	...
Atropine sulfate	●	...	...
Azithromycin	●	...	...
Aztreonam	●	...	...
Bleomycin sulfate	●	...	...
Carboplatin	●	...	...
Carmustine	●	...	...
Cefazolin sodium	●	...	...
Cefepime HCl	...	●	...
Cefotaxime sodium	●	...	...
Cefoxitin sodium	●	...	...
Ceftazidime	●	...	...
Ceftizoxime sodium	●	...	...
Cefuroxime sodium	●	...	...
Chlorpromazine HCl	●	...	...
Cimetidine HCl	●	...	...
Cisatracurium besylate	●	...	...
Cisplatin	●	...	...
Cladribine	●	...	...
Clindamycin phosphate	●	...	...
Cyclophosphamide	●	...	...
Cytarabine	●	...	...
Dacarbazine	●	...	...
Dactinomycin	●	...	...
Daunorubicin HCl	●	...	...
Dexamethasone sodium succinate	...	...	●
Dexmedetomidine HCl	●	...	...
Diphenhydramine HCl	●	...	...
Docetaxel	●	...	...
Dopamine HCl	●	...	...
Doxorubicin HCl	●	...	...
Doxorubicin HCl liposome injection	●	...	...
Doxycycline hyclate	●	...	...

Drugs	Compatible	Incompatible	Variable
Droperidol	...	...	•
Etoposide	•	...	...
Etoposide phosphate	•	...	...
Famotidine	•	...	...
Fenoldopam mesylate	•	...	...
Fentanyl citrate	•	...	...
Filgrastim	•	...	...
Floxuridine	•	...	...
Fluconazole	•	...	...
Fludarabine phosphate	•	...	...
Fluorouracil	...	•	...
Furosemide	...	•	...
Gallium nitrate	•	...	...
Ganciclovir sodium	...	•	...
Gemcitabine HCl	•	...	...
Gentamicin sulfate	•	...	...
Glycopyrrolate	•	...	...
Haloperidol lactate	•	...	...
Heparin sodium	•	...	...
Hextend	•	...	...
Hydrocortisone sodium phosphate	•	...	...
Hydrocortisone sodium succinate	•	...	...
Hydromorphone HCl	•	...	...
Hydroxyzine HCl	•	...	...
Ifosfamide	•	...	...
Imipenem–cilastatin sodium	•	...	...
Lansoprazole	...	•	...
Linezolid	•	...	...
Lorazepam	...	•	...
Magnesium sulfate	•	...	...
Mannitol	•	...	...
Mechlorethamine HCl	•	...	...
Melphalan HCl	•	...	...
Meperidine HCl	•	...	...
Meropenem	...	...	•
Mesna	•	...	...
Methotrexate sodium	•	...	...
Methylprednisolone sod. succ.	...	•	...
Metoclopramide HCl	•	...	...
Midazolam HCl	•	...	...

Drugs	Compatible	Incompatible	Variable
Mitomycin	●	...	...
Mitoxantrone HCl	●	...	...
Morphine sulfate	●	...	...
Naloxone HCl	●	...	...
Neostigmine methylsulfate	●	...	...
Oxaliplatin	●	...	...
Paclitaxel	●	...	...
Pemetrexed disodium	...	●	...
Pentostatin	●	...	...
Piperacillin sodium	...	●	...
Piperacillin sod.–tazobactam sod.	●	...	...
Potassium chloride	●	...	...
Prochlorperazine edisylate	●	...	...
Promethazine HCl	●	...	...
Propofol	●	...	...
Ranitidine HCl	●	...	...
Remifentanil HCl	●	...	...
Sargramostim	...	●	...
Sodium acetate	●	...	...
Sodium bicarbonate	...	●	...
Streptozocin	●	...	...
Teniposide	●	...	...
Thiotepa	●	...	...
Ticarcillin disod.–clavulanate pot.	●	...	...
Topotecan HCl	●	...	...
Vancomycin HCl	●	...	...
Vinblastine sulfate	●	...	...
Vincristine sulfate	●	...	...
Vinorelbine tartrate	●	...	...
Zidovudine	●	...	...

Oxaliplatin

Handbook on Injectable Drugs pp. 1261–1264.

Description: A platinum-containing antineoplastic drug.

Products: **Eloxatin;** 50- and 100-mg vials and 5-mg/mL concentrated solution.

Preparation: Reconstitute the vials with dextrose 5% to yield a concentration of 5 mg/mL. Chloride-containing solutions must not be used for reconstitution or dilution.

Administration: The reconstituted solution or liquid concentrated injection must be diluted in 250 to 500 mL of dextrose 5% for IV infusion. Chloride-containing solutions must not be used for dilution. Flush administration lines with dextrose 5%.

Stability: Store at controlled room temperature and protect from freezing and light. Reconstituted oxaliplatin has been reported to be stable for 48 hours refrigerated. The manufacturer indicates that oxaliplatin is stable diluted in dextrose 5% for six hours at room temperature and for 24 hours under refrigeration. Another report indicates the drug in dextrose 5% is stable for 24 hours at room temperature.

   Oxaliplatin is incompatible with alkaline drugs and solutions. Contact of oxaliplatin solutions with aluminum in needles or metal parts of administration equipment should be avoided. Aluminum has caused degradation of some platinum compounds.

Compatibility Table

Solutions	Compatible	Incompatible	Variable
Dextrose 5%	●	...	...
Ringer's injection, lactated	...	●	...
Sodium chloride 0.9%	...	●	...

Drugs	Compatible	Incompatible	Variable
Bumetanide	●	...	...
Buprenorphine HCl	●	...	...
Butorphanol tartrate	●	...	...
Calcium gluconate	●	...	...
Carboplatin	●	...	...

Drugs	Compatible	Incompatible	Variable
Chlorpromazine HCl	●	...	...
Cimetidine HCl	●	...	...
Cyclophosphamide	●	...	...
Dexamethasone sodium phosphate ...	●	...	...
Diazepam	...	●	...
Diphenhydramine HCl	●	...	...
Dobutamine HCl	●	...	...
Docetaxel	●	...	...
Dolasetron mesylate	●	...	...
Dopamine HCl	●	...	...
Doxorubicin HCl	●	...	...
Droperidol	●	...	...
Enalaprilat	●	...	...
Epirubicin HCl	●	...	...
Etoposide phosphate	●	...	...
Famotidine	●	...	...
Fentanyl citrate	●	...	...
Furosemide	●	...	...
Gemcitabine HCl	●	...	...
Granisetron HCl	●	...	...
Haloperidol lactate	●	...	...
Heparin sodium	●	...	...
Hydrocortisone sodium succinate	●	...	...
Hydromorphone HCl	●	...	...
Hydroxyzine HCl	●	...	...
Ifosfamide	●	...	...
Irinotecan HCl	●	...	...
Leucovorin calcium	●	...	...
Lorazepam	●	...	...
Magnesium sulfate	●	...	...
Mannitol	●	...	...
Methotrexate sodium	●	...	...
Meperidine HCl	●	...	...
Mesna	●	...	...
Methylprednisolone sod. succ.	●	...	...
Metoclopramide HCl	●	...	...
Mitoxantrone HCl	●	...	...
Morphine sulfate	●	...	...
Nalbuphine HCl	●	...	...
Ondansetron HCl	●	...	...

Drugs	Compatible	Incompatible	Variable
Paclitaxel	●	...	...
Palonosetron HCl	●	...	...
Potassium chloride	●	...	...
Prochlorperazine edisylate	●	...	...
Promethazine HCl	●	...	...
Ranitidine HCl	●	...	...
Theophylline	●	...	...
Topotecan HCl	●	...	...
Verapamil HCl	●	...	...
Vincristine sulfate	●	...	...
Vinorelbine tartrate	●	...	...

Paclitaxel

Handbook on Injectable Drugs pp. 1271–1279.

Description: A naturally occurring taxane antineoplastic.

Products: Onxol, Taxol; 6-mg/mL solution (as concentrate) in 5-mL (30-mg), 16.7-mL (100-mg), and 50-mL (300-mg) vials.

Preparation: Dilute the concentrate in a compatible infusion solution to 0.3 to 1.2 mg/mL. Use only non-PVC containers and administration sets (to avoid leaching of plasticizer) and an inline 0.22-μm filter.

Administration: Administer by IV infusion usually over three hours, although longer administration periods have also been investigated.

Stability: The clear, colorless to slight yellow, viscous concentrate should be stored between 20 and 25 °C and protected from light. Freezing does not adversely affect stability. Refrigeration may result in precipitate formation, but warming to room temperature should redissolve the precipitate. Discard the product if an insoluble precipitate forms. Observe all paclitaxel infusion solutions for potential precipitation over irregular and unpredictable time periods. Diluted infusion solutions may be hazy because of the surfactant in the formulation.

No sorption to any containers or sets has been found. However, the surfactant present in the formulation leaches DEHP plasticizer from PVC bags and administration sets.

Compatibility Table

Solutions	Compatible	Incompatible	Variable
Dextrose 5%	...	...	●
Sodium chloride 0.9%	●	...	...

Drugs			
Acyclovir sodium	●	...	...
Amikacin sulfate	●	...	...
Aminophylline	●	...	...
Amphotericin B......................	...	●	...
Amphotericin B cholesteryl sulfate complex	...	●	...

Drugs	Compatible	Incompatible	Variable
Ampicillin sod.–sulbactam sod.	●	...	...
Bleomycin sulfate	●	...	...
Butorphanol tartrate	●	...	...
Calcium chloride	●	...	...
Carboplatin	●	...	...
Cefepime HCl	●	...	...
Cefotetan disodium	●	...	...
Ceftazidime	●	...	...
Ceftriaxone sodium	●	...	...
Chlorpromazine HCl	...	●	...
Cimetidine HCl	●	...	...
Cisplatin	...	...	●
Cladribine	●	...	...
Cyclophosphamide	●	...	...
Cytarabine	●	...	...
Dacarbazine	●	...	...
Dexamethasone sodium phosphate ...	●	...	...
Diphenhydramine HCl	●	...	...
Doxorubicin HCl	●	...	...
Doxorubicin HCl liposome injection	...	●	...
Droperidol	●	...	...
Etoposide	●	...	...
Etoposide phosphate	●	...	...
Famotidine	●	...	...
Floxuridine	●	...	...
Fluconazole	●	...	...
Fluorouracil	●	...	...
Furosemide	●	...	...
Ganciclovir sodium	●	...	...
Gemcitabine HCl	●	...	...
Gentamicin sulfate	●	...	...
Granisetron HCl	●	...	...
Haloperidol lactate	●	...	...
Heparin sodium	●	...	...
Hydrocortisone sodium phosphate ...	●	...	...
Hydrocortisone sodium succinate	●	...	...
Hydromorphone HCl	●	...	...
Hydroxyzine HCl	...	●	...
Ifosfamide	●	...	...
Lansoprazole	●	...	...

Drugs	Compatible	Incompatible	Variable
Linezolid	●	...	...
Lorazepam	●	...	...
Magnesium sulfate	●	...	...
Mannitol	●	...	...
Meperidine HCl	●	...	...
Mesna	●	...	...
Methotrexate sodium	●	...	...
Methylprednisolone sod. succ.	...	●	...
Metoclopramide HCl	●	...	...
Mitoxantrone HCl	...	●	...
Morphine sulfate	●	...	...
Nalbuphine HCl	●	...	...
Ondansetron HCl	●	...	...
Oxaliplatin	●	...	...
Palonosetron HCl	●	...	...
Pemetrexed disodium	●	...	...
Pentostatin	●	...	...
Potassium chloride	●	...	...
Prochlorperazine edisylate	●	...	...
Propofol	●	...	...
Ranitidine HCl	●	...	...
Sodium bicarbonate	●	...	...
Thiotepa	●	...	...
Topotecan HCl	●	...	...
Vancomycin HCl	●	...	...
Vinblastine sulfate	●	...	...
Vincristine sulfate	●	...	...
Zidovudine	●	...	...

Palonosetron Hydrochloride

Handbook on Injectable Drugs pp. 1279–1281.

Description: A serotonin antagonist antiemetic.

Products: **Aloxi;** 0.05 mg/mL in 5-mL (0.25 mg) vials. *pH:* From 4.5 to 5.5.

Administration: Palonosetron hydrochloride is administered IV over 30 seconds. The manufacturer recommends that the infusion line be flushed with sodium chloride 0.9% before and after palonosetron hydrochloride is administered.

Stability: Store vials at controlled room temperature and protect from light and freezing.

Compatibility Table

Solutions	Compatible	Incompatible	Variable
Dextrose 5%	●	...	
Dextrose 5% in Ringer's Injection, lactated	●	...	...
Dextrose 5% in sodium chloride 0.45%	●	...	...
Sodium chloride 0.9%	●	...	...

Drugs			
Carboplatin	●	...	...
Cisplatin	●	...	...
Dexamethasone sodium phosphate	●	...	...
Docetaxel	●	...	...
Irinotecan HCl	●	...	...
Lorazepam	●	...	...
Midazolam HCl	●	...	...
Oxaliplatin	●	...	...
Paclitaxel	●	...	...
Topotecan HCl	●	...	...

Pancuronium Bromide

Handbook on Injectable Drugs pp. 1281–1283.

Description: A synthetic, nondepolarizing, neuromuscular blocking agent.

Products: 2 mg/mL in 2- and 5-mL ampuls and vials and 1 mg/mL in 10-mL vials. *pH:* The solution has been adjusted to pH 3.8 to 4.2.

Administration: Administer by direct IV injection or intermittent IV infusion.

Stability: Store intact containers under refrigeration. The drug is stable for six months at room temperature.

No sorption to glass or plastic containers has been observed.

Compatibility Table

Solutions	Compatible	Incompatible	Variable
Dextrose 5%	●	...	...
Dextrose 5% in sodium chloride 0.9%	●	...	...
Ringer's injection, lactated	●	...	...
Sodium chloride 0.9%	●	...	...

Drugs	Compatible	Incompatible	Variable
Aminophylline	●	...	...
Caffeine citrate	●	...	...
Cefazolin sodium	●	...	...
Cefuroxime sodium	●	...	...
Cimetidine HCl	●	...	...
Ciprofloxacin	●	...	...
Diazepam	...	●	...
Dobutamine HCl	●	...	...
Dopamine HCl	●	...	...
Epinephrine HCl	●	...	...
Esmolol HCl	●	...	...
Etomidate	●	...	...
Fenoldopam meyslate	●	...	...
Fentanyl citrate	●	...	...
Fluconazole	●	...	...

Drugs	Compatible	Incompatible	Variable
Gentamicin sulfate	●	...	...
Heparin sodium	●	...	...
Hextend	●	...	...
Hydrocortisone sodium succinate	●	...	...
Isoproterenol HCl	●	...	...
Levofloxacin	●	...	...
Lorazepam	●	...	...
Meperidine HCl	●	...	...
Midazolam HCl	●	...	...
Milrinone lactate	●	...	...
Morphine sulfate	●	...	...
Neostigmine methylsulfate	●	...	...
Nitroglycerin	●	...	...
Pantoprazole sodium	...	●	...
Promethazine HCl	●	...	...
Propofol	...	...	●
Ranitidine HCl	●	...	...
Sodium nitroprusside	●	...	...
Succinylcholine chloride	●	...	...
Thiopental sodium	...	●	...
Trimethoprim–sulfamethoxazole	●	...	...
Tubocurarine chloride	●	...	...
Vancomycin HCl	●	...	...
Verapamil HCl	●	...	...

Pantoprazole Sodium

Handbook on Injectable Drugs pp. 1283–1288.

Description: A proton-pump inhibitor used as a gastric antisecretory agent.

Products: **Protonix I.V.**; 40-mg vials. *pH:* From 9 to 10.5.

Preparation: Reconstitute the vials with 10 mL of sodium chloride 0.9% to a concentration of 4 mg/mL. For IV infusion, one vial of the reconstituted drug solution may be diluted further with 100 mL of sodium chloride 0.9%, dextrose 5%, or Ringer's injection, lactated to yield concentrations of about 0.4 mg/mL.

Administration: Pantoprazole sodium 4 mg/mL in sodium chloride 0.9% may be administered by IV injection over a period of at least two minutes. The reconstituted solution may also be diluted in a compatible infusion solution to a concentration about 0.4 mg/mL and administered by IV infusion over about 15 minutes.

Stability: Store vials at room temperature and protect from light. Reconstituted pantoprazole sodium may be stored for up to six hours at room temperature before use. The reconstituted solution should not be frozen. After dilution in a compatible infusion solution, the drug may be stored at room temperature for up to 24 hours prior to use. Protection from light exposure is not required.

Compatibility Table

Solutions	Compatible	Incompatible	Variable
Dextrose 5%	●	…	…
Ringer's injection, lactated	●	…	…
Sodium chloride 0.9%	●	…	…

Drugs	Compatible	Incompatible	Variable
Acetazolamide	●	…	…
Acyclovir sodium	…	●	…
Alprostadil	●	…	…
Amikacin sulfate	…	●	…
Aminophylline	●	…	…

Drugs	Compatible	Incompatible	Variable
Amiodarone HCl	...	●	...
Amphotericin B	...	●	...
Ampicillin sodium	●	...	...
Atropine sulfate	...	●	...
Caffeine citrate	...	●	...
Calcium chloride	...	●	...
Calcium gluconate	...	●	...
Cefazolin sodium	...	...	●
Cefotaxime sodium	...	●	...
Cefoxitin sodium	...	●	...
Ceftazidime	...	●	...
Ceftriaxone sodium	●	...	...
Cefuroxime sodium	...	●	...
Chlorpromazine HCl	...	●	...
Ciprofloxacin	...	●	...
Clindamycin phosphate	...	●	...
Cloxacillin sodium	...	●	...
Cyclosporine	...	●	...
Dexamethasone sodium phosphate	...	●	...
Diazepam	...	●	...
Digoxin	...	●	...
Dimenhydrinate	...	...	●
Diphenhydramine HCl	...	●	...
Dobutamine HCl	...	...	●
Dopamine HCl	...	●	...
Enalaprilat	...	●	...
Epinephrine HCl	...	...	●
Esmolol HCl	...	●	...
Estrogens, conjugated	...	●	...
Fentanyl citrate	...	●	...
Fluconazole	...	●	...
Furosemide	...	...	●
Gentamicin sulfate	...	●	...
Heparin sodium	...	●	...
Hydralazine HCl	...	●	...
Hydrocortisone sodium succinate	...	●	...
Hydromorphone HCl	...	●	...
Indomethacin sodium trihydrate	...	●	...
Insulin, regular	...	...	●
Isoproterenol HCl	...	●	...

Drugs	Compatible	Incompatible	Variable
Labetalol HCl	...	●	...
Lidocaine HCl	...	●	...
Lorazepam	...	●	...
Magnesium sulfate	...	●	...
Mannitol	...	●	...
Meperidine HCl	...	●	...
Meropenem	...	●	...
Methylprednisolone sod. succ.	...	●	...
Metoclopramide HCl	...	●	...
Metronidazole	...	●	...
Midazolam HCl	...	●	...
Morphine sulfate	...	...	●
Multivitamins	...	●	...
Naloxone HCl	...	●	...
Nitroglycerin	...	...	●
Norepinephrine bitartrate	...	...	●
Octreotide	...	...	●
Oxytocin	...	●	...
Pancuronium bromide	...	●	...
Penicillin G sodium	●	...	...
Phenobarbital sodium	...	●	...
Phenytoin sodium	...	●	...
Piperacillin sodium	●	...	...
Piperacillin sod.–tazobactam sod.	...	●	...
Potassium chloride	●	...	...
Potassium phosphates	...	●	...
Procainamide HCl	●	...	...
Prochlorperazine edisylate	...	●	...
Propofol	...	...	●
Propranolol HCl	...	●	...
Ranitidine HCl	...	●	...
Salbutamol	...	●	...
Sodium bicarbonate	...	●	...
Sodium nitroprusside	...	●	...
Thiopental sodium	...	●	...
Ticarcillin disod.–clavulanate pot.	●	...	...
Tobramycin sulfate	...	●	...
Trimethoprim–sulfamethoxazole	...	●	...
Vancomycin HCl	●	...	...
Vasopressin	●	...	...
Vecuronium bromide	...	●	...
Verapamil HCl	...	●	...
Zidovudine	●	...	...

Pemetrexed Disodium

Handbook on Injectable Drugs pp. 1294–1298.

Description: A folic acid antagonist antineoplastic agent.

Products: Alimta; 500-mg vials. *pH:* From 6.6 to 7.8.

Preparation: Reconstitute the vials with 20 mL of sodium chloride 0.9% (without preservatives) and swirl gently to yield a 25-mg/mL solution. Reconstituted pemetrexed disodium must be diluted to 100 mL with additional sodium chloride 0.9%.

Administration: IV infusion over 10 minutes.

Stability: Store vials at room temperature. The reconstituted solution is chemically and physically stable for up to 24 hours at room temperature and lighting and under refrigeration. Pemetrexed disodium diluted in sodium chloride 0.9% for IV infusion is also stable for 24 hours at room temperature and lighting and under refrigeration.

Compatibility Table

Solutions	Compatible	Incompatible	Variable
Ringer's injection	...	●	...
Ringer's injection, lactated	...	●	...
Sodium chloride 0.9%	●	...	...

Drugs			
Acyclovir sodium	●	...	...
Amifostine	●	...	...
Amikacin sulfate	●	...	...
Aminophylline	●	...	...
Amphotericin B	...	●	...
Ampicillin sodium	●	...	...
Ampicillin sod.–sulbactam sod.	●	...	...
Aztreonam	●	...	...
Bumetanide	●	...	...
Buprenorphine HCl	●	...	...
Butorphanol tartrate	●	...	...
Calcium gluconate	...	●	...
Carboplatin	●	...	...
Cefazolin sodium	...	●	...
Cefotaxime sodium	...	●	...

Drugs	Compatible	Incompatible	Variable
Cefotetan disodium	...	●	...
Cefoxitin sodium	...	●	...
Ceftazidime	...	●	...
Ceftizoxime sodium	●	...	...
Ceftriaxone sodium	●	...	...
Cefuroxime sodium	●	...	...
Chlorpromazine HCl	...	●	...
Cimetidine HCl	●	...	...
Ciprofloxacin	...	●	...
Cisplatin	●	...	...
Clindamycin phosphate	●	...	...
Cyclophosphamide	●	...	...
Cytarabine..........................	●	...	...
Dexamethasone sodium phosphate ...	●	...	...
Dexrazoxane	●	...	...
Diphenhydramine HCl	●	...	...
Dobutamine HCl	...	●	...
Docetaxel	●	...	...
Dopamine HCl	●	...	...
Doxorubicin HCl	...	●	...
Doxycycline hyclate	...	●	...
Droperidol	...	●	...
Enalaprilat	●	...	...
Famotidine	●	...	...
Fluconazole	●	...	...
Fluorouracil........................	●	...	...
Ganciclovir sodium	●	...	...
Gemcitabine HCl	...	●	...
Gentamicin sulfate	...	●	...
Granisetron HCl	●	...	...
Haloperidol lactate	●	...	...
Heparin sodium	●	...	...
Hydromorphone HCl	●	...	...
Hydroxyzine HCl	●	...	...
Ifosfamide..........................	●	...	...
Irinotecan HCl	...	●	...
Leucovorin calcium	●	...	...
Lorazepam	●	...	...
Mannitol	●	...	...
Meperidine HCl	●	...	...

Drugs	Compatible	Incompatible	Variable
Mesna	●	...	...
Methylprednisolone sod. succ.	●	...	...
Metoclopramide HCl	●	...	...
Metronidazole	...	●	...
Mitoxantrone HCl	...	●	...
Morphine sulfate	●	...	...
Nalbuphine HCl	...	●	...
Ondansetron HCl	...	●	...
Paclitaxel	●	...	...
Potassium chloride	●	...	...
Prochlorperazine edisylate	...	●	...
Promethazine HCl	●	...	...
Ranitidine HCl	●	...	...
Sodium bicarbonate	●	...	...
Ticarcillin disod.–clavulanate pot.	●	...	...
Tobramycin sulfate	...	●	...
Topotecan HCl	...	●	...
Trimethoprim–sulfamethoxazole	●	...	...
Vancomycin HCl	●	...	...
Vinblastine sulfate	●	...	...
Vincristine sulfate	●	...	...
Zidovudine	●	...	...

Penicillin G Potassium

Handbook on Injectable Drugs pp. 1299–1309.

Description: A natural penicillin which acts as a bactericidal antibiotic.

Products: Available from numerous manufacturers in vial sizes ranging from 1 to 20 million units and in frozen premixed infusion solutions of 1, 2, and 3 million units. *pH:* From 6 to 8.5 (reconstituted solution) and 5.5 to 8 (frozen premixed infusions).

Preparation: Depending on the route of administration, reconstitute the vials with sterile water for injection, dextrose 5%, or sodium chloride 0.9% according to label directions.

Administration: Administer by IM injection or continuous or intermittent IV infusion. It is also given by intrathecal, intraarticular, and intrapleural injections and other local instillations. High doses by the IV route should be given slowly to avoid electrolyte imbalance.

Stability: Reconstituted solutions are stable for seven days under refrigeration. Penicillin G potassium is most stable at about pH 7, with inactivation occurring more rapidly below pH 5.5 or above pH 8.

Compatibility Table

Solutions	Compatible	Incompatible	Variable
Dextrose 5%	●	...	...
Dextrose 5% in Ringer's injection	●	...	...
Dextrose 5% in Ringer's injection, lactated	●	...	...
Dextrose 5% in sodium chloride 0.2, 0.45, & 0.9%	●	...	...
Ringer's injection	●	...	...
Ringer's injection, lactated	●	...	...
Sodium chloride 0.9%	●	...	...

Drugs			
Acyclovir sodium	●	...	...
Amikacin sulfate	...	...	●
Aminophylline	...	●	...
Amiodarone HCl	●	...	...
Amphotericin B	...	●	...

Drugs	Compatible	Incompatible	Variable
Ascorbic acid injection	●	...	...
Barbiturates	...	●	...
Caffeine citrate	●	...	...
Calcium chloride & gluconate	●	...	...
Chloramphenicol sodium succinate	●	...	...
Chlorpromazine HCl	...	●	...
Cimetidine HCl	●	...	...
Clindamycin phosphate	●	...	...
Colistimethate sodium	●	...	...
Corticotropin	●	...	...
Cyclophosphamide	●	...	...
Diltiazem HCl	●	...	...
Dimenhydrinate	●	...	...
Diphenhydramine HCl	●	...	...
Dopamine HCl	...	●	...
Enalaprilat	●	...	...
Ephedrine sulfate	●	...	...
Erythromycin lactobionate	●	...	...
Esmolol HCl	●	...	...
Fluconazole ....,,,,,,,....	●	...	...
Foscarnet sodium	●	...	...
Furosemide	●	...	...
Heparin sodium	...	...	●
Hydrocortisone sodium succinate	...	...	●
Hydromorphone HCl	●	...	...
Hydroxyzine HCl	...	●	...
Kanamycin sulfate	●	...	...
Labetalol HCl	●	...	...
Lidocaine HCl	●	...	...
Lincomycin HCl	...	...	●
Magnesium sulfate	●	...	...
Meperidine HCl	●	...	...
Methylprednisolone sod. succ.	●	...	...
Metoclopramide HCl	...	●	...
Metronidazole	...	...	●
Morphine sulfate	●	...	...
Nicardipine HCl	●	...	...
Pentobarbital sodium	...	●	...
Phenytoin sodium	...	●	...
Polymyxin B sulfate	●	...	...

Drugs	Compatible	Incompatible	Variable
Potassium chloride	●	...	...
Procaine HCl	●	...	...
Prochlorperazine edisylate	...	...	●
Promethazine HCl	...	...	●
Ranitidine HCl	●	...	...
Sodium bicarbonate	...	●	...
Tacrolimus	●	...	...
Theophylline	●	...	...
Thiopental sodium	...	●	...
Vancomycin HCl	...	●	...
Verapamil HCl	●	...	...

Penicillin G Sodium

Handbook on Injectable Drugs pp. 1309–1314.

Description: A natural penicillin which acts as a bactericidal antibiotic.

Products: 5 million units/vial. *pH:* From 5 to 7.5 when reconstituted.

Preparation: Depending on the route of administration, reconstitute the 5 million-unit vial with sterile water for injection, dextrose 5%, or sodium chloride 0.9% in the following amounts:

Diluent Volume	Concentration
8 mL	500,000 units/mL
3 mL	1 million units/mL

Administration: Administer by IM injection or continuous or intermittent IV infusion. High doses by the IV route should be given slowly to avoid electrolyte imbalance.

Stability: Store intact vials at room temperature. Reconstituted solutions are stable for one week under refrigeration. IV infusions of this drug are stable for at least 24 hours at room temperature.

At room temperature, a maximum stability is attained at pH 6.8. No more than a 10% loss of activity occurs in 24 hours at a pH of approximately 5.4 to 8.5.

Compatibility Table

Solutions	Compatible	Incompatible	Variable
Dextrose 5%	...	...	●
Fat emulsion 10%, IV	...	●	...
Sodium chloride 0.9%	●	...	...

Drugs	Compatible	Incompatible	Variable
Amphotericin B	...	●	...
Bleomycin sulfate	...	●	...
Caffeine citrate	●	...	...
Calcium chloride & gluconate	●	...	...
Chloramphenicol sodium succinate	●	...	...

Drugs	Compatible	Incompatible	Variable
Chlorpromazine HCl	...	●	...
Cimetidine HCl	●	...	...
Clindamycin phosphate	●	...	...
Colistimethate sodium	●	...	...
Cytarabine........................	...	●	...
Dimenhydrinate....................	●	...	...
Diphenhydramine HCl	●	...	...
Erythromycin lactobionate	●	...	...
Furosemide	●	...	...
Gentamicin sulfate	...	...	●
Heparin sodium	...	...	●
Hydrocortisone sodium succinate	●	...	...
Hydroxyzine HCl	...	●	...
Kanamycin sulfate	...	...	●
Levofloxacin	●	...	...
Lincomycin HCl	...	...	●
Methylprednisolone sod. succ.	...	●	...
Pantoprazole sodium	●	...	...
Polymyxin B sulfate	●	...	...
Potassium chloride	...	...	●
Procaine HCl	●	...	...
Prochlorperazine mesylate	...	●	...
Promethazine HCl	...	●	...
Ranitidine HCl	●	...	...
Streptomycin sulfate	●	...	...
Vancomycin HCl	...	●	...
Verapamil HCl	●	...	...

Pentazocine Lactate

Handbook on Injectable Drugs pp. 1316–1319.

Description: A potent synthetic opiate analgesic.

Products: **Talwin;** 30 mg/mL in 1- and 2-mL ampuls and disposable syringe cartridges and also 10-mL vials. *pH:* From 4 to 5.

Administration: Administer by IM, SC, or IV injection. Because of possible tissue damage upon multiple IM or SC injections, constant rotation of the injection sites is required. Because of possible tissue damage, SC injection should be used only when necessary.

Stability: Store at room temperature and protect from freezing and temperatures above 40 °C.

Compatibility Table

Drugs	Compatible	Incompatible	Variable
Aminophylline	...	●	...
Amobarbital sodium	...	●	...
Atropine sulfate	●	...	...
Butorphanol tartrate	●	...	...
Chlorpromazine HCl	●	...	...
Cimetidine HCl	●	...	...
Dimenhydrinate	●	...	...
Diphenhydramine HCl	●	...	...
Droperidol	●	...	...
Fentanyl citrate	●	...	...
Glycopyrrolate	...	●	...
Heparin sodium	...	...	●
Hydrocortisone sodium succinate	●	...	...
Hydromorphone HCl	●	...	...
Hydroxyzine HCl	●	...	...
Meperidine HCl	●	...	...
Metoclopramide HCl	●	...	...
Morphine sulfate	●	...	...
Nafcillin sodium	...	●	...
Pentobarbital sodium	...	●	...
Phenobarbital sodium	...	●	...
Potassium chloride	●	...	...
Prochlorperazine edisylate	●	...	...
Promethazine HCl	●	...	...
Ranitidine HCl	●	...	...
Scopolamine HBr	●	...	...
Sodium bicarbonate	...	●	...

Pentobarbital Sodium

Handbook on Injectable Drugs pp. 1319–1325.

Description: A short-acting barbiturate sedative-hypnotic.

Products: Nembutal; 50 mg/mL in 20-mL (1 g) and 50-mL (2.5 g) multiple-dose vials. *pH:* About 9.5.

Administration: Administer by deep IM or slow IV injection, usually in a concentration of 50 mg/mL. The rate of IV administration should not exceed 50 mg/min. No more than 5 mL (250 mg) should be injected IM at any one site.

Stability: Store intact containers at room temperature protected from heat and freezing. Aqueous solutions of pentobarbital sodium are not stable. The commercially available pentobarbital sodium in a propylene glycol vehicle is more stable. In an acidic medium, pentobarbital may precipitate. No sorption to plastic IV bags or filters has been noted.

Compatibility Table

Solutions	Compatible	Incompatible	Variable
Dextrose 5%	●	...	...
Dextrose 5% in Ringer's injection, lactated	●	...	...
Dextrose 5% in sodium chloride 0.2, 0.45, & 0.9%	●	...	...
Ringer's injection, lactated	●	...	...
Sodium chloride 0.45 & 0.9%	●	...	...

Drugs			
Acyclovir sodium	●	...	...
Amikacin sulfate	●	...	...
Aminophylline	●	...	...
Amphotericin B cholesteryl sulfate complex	...	●	...

Drugs	Compatible	Incompatible	Variable
Atropine sulfate	...	...	●
Butorphanol tartrate	...	●	...
Calcium chloride	●	...	...
Cefazolin sodium	...	●	...
Chloramphenicol sodium succinate	●	...	...
Chlorpromazine HCl	...	...	●
Cimetidine HCl	...	●	...
Clindamycin phosphate	...	●	...
Dimenhydrinate	...	...	●
Diphenhydramine HCl	...	●	...
Droperidol	...	●	...
Ephedrine sulfate	...	...	●
Erythromycin lactobionate	●	...	...
Fenoldopam mesylate	...	●	...
Fentanyl citrate	...	●	...
Glycopyrrolate	...	●	...
Hyaluronidase	●	...	...
Hydrocortisone sodium succinate	...	...	●
Hydromorphone HCl	●	...	...
Hydroxyzine HCl	...	●	...
Insulin, regular	...	...	●
Isoproterenol HCl	...	●	...
Lansoprazole	...	●	...
Lidocaine HCl	●	...	...
Linezolid	●	...	...
Meperidine HCl	...	●	...
Methyldopate HCl	...	●	...
Midazolam HCl	...	●	...
Morphine sulfate	...	...	●
Nalbuphine HCl	...	●	...
Neostigmine methylsulfate	●	...	...
Norepinephrine bitartrate	...	●	...
Pancuronium bromide	...	●	...
Penicillin G potassium	...	●	...
Pentazocine lactate	...	●	...

Drugs	Compatible	Incompatible	Variable
Phenytoin sodium	...	●	...
Prochlorperazine edisylate	...	●	...
Promethazine HCl	...	...	●
Propofol	●	...	...
Ranitidine HCl	...	●	...
Scopolamine HBr	●	...	...
Sodium bicarbonate	...	...	●
Streptomycin sulfate	...	●	...
Succinylcholine chloride	...	...	●
Thiopental sodium	●	...	...
Vancomycin HCl	...	●	...
Verapamil HCl	●	...	...

Phenobarbital Sodium

Handbook on Injectable Drugs pp. 1331–1335.

Description: A long-acting barbiturate used primarily as a sedative and an anticonvulsant.

Products: Available from various manufacturers in concentrations from 30 to 130 mg/mL. The vehicle is a mixture of propylene glycol, alcohol, and water. *pH:* From 9.2 to 10.2.

Administration: Administer by IM or slow IV injection. When given IV, the rate should not exceed 60 mg/min. The injection is highly alkaline and may cause local tissue damage. Do not administer by SC injection.

Stability: Store intact containers at room temperature and protect from light. Aqueous solutions are not generally considered to be stable. However, a test of phenobarbital sodium 10% in aqueous solution showed 7% decomposition in four weeks at room temperature. The drug may precipitate from solutions, depending on concentration and pH. No solution containing a precipitate should be used.

Compatibility Table

Solutions	Compatible	Incompatible	Variable
Dextrose 5%	●	...	...
Dextrose 5% in Ringer's injection	●	...	...
Dextrose 5% in Ringer's injection, lactated	●	...	...
Dextrose 5% in sodium chloride 0.2, 0.45, & 0.9%	●	...	...
Ringer's injection	●	...	...
Ringer's injection, lactated	●	...	...
Sodium chloride 0.45 & 0.9%	●	...	...

Drugs	Compatible	Incompatible	Variable
Amikacin sulfate	●	...	...
Aminophylline	●	...	...
Amphotericin B cholesteryl sulfate complex	...	●	...
Atracurium besylate	...	●	...
Caffeine citrate	●	...	...
Calcium chloride & gluconate	●	...	...
Chlorpromazine HCl	...	●	...
Cimetidine HCl	...	●	...
Clindamycin phosphate	...	●	...
Colistimethate sodium	●	...	...
Dimenhydrinate.....................	...	...	●
Diphenhydramine HCl	...	●	...
Doxapram hydrochloride	●	...	...
Droperidol	...	●	...
Enalaprilat	●	...	...
Ephedrine sulfate	...	●	...
Fentanyl citrate	●	...	...
Fosphenytoin sodium	●	...	...
Heparin sodium	●	...	...
Hydralazine HCl	...	●	...
Hydrocortisone sodium succinate	...	●	...
Hydromorphone HCl	...	...	●
Hydroxyzine HCl	...	●	...
Insulin, regular	...	●	...
Isoproterenol HCl	...	●	...
Kanamycin sulfate	...	●	...
Lansoprazole	...	●	...
Levofloxacin	●	...	...
Linezolid	●	...	...
Meperidine HCl	...	●	...
Meropenem	●	...	...
Methadone HCl	●	...	...
Morphine sulfate	...	...	●
Norepinephrine bitartrate	...	●	...
Pancuronium bromide	...	●	...
Pantoprazole sodium	...	●	...
Pentazocine lactate	...	●	...
Phenytoin sodium	...	●	...
Polymyxin B sulfate	●	...	...

Drugs	Compatible	Incompatible	Variable
Procaine HCl	...	●	...
Prochlorperazine edisylate	...	●	...
Promethazine HCl	...	●	...
Propofol	●	...	...
Ranitidine HCl	...	●	...
Streptomycin sulfate	...	●	...
Succinylcholine chloride	...	●	...
Sufentanil citrate	...	...	●
Thiopental sodium	●	...	...
Vancomycin HCl	...	●	...
Verapamil HCl	●	...	...

Phenytoin Sodium

Handbook on Injectable Drugs pp. 1340–1347.

Description: An anticonvulsant compound chemically related to the barbiturates.

Products: 100-mg (2 mL) and 250-mg (5 mL) vials. *pH:* Adjusted to 12.

Administration: Administration may be by direct IV or IM injection, but the IV route is preferred because of delayed absorption by the IM route. Do not give by SC injection. The rate of IV injection is not to exceed 50 mg/min in adults or 1 to 3 mg/kg/min in neonates. Following IV injection, flush with sodium chloride 0.9% to reduce irritation.

Stability: Phenytoin sodium is stable as long as it remains free of haziness and precipitation. If refrigerated or frozen, a precipitate may form, but it dissolves on standing at room temperature. Upon dissolution of the precipitate, the product is suitable for use. Also, a faint yellow color, which has no effect on potency, may develop in the injection.

No sorption to plastic IV bags, sets, or syringes has been noted.

Compatibility Table

Solutions	Compatible	Incompatible	Variable
Dextrose 5%	...	●	...
Dextrose 5% in sod. chloride 0.9% ...	...	●	...
Fat emulsion 10%, IV	...	●	...
Ringer's injection, lactated*	...	●	...
Sodium chloride 0.9%*	...	...	●

*Depending on drug concentration and solution pH, crystallization of phenytoin may not occur immediately but will occur up to several hours after mixture.

Drugs			
Amikacin sulfate	...	●	...
Aminophylline	...	●	...
Amphotericin B cholesteryl sulfate complex	...	●	...
Barbiturates	...	●	...

Drugs	Compatible	Incompatible	Variable
Cefepime HCl	...	●	...
Ceftazidime	...	●	...
Ciprofloxacin	...	●	...
Clindamycin phosphate	...	●	...
Diltiazem HCl	...	●	...
Dimenhydrinate	...	●	...
Diphenhydramine HCl	...	●	...
Dobutamine HCl	...	●	...
Enalaprilat	...	●	...
Esmolol HCl	●	...	...
Famotidine	●	...	...
Fenoldopam mesylate	...	●	...
Fentanyl citrate	...	●	...
Fluconazole	●	...	...
Foscarnet sodium	●	...	...
Gentamicin sulfate	...	●	...
Heparin sodium	...	●	...
Hydromorphone HCl	...	●	...
Hydroxyzine HCl	...	●	...
Insulin, regular	...	●	...
Kanamycin sulfate	...	●	...
Lansoprazole	...	●	...
Lidocaine HCl	...	●	...
Lincomycin HCl	...	●	...
Linezolid	...	●	...
Meperidine HCl	...	●	...
Methadone HCl	...	●	...
Morphine sulfate	...	●	...
Nitroglycerin	...	●	...
Norepinephrine bitartrate	...	●	...
Pantoprazole sodium	...	●	...
Penicillin G potassium	...	●	...
Pentobarbital sodium	...	●	...
Phenobarbital sodium	...	●	...
Phenylephrine HCl	...	●	...
Phytonadione	...	●	...
Potassium chloride	...	●	...
Procainamide HCl	...	●	...
Procaine HCl	...	●	...
Prochlorperazine edisylate	...	●	...

Drugs	Compatible	Incompatible	Variable
Promethazine HCl	...	●	...
Propofol	...	●	...
Sodium bicarbonate	●	...	...
Streptomycin sulfate	...	●	...
Sufentanil citrate	...	●	...
Tacrolimus	●	...	...
Theophylline	...	●	...
Vancomycin HCl	...	●	...
Verapamil HCl	●	...	...

Piperacillin Sodium

Handbook on Injectable Drugs pp. 1351–1359.

Description: A semisynthetic, extended-spectrum penicillin.

Products: **Pipracil**; 2-, 3-, and 4-g vials and infusion bottles. *pH:* From 5.5 to 7.5 when reconstituted.

Preparation: For IM use, reconstitute with 2 mL of diluent per gram of drug to yield 1 g/2.5 mL. Recommended diluents are sterile or bacteriostatic water for injection, lidocaine hydrochloride 0.5 to 1%, and the diluents used for IV administration.

For IV use, reconstitute with 5 mL of diluent per gram of drug. Recommended diluents are sterile or bacteriostatic water for injection or sodium chloride 0.9%, dextrose 5%, and dextrose 5% in sodium chloride 0.9%.

Administration: Administer by IM injection with no more than 2 g at any one site, direct IV injection over three to five minutes, or intermittent IV infusion in at least 50 mL of compatible diluent over 20 to 30 minutes.

Stability: Store intact containers at room temperature. Reconstituted solutions are colorless to pale yellow. Both the reconstituted vials and piggyback infusion bottles are stable for 24 hours at room temperature, one week under refrigeration, and one month if frozen. Slight darkening of the powder or solution does not indicate a potency loss. No sorption to filters or infusion containers has been reported.

Compatibility Table

Solutions	Compatible	Incompatible	Variable
Dextrose 5%	●	...	...
Dextrose 5% in sodium chloride 0.9%	●	...	...
Ringer's injection, lactated	●	...	...
Sodium chloride 0.9%	●	...	...

Drugs	Compatible	Incompatible	Variable
Acyclovir sodium	●	. . .	. . .
Aldesleukin	●	. . .	. . .
Allopurinol sodium	●	. . .	. . .
Amifostine	●	. . .	. . .
Aminoglycosides	. . .	. . .	●
Amiodarone HCl	. . .	●	. . .
Amphotericin B cholesteryl sulfate complex	. . .	●	. . .
Anakinra	. . .	. . .	●
Aztreonam	●	. . .	. . .
Bivalirudin	●	. . .	. . .
Ciprofloxacin	. . .	. . .	●
Cisatracurium besylate	. . .	. . .	●
Clindamycin phosphate	●	. . .	. . .
Cyclophosphamide	●	. . .	. . .
Dexmedetomidine HCl	●	. . .	. . .
Diltiazem HCl	●	. . .	. . .
Dimenhydrinate	●	. . .	. . .
Docetaxel	●	. . .	. . .
Doxorubicin HCl liposome injection	●	. . .	. . .
Enalaprilat	●	. . .	. . .
Esmolol HCl	●	. . .	. . .
Etoposide phosphate	●	. . .	. . .
Famotidine	●	. . .	. . .
Fenoldopam mesylate	●	. . .	. . .
Filgrastim	. . .	●	. . .
Fluconazole	. . .	. . .	●
Fludarabine phosphate	●	. . .	. . .
Foscarnet sodium	●	. . .	. . .
Gallium nitrate	●	. . .	. . .
Gemcitabine HCl	. . .	●	. . .
Granisetron HCl	●	. . .	. . .
Heparin sodium	●	. . .	. . .
Hextend	●	. . .	. . .
Hydrocortisone sodium succinate	●	. . .	. . .
Hydromorphone HCl	●	. . .	. . .
Labetalol HCl	●	. . .	. . .
Lansoprazole	●	. . .	. . .
Linezolid	●	. . .	. . .
Lorazepam	●	. . .	. . .

Drugs	Compatible	Incompatible	Variable
Magnesium sulfate	●	...	...
Melphalan hydrochloride	●	...	...
Meperidine HCl	●	...	...
Midazolam HCl	●	...	...
Milrinone lactate	●	...	...
Morphine sulfate	●	...	...
Nicardipine HCl.....................	●	...	...
Ondansetron HCl	...	●	...
Pantoprazole sodium	●	...	...
Potassium chloride	●	...	...
Propofol	●	...	...
Ranitidine HCl	●	...	...
Remifentanil HCl	●	...	...
Sargramostim	...	●	...
Tacrolimus	●	...	...
Teniposide	●	...	...
Theophylline	●	...	...
Thiotepa	●	...	...
Vancomycin HCl	...	...	●
Verapamil HCl	●	...	...
Vinorelbine tartrate	...	●	...
Zidovudine	●	...	...

Piperacillin Sodium–Tazobactam Sodium

Handbook on Injectable Drugs pp. 1359–1366.

Description: A fixed combination of an extended-spectrum penicillin and an inhibitor of penicillin inactivation.

Products: Zosyn; Vials containing piperacillin 2, 3, and 4 g with tazobactam 250, 375, and 500 mg, respectively, as the sodium salts. *pH:* From 4.5 to 6.8.

Preparation: Reconstitute each gram of piperacillin with at least 5 mL of sterile water for injection or another compatible diluent and shake well. For IV infusion, dilute the dose further in at least 50 mL of compatible infusion solution.

Administration: Administer by intermittent IV infusion over at least 30 minutes.

Stability: The white to off-white powder may be stored at room temperature. Discard reconstituted solutions after 24 hours at room temperature or 48 hours under refrigeration. In compatible infusion solutions, the drug is stable for 24 hours at room temperature or one week under refrigeration. Piperacillin sodium–tazobactam sodium 80 + 10 mg/mL in PVC bags of dextrose 5% and sodium chloride 0.9% frozen at −15 °C for 30 days and thawed by microwave radiation showed no loss of either component.

Compatibility Table

Solutions	Compatible	Incompatible	Variable
Dextrose 5%	●	...	...
Ringer's injection, lactated	...	●	...
Sodium chloride 0.9%	●	...	...

Drugs			
Acyclovir sodium	...	●	...
Aminoglycosides	...	...	●
Aminophylline	●	...	...
Amiodarone HCl	...	●	...
Amphotericin B	...	●	...

Drugs	Compatible	Incompatible	Variable
Amphotericin B cholesteryl sulfate complex	...	●	...
Azithromycin	...	●	...
Aztreonam	●	...	...
Bivalirudin	●	...	...
Bleomycin sulfate	●	...	...
Bumetanide	●	...	...
Buprenorphine HCl	●	...	...
Butorphanol tartrate	●	...	...
Calcium gluconate	●	...	...
Carboplatin	●	...	...
Carmustine	●	...	...
Cefepime HCl	●	...	...
Chlorpromazine HCl	...	●	...
Cimetidine HCl	●	...	...
Cisatracurium besylate	...	...	●
Cisplatin	...	●	...
Clindamycin phosphate	●	...	...
Cyclophosphamide	●	...	...
Cytarabine	●	...	...
Dacarbazine	...	●	...
Daunorubicin HCl	...	●	...
Dexamethasone sodium phosphate	●	...	...
Dexmedetomidine HCl	●	...	...
Dimenhydrinate	●	...	...
Diphenhydramine HCl	●	...	...
Dobutamine HCl	...	●	...
Docetaxel	●	...	...
Dopamine HCl	●	...	...
Doxorubicin HCl	...	●	...
Doxorubicin HCl liposome injection	...	●	...
Doxycycline hyclate	...	●	...
Droperidol	...	●	...
Drotrecogin alfa (activated)	...	●	...
Enalaprilat	●	...	...
Etoposide	●	...	...
Etoposide phosphate	●	...	...
Famotidine	...	●	...
Fenoldopam mesylate	●	...	...

Drugs	Compatible	Incompatible	Variable
Floxuridine	●	...	...
Fluconazole	●	...	...
Fludarabine phosphate	●	...	...
Fluorouracil	●	...	...
Furosemide	●	...	...
Gallium nitrate	●	...	...
Ganciclovir sodium	...	●	...
Gemcitabine HCl	...	●	...
Granisetron HCl	●	...	...
Haloperidol lactate	...	●	...
Heparin sodium	●	...	...
Hextend	●	...	...
Hydrocortisone sodium phosphate	●	...	...
Hydrocortisone sodium succinate	●	...	...
Hydromorphone HCl	●	...	...
Hydroxyzine HCl	...	●	...
Idarubicin HCl	...	●	...
Ifosfamide	●	...	...
Lansoprazole	●	...	...
Leucovorin calcium	●	...	...
Linezolid	●	...	...
Lorazepam	●	...	...
Magnesium sulfate	●	...	...
Mannitol	●	...	...
Meperidine HCl	●	...	...
Mesna	●	...	...
Methotrexate sodium	●	...	...
Methylprednisolone sod. succ.	●	...	...
Metoclopramide HCl	●	...	...
Metronidazole	●	...	...
Milrinone lactate	●	...	...
Mitomycin	...	●	...
Mitoxantrone HCl	...	●	...
Morphine sulfate	●	...	...
Nalbuphine HCl	...	●	...
Ondansetron HCl	●	...	...
Pantoprazole sodium	...	●	...
Potassium chloride	●	...	...
Prochlorperazine edisylate	...	●	...
Promethazine HCl	...	●	...

Drugs	Compatible	Incompatible	Variable
Ranitidine HCl	●	...	...
Remifentanil HCl	●	...	...
Sargramostim	●	...	...
Sodium bicarbonate	●	...	...
Streptozocin	...	●	...
Thiotepa	●	...	...
Trimethoprim–sulfamethoxazole	●	...	...
Vancomycin HCl	...	...	●
Vinblastine sulfate	●	...	...
Vincristine sulfate	●	...	...
Zidovudine	●	...	...

Potassium Chloride

Handbook on Injectable Drugs pp. 1370–1384.

Description: A potassium salt used for the prevention and treatment of potassium deficiencies.

Products: 10-, 20-, 30-, and 40-mEq sizes, as concentrate, in ampuls, vials, and syringes. *pH:* From 4 to 8.

Preparation: The concentrate must be diluted before use. Mix thoroughly before administration to prevent pooling.

Administration: Administer by slow dilute IV infusion; avoid extravasation. The usual maximum concentration is 40 mEq/L of IV solution. The rate of administration is generally not greater than 10 to 20 mEq/hr.

Stability: Store at controlled room temperature, and use only if the solution is clear.

Compatibility Table

Solutions	Compatible	Incompatible	Variable
Dextrose 5 & 10%	●	...	...
Dextrose 5% in Ringer's injection	●	...	...
Dextrose 5% in Ringer's injection, lactated	●	...	...
Dextrose 5% in sodium chloride 0.2, 0.45, & 0.9%	●	...	...
Fat emulsion 10%, IV	...	...	●
Ionosol products	●	...	...
Mannitol 20 & 25%	...	●	...
Ringer's injection	●	...	...
Ringer's injection, lactated	●	...	...
Sodium chloride 0.45 & 0.9%	●	...	...

Drugs	Compatible	Incompatible	Variable
Acyclovir sodium	●	...	...
Aldesleukin	...	...	●
Allopurinol sodium	●	...	...
Amifostine	●	...	...
Amikacin sulfate	...	...	●

Drugs	Compatible	Incompatible	Variable
Aminophylline	●	...	...
Amiodarone HCl	●	...	...
Amphotericin B	...	●	...
Amphotericin B cholesteryl sulfate complex	...	●	...
Ampicillin sodium	●	...	...
Atracurium besylate	●	...	...
Atropine sulfate	●	...	...
Azithromycin	...	●	...
Aztreonam	●	...	...
Betamethasone sodium phosphate	●	...	...
Bivalirudin	●	...	...
Calcium gluconate	●	...	...
Cefepime HCl	●	...	...
Chloramphenicol sodium succinate	●	...	...
Chlordiazepoxide HCl	●	...	...
Chlorpromazine HCl	●	...	...
Cimetidine HCl	●	...	...
Ciprofloxacin	●	...	...
Cisatracurium besylate	●	...	...
Cladribine	●	...	...
Clindamycin phosphate	●	...	...
Cloxacillin sodium	●	...	...
Corticotropin	●	...	...
Cyanocobalamin	●	...	...
Cytarabine	●	...	...
Dexamethasone sodium phosphate	●	...	...
Dexmedetomidine HCl	●	...	...
Diazepam	...	●	...
Digoxin	●	...	...
Diltiazem HCl	●	...	...
Dimenhydrinate	...	...	●
Diphenhydramine HCl	●	...	...
Dobutamine HCl	...	...	●
Docetaxel	●	...	...
Dopamine HCl	●	...	...
Doxorubicin HCl liposome injection	●	...	...
Droperidol	●	...	...
Drotrecogin alfa (activated)	●	...	...

Drugs	Compatible	Incompatible	Variable
Edrophonium chloride	●	...	...
Enalaprilat	●	...	...
Epinephrine HCl	●	...	...
Ergotamine tartrate	...	●	...
Ertapenem	●	...	...
Erythromycin lactobionate	●	...	...
Esmolol HCl	●	...	...
Estrogens, conjugated	●	...	...
Ethacrynate sodium	●	...	...
Etoposide phosphate	●	...	...
Famotidine	●	...	...
Fenoldopam mesylate	●	...	...
Fentanyl citrate	●	...	...
Filgrastim	●	...	...
Fluconazole	●	...	...
Fludarabine phosphate	●	...	...
Fluorouracil	●	...	...
Foscarnet sodium	●	...	...
Fosphenytoin sodium	●	...	...
Furosemide	●	...	...
Gallium nitrate	●	...	...
Gemcitabine HCl	●	...	...
Granisetron HCl	●	...	...
Heparin sodium	●	...	...
Hextend	●	...	...
Hydralazine HCl	●	...	...
Hydrocortisone sodium succinate	●	...	...
Hydromorphone HCl	●	...	...
Idarubicin HCl	●	...	...
Indomethacin sodium trihydrate	●	...	...
Insulin, regular	●	...	...
Isoproterenol HCl	●	...	...
Kanamycin sulfate	●	...	...
Labetalol HCl	●	...	...
Lansoprazole	...	●	...
Lidocaine HCl	●	...	...
Linezolid	●	...	...
Lorazepam	●	...	...
Magnesium sulfate	●	...	...
Melphalan HCl	●	...	...

Drugs	Compatible	Incompatible	Variable
Meperidine HCl	●	...	...
Meropenem	●	...	...
Methyldopate HCl	●	...	...
Methylprednisolone sod. succ.	...	...	●
Metoclopramide HCl	●	...	...
Midazolam HCl	●	...	...
Milrinone lactate	●	...	...
Mitoxantrone HCl	●	...	...
Morphine sulfate	●	...	...
Nafcillin sodium	●	...	...
Neostigmine methylsulfate	●	...	...
Nicardipine HCl	●	...	...
Norepinephrine bitartrate	●	...	...
Ondansetron HCl	●	...	...
Oxacillin sodium	●	...	...
Oxaliplatin	●	...	...
Oxytocin	●	...	...
Paclitaxel	●	...	...
Pantoprazole sodium	●	...	...
Pemetrexed disodium	●	...	...
Penicillin G potassium & sodium	●	...	...
Pentazocine lactate	●	...	...
Phenylephrine HCl	●	...	...
Phenytoin sodium	...	●	...
Phytonadione	●	...	...
Piperacillin sodium	●	...	...
Piperacillin sod.–tazobactam sod.	●	...	...
Procainamide HCl	●	...	...
Prochlorperazine edisylate	●	...	...
Promethazine HCl	...	...	●
Propofol	●	...	...
Propranolol HCl	●	...	...
Pyridostigmine bromide	●	...	...
Quinupristin–dalfopristin	●	...	...
Ranitidine HCl	●	...	...
Remifentanil HCl	●	...	...
Sargramostim	●	...	...
Scopolamine HBr	●	...	...
Sodium bicarbonate	●	...	...
Sodium nitroprusside	●	...	...

Drugs	Compatible	Incompatible	Variable
Succinylcholine chloride	●	...	...
Tacrolimus	●	...	...
Teniposide	●	...	...
Theophylline	●	...	...
Thiopental sodium	●	...	...
Thiotepa	●	...	...
Tirofiban HCl	●	...	...
Trimethobenzamide HCl	●	...	...
Vancomycin HCl	●	...	...
Verapamil HCl	●	...	...
Vinorelbine tartrate	●	...	...
Warfarin sodium	●	...	...
Zidovudine	●	...	...

Potassium Chloride

Prochlorperazine Edisylate

Handbook on Injectable Drugs pp. 1397–1404.

Description: A phenothiazine tranquilizer and antiemetic.

Products: Compazine; 5 mg/mL in 2-mL vials and disposable syringes and 10-mL multiple-dose vials. *pH:* From 4.2 to 6.2.

Preparation: For IV infusion, dilution of 20 mg in a liter of compatible infusion solution is recommended.

Administration: IM injections should be made deep into a large muscle mass.

By direct IV injection, the drug can be given undiluted or diluted in a compatible diluent. It should not be given as a bolus IV injection. The rate should not exceed 5 mg/min. The drug may also be given by IV infusion after dilution in a compatible infusion solution.

SC injection is not recommended due to local irritation.

Stability: Store intact containers at room temperature protected from heat and freezing. Solutions should be protected from light. A slightly yellowed solution has not had its potency altered, but discard a markedly discolored solution.

Compatibility Table

Solutions	Compatible	Incompatible	Variable
Dextrose 5%	●	...	...
Dextrose 5% in Ringer's injection	●	...	...
Dextrose 5% in Ringer's injection, lactated	●	...	...
Dextrose 5% in sodium chloride 0.2, 0.45, & 0.9%	●	...	...
Ringer's injection	●	...	...
Ringer's injection, lactated	●	...	...
Sodium chloride 0.45 & 0.9%	●	...	...

Drugs	Compatible	Incompatible	Variable
Aldesleukin	...	●	...
Allopurinol sodium	...	●	...
Amifostine	...	●	...
Amikacin sulfate	●	...	...
Aminophylline	...	●	...
Amphotericin B cholesteryl sulfate complex	...	●	...
Ascorbic acid injection	●	...	...
Atropine sulfate	●	...	...
Aztreonam	...	●	...
Bivalirudin	...	●	...
Butorphanol tartrate	●	...	...
Calcium gluconate	...	...	●
Cefepime HCl	...	●	...
Chloramphenicol sodium succinate	...	●	...
Chlorothiazide sodium	...	●	...
Chlorpromazine HCl	●	...	...
Cimetidine HCl	●	...	...
Cisatracurium besylate	●	...	...
Cisplatin	●	...	...
Cladribine	●	...	...
Cyclophosphamide	●	...	...
Cytarabine	●	...	...
Dexamethasone sodium phosphate	...	...	●
Dexmedetomidine HCl	●	...	...
Dimenhydrinate	...	...	●
Diphenhydramine HCl	●	...	...
Docetaxel	●	...	...
Doxorubicin HCl	●	...	...
Doxorubicin HCl liposome injection	●	...	...
Droperidol	●	...	...
Erythromycin lactobionate	●	...	...
Ethacrynate sodium	●	...	...
Etoposide phosphate	...	●	...
Fenoldopam mesylate	...	●	...

Drugs	Compatible	Incompatible	Variable
Fentanyl citrate	●	...	...
Filgrastim	...	●	...
Fluconazole	●	...	...
Fludarabine phosphate	...	●	...
Foscarnet sodium	...	●	...
Furosemide	...	●	...
Gallium nitrate	...	●	...
Gemcitabine HCl	...	●	...
Glycopyrrolate	●	...	...
Granisetron HCl	●	...	...
Heparin sodium	...	...	●
Hextend	●	...	...
Hydrocortisone sodium succinate	...	...	●
Hydromorphone HCl	...	...	●
Hydroxyzine HCl	●	...	...
Ketorolac tromethamine	...	●	...
Lansoprazole	...	●	...
Lidocaine HCl	●	...	...
Linezolid	●	...	...
Melphalan HCl	●	...	...
Meperidine HCl	●	...	...
Methotrexate sodium	●	...	...
Metoclopramide HCl	●	...	...
Midazolam HCl	...	●	...
Morphine sulfate	...	...	●
Nafcillin sodium	●	...	...
Nalbuphine HCl	●	...	...
Ondansetron HCl	●	...	...
Oxaliplatin	●	...	...
Paclitaxel	●	...	...
Pemetrexed disodium	...	●	...
Penicillin G potassium	...	...	●
Pentazocine lactate	●	...	...
Pentobarbital sodium	...	●	...
Phenytoin sodium	...	●	...

Drugs	Compatible	Incompatible	Variable
Piperacillin sod.–tazobactam sod.	...	●	...
Potassium chloride	●	...	...
Prednisolone sodium phosphate	...	●	...
Promethazine HCl	●	...	...
Propofol	●	...	...
Ranitidine HCl	●	...	...
Remifentanil HCl	●	...	...
Sargramostim	●	...	...
Scopolamine HBr	●	...	...
Sodium bicarbonate	●	...	...
Sufentanil citrate	●	...	...
Teniposide	●	...	...
Thiopental sodium	...	●	...
Thiotepa	●	...	...
Topotecan HCl	●	...	...
Vinorelbine tartrate	●	...	...

Prochlorperazine Edisylate

Promethazine Hydrochloride

Handbook on Injectable Drugs pp. 1410–1419.

Description: A phenothiazine derivative with antihistamine, antiemetic, and sedative properties.

Products: Phenergan; 25 and 50 mg/mL in ampuls and syringe cartridges. *pH:* From 4 to 5.5.

Administration: Administer by deep IM or IV injection. By direct IV injection, a concentration not exceeding 25 mg/mL should be given into the tubing of a running infusion solution at a rate not exceeding 25 mg/min. It has also been given by continuous or intermittent IV infusion. Avoid extravasation. Do not administer SC or intraarterially.

Stability: Store intact containers at room temperature protected from freezing and light. Contact of promethazine hydrochloride with plastic IV infusion bags and infusion sets and tubing results in significant drug loss due to sorption.

Compatibility Table

Solutions	Compatible	Incompatible	Variable
Dextrose 5%	●	...	...
Dextrose 5% in sodium chloride 0.2, 0.45, & 0.9%	●	...	...
Ringer's injection	●	...	...
Ringer's injection, lactated	●	...	...
Sodium chloride 0.45 & 0.9%	●	...	...

Drugs			
Aldesleukin	...	●	...
Allopurinol sodium	...	●	...
Amifostine	●	...	...
Amikacin sulfate	●	...	...
Aminophylline	...	●	...
Amphotericin B cholesteryl sulfate complex	...	●	...
Ascorbic acid injection	●	...	...
Atropine sulfate	●	...	...
Aztreonam	●	...	...

Drugs	Compatible	Incompatible	Variable
Bivalirudin	●	...	...
Butorphanol tartrate	●	...	...
Cefazolin sodium	...	...	●
Cefepime HCl	...	●	...
Cefotetan disodium	...	●	...
Ceftizoxime sodium	...	...	●
Chloramphenicol sodium succinate	...	●	...
Chlorothiazide sodium	...	●	...
Chlorpromazine HCl	●	...	...
Cimetidine HCl	●	...	...
Ciprofloxacin	●	...	...
Cisatracurium besylate	●	...	...
Cisplatin	●	...	...
Cladribine	●	...	...
Cyclophosphamide	●	...	...
Cytarabine	●	...	...
Dexmedetomidine HCl	●	...	...
Diatrizoate meglumine & sodium	...	●	...
Dihydroergotamine mesylate	●	...	...
Dimenhydrinate	...	●	...
Diphenhydramine HCl	●	...	...
Docetaxel	●	...	...
Doxorubicin HCl	●	...	...
Doxorubicin HCl liposome injection	...	●	...
Droperidol	●	...	...
Etoposide phosphate	●	...	...
Fenoldopam mesylate	●	...	...
Fentanyl citrate	●	...	...
Filgrastim	●	...	...
Fluconazole	●	...	...
Fludarabine phosphate	●	...	...
Foscarnet sodium	...	●	...
Furosemide	...	●	...
Gemcitabine HCl	●	...	...
Glycopyrrolate	●	...	...
Granisetron HCl	●	...	...
Heparin sodium	...	...	●
Hextend	●	...	...
Hydrocortisone sodium succinate	...	...	●

Drugs	Compatible	Incompatible	Variable
Hydromorphone HCl	•	...	...
Hydroxyzine HCl	•	...	...
Iodipamide meglumine	...	•	...
Iothalamate meglumine & sodium	...	•	...
Ketorolac tromethamine	...	•	...
Lansoprazole	...	•	...
Linezolid	•	...	...
Melphalan HCl	•	...	...
Meperidine HCl	•	...	...
Methohexital sodium	...	•	...
Methotrexate sodium	...	•	...
Metoclopramide HCl	•	...	...
Midazolam HCl	•	...	...
Morphine sulfate	...	...	•
Nalbuphine HCl	...	...	•
Ondansetron HCl	•	...	...
Oxaliplatin	•	...	...
Pemetrexed disodium	•	...	...
Penicillin G potassium	...	...	•
Penicillin G sodium	...	...	•
Pentazocine lactate	•	...	...
Pentobarbital sodium	...	...	•
Phenobarbital sodium	...	•	...
Phenytoin sodium	...	•	...
Piperacillin sod.–tazobactam sod.	...	•	...
Potassium chloride	...	...	•
Prochlorperazine edisylate	•	...	...
Ranitidine HCl	•	...	...
Remifentanil HCl	•	...	...
Sargramostim	•	...	...
Scopolamine HBr	•	...	...
Teniposide	•	...	...
Thiopental sodium	...	•	...
Thiotepa	•	...	...
Vinorelbine tartrate	•	...	...

Propofol

Handbook on Injectable Drugs pp. 1421–1429.

Description: An anesthetic formulated as an opaque emulsion.

Products: Diprivan; Available as a 1% (10-mg/mL) ready-to-use oil-in-water emulsion. *pH:* Diprivan from 7 to 8.5; generic from 4.5 to 6.6.

Administration: Shake well before use. Administer undiluted by IV injection or infusion or diluted with dextrose 5% at a concentration of no less than 2 mg/mL. Strict aseptic procedures, including wiping containers with isopropanol 70%, are required during preparation because the product's lipid content supports microbiological growth.

Stability: Store intact containers at room temperatures up to 22 °C protected from light. Do not use the emulsion if phase separation is evident. If propofol is administered directly from the vial, administration should be completed within 12 hours due to degradation. If the drug is transferred to a syringe or other container, the manufacturer recommends that administration be begun promptly and completed within six hours.

Filters having a pore size of less than 5 μm should not be used with propofol emulsion.

Compatibility Table

Solutions	Compatible	Incompatible	Variable
Dextrose 5%	●	...	...
Dextrose 5% in Ringer's injection, lactated	●	...	...
Dextrose 5% in sodium chloride 0.2 & 0.45%	●	...	...
Ringer's injection, lactated	●	...	...

Drugs	Compatible	Incompatible	Variable
Acyclovir sodium	●	...	...
Alfentanil HCl	●	...	...
Amikacin sulfate	...	●	...
Aminophylline	●	...	...
Amphotericin B	...	●	...

Drugs	Compatible	Incompatible	Variable
Ampicillin sodium	●	...	...
Ascorbic acid injection	...	...	●
Atracurium besylate	...	●	...
Atropine sulfate	...	...	●
Aztreonam	●	...	...
Bumetanide	●	...	...
Buprenorphine HCl	●	...	...
Butorphanol tartrate	●	...	...
Calcium chloride	...	●	...
Calcium gluconate	●	...	...
Carboplatin........................	●	...	...
Cefazolin sodium	●	...	...
Cefepime HCl	...	...	●
Cefotaxime sodium	●	...	...
Cefotetan disodium	●	...	...
Cefoxitin sodium	●	...	...
Ceftazidime........................	...	...	●
Ceftizoxime sodium	●	...	...
Ceftriaxone sodium	●	...	...
Cefuroxime sodium	●	...	...
Chlorpromazine HCl	●	...	...
Cimetidine HCl	●	...	...
Ciprofloxacin	...	●	...
Cisatracurium besylate	...	●	...
Cisplatin	●	...	...
Clindamycin phosphate	●	...	...
Cyclophosphamide	●	...	...
Cyclosporine	●	...	...
Cytarabine	●	...	...
Dexamethasone sodium phosphate ...	●	...	...
Dexmedetomidine	●	...	...
Diazepam	...	●	...
Digoxin	...	●	...
Diphenhydramine HCl	●	...	...
Dobutamine HCl	●	...	...
Dopamine HCl	●	...	...
Doxorubicin HCl	...	●	...
Doxycycline hyclate	●	...	...
Droperidol	●	...	...
Enalaprilat	●	...	...

Drugs	Compatible	Incompatible	Variable
Ephedrine sulfate	●	...	...
Epinephrine HCl	●	...	...
Esmolol HCl	●	...	...
Famotidine	●	...	...
Fenoldopam mesylate	●	...	...
Fentanyl citrate	●	...	...
Fluconazole	●	...	...
Fluorouracil	●	...	...
Furosemide	●	...	...
Ganciclovir sodium	●	...	...
Gentamicin sulfate	...	●	...
Glycopyrrolate	●	...	...
Granisetron HCl	●	...	...
Haloperidol lactate	●	...	...
Heparin sodium	●	...	...
Hydrocortisone sodium succinate	●	...	...
Hydromorphone HCl	●	...	...
Hydroxyzine HCl	●	...	...
Ifosfamide	●	...	...
Imipenem–cilastatin sodium	●	...	...
Insulin, regular	●	...	...
Isoproterenol HCl	●	...	...
Ketamine HCl	●	...	...
Labetalol HCl	●	...	...
Levofloxacin	...	●	...
Lidocaine HCl	...	...	●
Lorazepam	●	...	...
Magnesium sulfate	●	...	...
Mannitol	●	...	...
Meperidine HCl	●	...	...
Methotrexate sodium	...	●	...
Methylprednisolone sod. succ.	...	●	...
Metoclopramide HCl	...	●	...
Midazolam HCl	...	...	●
Milrinone lactate	●	...	...
Mitoxantrone HCl	...	●	...
Morphine sulfate	...	...	●
Nafcillin sodium	●	...	...
Nalbuphine HCl	●	...	...
Naloxone HCl	●	...	...

Drugs	Compatible	Incompatible	Variable
Nitroglycerin	●	...	...
Norepinephrine bitartrate	●	...	...
Ondansetron HCl	●	...	...
Paclitaxel	●	...	...
Pancuronium bromide	...	...	●
Pantoprazole sodium	...	...	●
Pentobarbital sodium	●	...	...
Phenobarbital sodium	●	...	...
Phenylephrine HCl	...	...	●
Phenytoin sodium	...	●	...
Piperacillin sodium	●	...	...
Potassium chloride	●	...	...
Prochlorperazine edisylate	●	...	...
Propranolol HCl	●	...	...
Ranitidine HCl	●	...	...
Scopolamine HBr	●	...	...
Sodium bicarbonate	●	...	...
Sodium nitroprusside	●	...	...
Succinylcholine chloride	●	...	...
Sufentanil citrate	●	...	...
Thiopental sodium	●	...	...
Ticarcillin disod.–clavulanate pot.	●	...	...
Tobramycin sulfate	...	●	...
Vancomycin HCl	...	...	●
Vecuronium bromide	●	...	...
Verapamil HCl	...	●	...

Ranitidine Hydrochloride

Handbook on Injectable Drugs pp. 1439–1455.

Description: A histamine H$_2$ receptor antagonist.

Products: Zantac; 25-mg/mL solution in 2-mL vials, 6-mL multiple-dose vials, 40-mL bulk packages, and 50-mg/50-mL pre-mixed infusion solutions. *pH:* From 6.7 to 7.3.

Administration: Administer IM or IV. By direct IV injection, 50 mg is usually diluted to a total of 20 mL with compatible infusion solution and given over at least five minutes. For intermittent infusion, 50 mg may be added to 100 mL of an appropriate solution and infused over 15 to 20 minutes. For continuous IV infusion, 150 mg may be diluted in 250 mL of compatible IV fluid and infused at 6.25 mg/hr for 24 hours.

Stability: Store below 30 °C; protect from light. The product is a clear, colorless to yellow solution. Slight darkening does not affect potency.

Compatibility Table

Solutions	Compatible	Incompatible	Variable
Dextrose 5 & 10%	●	...	...
Dextrose 5% in Ringer's injection, lactated	...	...	●
Dextrose 5% in sodium chloride 0.45%	●	...	...
Ringer's injection, lactated	●	...	...
Sodium bicarbonate 5%	●	...	...
Sodium chloride 0.9%	●	...	...

Drugs	Compatible	Incompatible	Variable
Acetazolamide HCl	●	...	...
Acyclovir sodium	●	...	...
Aldesleukin	●	...	...
Allopurinol sodium	●	...	...
Amifostine	●	...	...

Drugs	Compatible	Incompatible	Variable
Amikacin sulfate	●	...	...
Aminophylline	●	...	...
Amphotericin B	...	●	...
Amphotericin B cholesteryl sulfate complex	...	●	...
Ampicillin sodium	...	...	●
Atracurium besylate	...	...	●
Atropine sulfate	●	...	...
Aztreonam	●	...	...
Bivalirudin	●	...	...
Cefamandole nafate	...	●	...
Cefazolin sodium	...	...	●
Cefepime HCl	●	...	...
Cefoxitin sodium	...	...	●
Ceftazidime	...	...	●
Ceftizoxime sodium	●	...	...
Cefuroxime sodium	...	...	●
Chloramphenicol sodium succinate	●	...	...
Chlorothiazide sodium	●	...	...
Chlorpromazine HCl	...	...	●
Ciprofloxacin	●	...	...
Cisatracurium besylate	●	...	...
Cisplatin	●	...	...
Cladribine	●	...	...
Clindamycin phosphate	...	...	●
Colistimethate sodium	●	...	...
Cyclophosphamide	●	...	...
Cytarabine	●	...	...
Dexamethasone sodium phosphate ...	●	...	...
Dexmedetomidine HCl	●	...	...
Diazepam	...	...	●
Digoxin	●	...	...
Diltiazem HCl	●	...	...
Dimenhydrinate	●	...	...
Diphenhydramine HCl	●	...	...
Dobutamine HCl	●	...	...
Docetaxel	●	...	...
Dopamine HCl	●	...	...
Doxapram HCl	●	...	...

Drugs	Compatible	Incompatible	Variable
Doxorubicin HCl	●	…	…
Doxorubicin HCl liposome injection	●	…	…
Doxycycline hyclate	●	…	…
Drotrecogin alfa (activated)	…	…	●
Enalaprilat	●	…	…
Epinephrine HCl	●	…	…
Erythromycin lactobionate	●	…	…
Esmolol HCl	●	…	…
Ethacrynate sodium	…	●	…
Etoposide phosphate	●	…	…
Fenoldopam mesylate	●	…	…
Fentanyl citrate	●	…	…
Filgrastim	●	…	…
Floxacillin sodium	●	…	…
Fluconazole	●	…	…
Fludarabine phosphate	●	…	…
Flumazenil	●	…	…
Foscarnet sodium	●	…	…
Furosemide	●	…	…
Gallium nitrate	●	…	…
Gemcitabine HCl	●	…	…
Gentamicin sulfate	●	…	…
Glycopyrrolate	●	…	…
Granisetron HCl	●	…	…
Heparin sodium	●	…	…
Hetastarch in sodium chloride 0.9%	…	…	●
Hextend	●	…	…
Hydromorphone HCl	●	…	…
Hydroxyzine HCl	…	●	…
Idarubicin HCl	●	…	…
Insulin, regular	…	…	●
Isoproterenol HCl	●	…	…
Labetalol HCl	●	…	…
Lansoprazole	…	●	…
Lidocaine HCl	●	…	…
Lincomycin HCl	●	…	…
Linezolid	●	…	…
Lorazepam	…	…	●

Drugs	Compatible	Incompatible	Variable
Melphalan HCl	●	...	...
Meperidine HCl	●	...	...
Meropenem	●	...	...
Methotrexate sodium	●	...	...
Methylprednisolone sod. succ.	●	...	...
Metoclopramide HCl	●	...	...
Midazolam HCl	...	...	●
Milrinone lactate	●	...	...
Morphine sulfate	●	...	...
Nalbuphine sulfate	●	...	...
Nicardipine HCl	●	...	...
Nitroglycerin	●	...	...
Norepinephrine bitartrate	...	...	●
Ondansetron HCl	●	...	...
Oxaliplatin	●	...	...
Oxymorphone HCl	●	...	...
Paclitaxel	●	...	...
Pancuronium bromide	●	...	...
Pantoprazole sodium	...	●	...
Pemetrexed disodium	●	...	...
Penicillin G potassium	●	...	...
Penicillin G sodium	●	...	...
Pentazocine lactate	●	...	...
Pentobarbital sodium	...	●	...
Phenobarbital sodium	...	●	...
Phytonadione	...	●	...
Piperacillin sodium	●	...	...
Piperacillin sod.–tazobactam sod.	●	...	...
Polymyxin B sulfate	●	...	...
Potassium chloride	●	...	...
Procainamide HCl	●	...	...
Prochlorperazine edisylate	●	...	...
Promethazine HCl	●	...	...
Propofol	●	...	...
Protamine sulfate	●	...	...
Quinidine gluconate	●	...	...
Remifentanil HCl	●	...	...
Sargramostim	●	...	...
Scopolamine HBr	●	...	...
Sodium nitroprusside	●	...	...

Drugs	Compatible	Incompatible	Variable
Tacrolimus	●	...	...
Teniposide	●	...	...
Theophylline	●	...	...
Thiethylperazine malate	●	...	...
Thiopental sodium	●	...	...
Thiotepa	●	...	...
Tobramycin sulfate	●	...	...
Vancomycin sulfate	●	...	...
Vecuronium bromide	●	...	...
Vinorelbine tartrate	●	...	...
Warfarin sodium	●	...	...
Zidovudine	●	...	...

Sargramostim

Handbook on Injectable Drugs pp. 1466–1470.

Description: A recombinant human granulocyte-macrophage colony stimulating factor.

Products: Leukine; 250-mcg in dry form and 500-mcg/1-mL liquid injection. *pH:* From 7.1 to 7.7.

Preparation: Reconstitute the dry product by directing 1 mL of sterile water for injection or bacteriostatic water for injection containing benzyl alcohol 0.9% at the sides of the vial. Gently swirl to avoid foaming during dissolution, and do not shake. For IV infusion, dilute the dose in sodium chloride 0.9%. For sargramostim concentrations below 10 mcg/mL, normal human serum albumin at a final concentration of 0.1% (1 mg/mL) should be added to prevent adsorption.

Administration: Administer the reconstituted solution by SC injection undiluted or by IV infusion usually over two to four hours after dilution in sodium chloride 0.9%.

Stability: Store intact vials and solutions under refrigeration and protected from freezing. The reconstituted solution is clear and colorless and should be used within six hours following reconstitution with sterile water for injection or within 20 days if reconstituted with bacteriostatic water for injection and stored under refrigeration.

Sargramostim will adsorb to containers and tubing if the concentration is below 10 mcg/mL. Albumin at a final concentration of 0.1% should be added to the IV solution to prevent this adsorption.

Compatibility Table

Solutions	Compatible	Incompatible	Variable
Sodium chloride 0.9%	●	...	...

Drugs	Compatible	Incompatible	Variable
Acyclovir sodium	...	●	...
Amikacin sulfate	●	...	...
Aminophylline	●	...	...
Amphotericin B	...	...	●
Ampicillin sodium	...	●	...

Drugs	Compatible	Incompatible	Variable
Ampicillin sod.–sulbactam sod.	...	●	...
Aztreonam	●	...	...
Bleomycin sulfate	●	...	...
Butorphanol tartrate	●	...	...
Calcium gluconate	●	...	...
Carboplatin........................	●	...	...
Carmustine	●	...	...
Cefazolin sodium	●	...	...
Cefepime HCl	●	...	...
Cefotaxime sodium	●	...	...
Cefotetan disodium	●	...	...
Ceftazidime	...	...	●
Ceftizoxime sodium	●	...	...
Ceftriaxone sodium	●	...	...
Cefuroxime sodium	●	...	...
Chlorpromazine HCl	...	●	...
Cimetidine HCl	●	...	...
Cisplatin	●	...	...
Clindamycin phosphate	●	...	...
Cyclophosphamide	●	...	...
Cyclosporine	●	...	...
Cytarabine	●	...	...
Dacarbazine	●	...	...
Dactinomycin	●	...	...
Dexamethasone sodium phosphate ...	●	...	...
Diphenhydramine HCl	●	...	...
Dopamine HCl	●	...	...
Doxorubicin HCl	●	...	...
Doxycycline hyclate	●	...	...
Droperidol	●	...	...
Etoposide	●	...	...
Famotidine	●	...	...
Fentanyl citrate	●	...	...
Floxuridine	●	...	...
Fluconazole	●	...	...
Fluorouracil	●	...	...
Furosemide	●	...	...
Ganciclovir sodium	...	●	...
Gentamicin sulfate	●	...	...
Granisetron HCl	●	...	...

Drugs	Compatible	Incompatible	Variable
Haloperidol lactate	...	●	...
Heparin sodium	●	...	...
Hydrocortisone sodium phosphate ...	...	●	...
Hydrocortisone sodium succinate	...	●	...
Hydromorphone HCl	...	●	...
Hydroxyzine HCl	...	●	...
Idarubicin HCl	●	...	...
Ifosfamide	●	...	...
Imipenem–cilastatin sodium	...	●	...
Immune globulin IV	●	...	...
Lorazepam	...	●	...
Magnesium sulfate	●	...	...
Mannitol	●	...	...
Mechlorethamine HCl	●	...	...
Meperidine HCl	●	...	...
Mesna	●	...	...
Methotrexate sodium	●	...	...
Methylprednisolone sod. succ.	...	●	...
Metoclopramide HCl	●	...	...
Metronidazole	●	...	...
Mitomycin	...	●	...
Mitoxantrone HCl	●	...	...
Morphine sulfate	...	●	...
Nalbuphine HCl	...	●	...
Ondansetron HCl	...	●	...
Pentostatin	●	...	...
Piperacillin sodium	...	●	...
Piperacillin sod.–tazobactam sod.	●	...	...
Potassium chloride	●	...	...
Prochlorperazine edisylate	●	...	...
Promethazine HCl	●	...	...
Ranitidine HCl	●	...	...
Sodium bicarbonate	...	●	...
Teniposide	●	...	...
Ticarcillin disod.–clavulanate pot.	●	...	...
Tobramycin sulfate	...	●	...
Trimethoprim–sulfamethoxazole	●	...	...
Vancomycin HCl	...	...	●
Vinblastine sulfate	●	...	...
Vincristine sulfate	●	...	...
Zidovudine	●	...	...

Scopolamine Hydrobromide

Handbook on Injectable Drugs pp. 1472–1476.

Description: An alkaloid, obtained from the plant *Atropa bella-donna*, that is a parasympatholytic agent.

Products: In concentrations of 0.4 and 1 mg/mL in 1-mL vials. *pH:* From 3.5 to 6.5.

Administration: Administer by SC, IM, or IV injection after dilution with sterile water for injection.

Stability: Store at controlled room temperature with protection from light. The minimum rate of decomposition occurs at pH 3.5.

Compatibility Table

Drugs	Compatible	Incompatible	Variable
Atropine sulfate	●	. . .	. . .
Buprenorphine HCl	●	. . .	. . .
Butorphanol tartrate	●	. . .	. . .
Chlorpromazine HCl	●	. . .	. . .
Cimetidine HCl	●	. . .	. . .
Dimenhydrinate	●	. . .	. . .
Diphenhydramine HCl	●	. . .	. . .
Droperidol	●	. . .	. . .
Fentanyl citrate	●	. . .	. . .
Furosemide	●	. . .	. . .
Glycopyrrolate	●	. . .	. . .
Heparin sodium	●	. . .	. . .
Hydrocortisone sodium succinate	●	. . .	. . .
Hydromorphone HCl	●	. . .	. . .
Hydroxyzine HCl	●	. . .	. . .
Meperidine HCl	●	. . .	. . .
Methadone HCl	●	. . .	. . .
Methohexital sodium	. . .	●	. . .
Metoclopramide HCl	●	. . .	. . .
Midazolam HCl	●	. . .	. . .

Drugs	Compatible	Incompatible	Variable
Morphine sulfate	●	...	...
Nalbuphine HCl	●	...	...
Pentazocine lactate	●	...	...
Pentobarbital sodium	●	...	...
Potassium chloride	●	...	...
Prochlorperazine edisylate	●	...	...
Promethazine HCl	●	...	...
Propofol	●	...	...
Ranitidine HCl	●	...	...
Succinylcholine chloride	●	...	...
Sufentanil citrate	●	...	...
Thiopental sodium	●	...	...

Sodium Bicarbonate

Handbook on Injectable Drugs pp. 1477–1490.

Description: Indicated as a parenteral electrolyte for the correction of metabolic acidosis and other conditions requiring alkalinization.

Products: 8.4%—50 mEq/50 mL, 10 mEq/10 mL
7.5%—44.6 mEq/50 mL
4.2%—5 mEq/10 mL

Also as a 5% solution in 500-mL (297.5 mEq) containers. *pH:* From 7 to 8.5.

Administration: Administer IV, either undiluted or diluted in other infusion fluids. It may also be given by SC injection if diluted to isotonicity.

Stability: The clear, colorless solution in intact containers should be stored at room temperature protected from freezing and heat. Do not use solutions that are not clear or that contain a precipitate.

Compatibility Table

Solutions	Compatible	Incompatible	Variable
Dextrose 5%	●	...	...
Dextrose 5% in Ringer's injection	●	...	...
Dextrose 5% in Ringer's injection, lactated	...	...	●
Dextrose 5% in sodium chloride 0.2, 0.45, & 0.9%	●	...	...
Ringer's injection	...	...	●
Ringer's injection, lactated	...	...	●
Sodium chloride 0.45 & 0.9%	●	...	...
Sodium lactate 1/6 M	...	...	●

Drugs			
Acyclovir sodium	●	...	...
Allopurinol sodium	...	●	...
Amifostine	●	...	...
Amikacin sulfate	●	...	...
Aminophylline	●	...	...

Drugs	Compatible	Incompatible	Variable
Amiodarone HCl	...	●	...
Amobarbital sodium	●	...	...
Amphotericin B	...	...	●
Amphotericin B cholesteryl sulfate complex	...	●	...
Ampicillin sodium	...	...	●
Ascorbic acid injection	...	●	...
Asparaginase	●	...	...
Atropine sulfate	●	...	...
Aztreonam	●	...	...
Bivalirudin	●	...	...
Bupivacaine HCl	...	...	●
Caffeine citrate	●	...	...
Calcium chloride	...	...	●
Calcium gluconate	...	...	●
Carboplatin........................	...	●	...
Carmustine	...	●	...
Cefepime HCl	●	...	...
Cefotaxime sodium	...	●	...
Cefoxitin sodium	●	...	...
Ceftazidime........................	●	...	...
Ceftriaxone sodium	●	...	...
Chloramphenicol sodium succinate	●	...	...
Chlorothiazide sodium	●	...	...
Chloroprocaine HCl	...	...	●
Cimetidine HCl	●	...	...
Ciprofloxacin	...	...	●
Cisatracurium besylate	...	...	●
Cisplatin	...	●	...
Cladribine	●	...	...
Clindamycin phosphate	●	...	...
Corticotropin	...	...	●
Cyclophosphamide	●	...	...
Cytarabine........................	●	...	...
Daunorubicin HCl	●	...	...
Dexamethasone sodium phosphate ...	●	...	...
Dexmedetomidine HCl	●	...	...
Diltiazem HCl	...	...	●
Dimenhydrinate	...	●	...

Drugs	Compatible	Incompatible	Variable
Dobutamine HCl	...	●	...
Docetaxel	●	...	...
Dopamine HCl	...	●	...
Doxorubicin HCl	●	...	...
Doxorubicin HCl liposome injection	...	●	...
Epinephrine HCl	...	●	...
Ergonovine maleate	●	...	...
Erythromycin lactobionate	●	...	...
Esmolol HCl	●	...	...
Etoposide	●	...	...
Etoposide phosphate	●	...	...
Famotidine	●	...	...
Fenoldopam mesylate	...	●	...
Filgrastim	●	...	...
Fludarabine phosphate	●	...	...
Furosemide	●	...	...
Gallium nitrate	●	...	...
Gemcitabine HCl	●	...	...
Glycopyrrolate	...	●	...
Granisetron HCl	●	...	...
Heparin sodium	●	...	...
Hextend	...	●	...
Hyaluronidase	●	...	...
Hydrocortisone sodium phosphate ...	●	...	...
Hydrocortisone sodium succinate	●	...	...
Hydromorphone HCl	...	●	...
Idarubicin HCl	...	●	...
Ifosfamide	●	...	...
Imipenem–cilastatin sodium	...	●	...
Indomethacin sodium trihydrate	●	...	...
Insulin, regular	●	...	...
Isoproterenol HCl	...	●	...
Kanamycin sulfate	●	...	...
Labetalol HCl	...	●	...
Lansoprazole	...	●	...
Leucovorin calcium	...	●	...
Levofloxacin	●	...	...
Lidocaine HCl	...	...	●
Linezolid	●	...	...
Magnesium sulfate	...	●	...

Drugs	Compatible	Incompatible	Variable
Mannitol	●	...	...
Melphalan HCl	●	...	...
Meperidine HCl	...	...	●
Mepivacaine HCl	...	●	...
Meropenem	...	●	...
Mesna	●	...	...
Methotrexate sodium	●	...	...
Methyldopate HCl	●	...	...
Methylprednisolone sod. succ.	...	...	●
Metoclopramide HCl	...	●	...
Midazolam HCl	...	●	...
Milrinone lactate	●	...	...
Morphine sulfate	...	...	●
Nafcillin sodium	●	...	...
Nalbuphine HCl	...	●	...
Nalmefene HCl	●	...	...
Nicardipine HCl	...	●	...
Norepinephrine bitartrate	...	●	...
Ondansetron HCl	...	●	...
Oxacillin sodium	...	...	●
Oxytocin	●	...	...
Paclitaxel	●	...	...
Pantoprazole sodium	...	●	...
Pemetrexed disodium	●	...	...
Penicillin G potassium	...	●	...
Pentazocine lactate	...	●	...
Pentobarbital sodium	...	...	●
Phenobarbital sodium	●	...	...
Phenylephrine HCl	●	...	...
Phenytoin sodium	●	...	...
Phytonadione	●	...	...
Piperacillin sod.–tazobactam sod.	●	...	...
Potassium chloride	●	...	...
Procaine HCl	...	●	...
Prochlorperazine edisylate	●	...	...
Propofol	●	...	...
Remifentanil HCl	●	...	...
Sargramostim	...	●	...
Sodium lactate	...	...	●
Streptomycin sulfate	...	●	...

Drugs	Compatible	Incompatible	Variable
Succinylcholine chloride	...	●	...
Tacrolimus	●	...	...
Teniposide	●	...	...
Thiopental sodium	...	...	●
Thiotepa	●	...	...
Ticarcillin disod.–clavulanate pot.	...	●	...
Vancomycin HCl	...	...	●
Verapamil HCl	...	...	●
Vincristine sulfate	...	●	...
Vinorelbine tartrate	...	●	...

Sufentanil Citrate

Handbook on Injectable Drugs pp. 1513–1518.

Description: A synthetic opiate agonist.

Products: **Sufenta;** 50 mcg/mL in 1-, 2-, and 5-mL ampuls. *pH:* From 3.5 to 6.

Preparation: By IV injection undiluted or as an infusion in a compatible diluent.

Administration: Administer by slow direct IV injection or IV infusion. It is also administered epidurally and by IM injection.

Stability: Sufentanil citrate is a clear, colorless liquid. It should be stored at room temperature and protected from light. The drug is slowly hydrolyzed in acidic solutions with a pH of 3 or below.

Sufentanil citrate sorbs to PVC/Kalex CADD pump plastic reservoirs.

Compatibility Table

Solutions	Compatible	Incompatible	Variable
Dextrose 5%	●	...	...
Sodium chloride 0.9%	...	...	●

Drugs			
Amphotericin B cholesteryl sulfate complex	●	...	...
Atracurium besylate	●	...	...
Atropine sulfate	●	...	...
Bivalirudin	●	...	...
Bupivacaine HCl	●	...	...
Cefepime HCl	●	...	...
Ceftazidime	●	...	...
Cisatracurium besylate	●	...	...
Dexamethasone sodium phosphate ...	●	...	...
Dexmedetomidine HCl	●	...	...
Diazepam	...	...	●
Diphenhydramine HCl	●	...	...
Etomidate	●	...	...
Fenoldopam mesylate	●	...	...

Drugs	Compatible	Incompatible	Variable
Haloperidol lactate	●	...	...
Hextend	●	...	...
Hydroxyzine HCl	●	...	...
Ketorolac tromethamine	●	...	...
Lansoprazole	●	...	...
Levobupivacaine HCl	●	...	...
Linezolid	●	...	...
Lorazepam	...	●	...
Metoclopramide HCl	●	...	...
Midazolam HCl	●	...	...
Phenobarbital sodium	...	...	●
Phenytoin sodium	...	●	...
Prochlorperazine edisylate	●	...	...
Propofol	●	...	...
Remifentanil HCl	●	...	...
Ropivacaine HCl	●	...	...
Scopolamine HBr	●	...	...
Thiopental sodium	...	●	...

Tacrolimus

Handbook on Injectable Drugs pp. 1519–1522.

Description: A potent immunosuppressive agent used in the prevention of liver allograft rejection.

Products: Prograf; 5 mg/mL as a concentrate in 1-mL ampuls.

Preparation: By IV infusion, the concentrate must be diluted to 0.004 to 0.02 mg/mL in dextrose 5% or sodium chloride 0.9% in a glass or polyethylene container. *Do not use DEHP-plasticized PVC containers or administration sets.*

Administration: Administer by IV infusion after appropriate dilution.

Stability: Store intact containers between 5 and 25 °C. Tacrolimus is most stable between pH 2 and 6; the rate of decomposition increases substantially at higher pH values. Dilutions to concentrations of 0.004 to 0.02 mg/mL in dextrose 5% or sodium chloride 0.9% in glass or polyethylene containers are stable for 24 hours at room temperature. Tacrolimus undergoes sorption to PVC plastic IV bags.

The tacrolimus formulation contains a surfactant which causes extraction of DEHP plasticizer from PVC bags of solutions and PVC administration sets. Consequently, glass or polyethylene containers and non-DEHP plasticized administration sets are recommended. PVC containers and administration sets should be avoided.

Compatibility Table

Solutions	Compatible	Incompatible	Variable
Dextrose 5%	●	...	...
Sodium chloride 0.9%	●	...	...

Drugs	Compatible	Incompatible	Variable
Acyclovir sodium	...	●	...
Aminophylline	●	...	...
Amphotericin B	●	...	...
Ampicillin sodium	●	...	...
Ampicillin sod.–sulbactam sod.	●	...	...

Drugs	Compatible	Incompatible	Variable
Calcium gluconate	●	…	…
Cefazolin sodium	●	…	…
Cefotetan disodium	●	…	…
Ceftazidime	●	…	…
Ceftriaxone sodium	●	…	…
Cefuroxime sodium	●	…	…
Chloramphenicol sodium succinate	●	…	…
Cimetidine HCl	●	…	…
Ciprofloxacin	●	…	…
Clindamycin phosphate	●	…	…
Dexamethasone sodium phosphate	●	…	…
Digoxin	●	…	…
Diphenhydramine HCl	●	…	…
Dobutamine HCl	●	…	…
Dopamine HCl	●	…	…
Doxycycline hyclate	●	…	…
Erythromycin lactobionate	●	…	…
Esmolol HCl	●	…	…
Fluconazole	●	…	…
Furosemide	●	…	…
Ganciclovir sodium	…	●	…
Gentamicin sulfate	●	…	…
Haloperidol lactate	●	…	…
Heparin sodium	●	…	…
Hydrocortisone sodium succinate	●	…	…
Hydromorphone HCl	●	…	…
Imipenem–cilastatin sodium	●	…	…
Insulin, regular	●	…	…
Isoproterenol HCl	●	…	…
Leucovorin calcium	●	…	…
Lorazepam	●	…	…
Methylprednisolone sod. succ.	●	…	…
Metoclopramide HCl	●	…	…
Metronidazole	●	…	…
Morphine sulfate	●	…	…
Multivitamins	●	…	…
Nitroglycerin	●	…	…
Oxacillin sodium	●	…	…
Penicillin G potassium	●	…	…

Drugs	Compatible	Incompatible	Variable
Phenytoin sodium	●	...	...
Piperacillin sodium	●	...	...
Potassium chloride	●	...	...
Propranolol HCl	●	...	...
Ranitidine HCl	●	...	...
Sodium bicarbonate	●	...	...
Sodium nitroprusside	●	...	...
Tobramycin sulfate	●	...	...
Trimethoprim–sulfamethoxazole	●	...	...
Vancomycin HCl	●	...	...

Teniposide

Handbook on Injectable Drugs pp. 1524–1532.

Description: A semisynthetic podophyllotoxin-derivative antineoplastic agent.

Products: Vumon; 10 mg/mL as a concentrate in 5-mL ampuls. *pH:* Approximately 5.

Preparation: By IV infusion, the concentrate must be diluted to 0.1 to 1 mg/mL in dextrose 5% or sodium chloride 0.9% in a glass or polyolefin container. *Do not use DEHP-plasticized PVC containers or administration sets.*

Administration: Administer by IV infusion over 30 to 60 minutes after appropriate dilution. Avoid extravasation because of possible tissue irritation and phlebitis.

Stability: Teniposide in intact ampuls should be stored under refrigeration in the original package to protect from light. The concentrate is clear, but after dilution in infusion solutions, a slight opalescence may be present. Dilutions to concentrations of 0.1 to 0.4 mg/mL in dextrose 5% or sodium chloride 0.9% in glass or polyolefin containers are stable for 24 hours at room temperature. At 1 mg/mL, the potential for precipitation is greater so that administration should be completed within four hours. Although chemically stable, teniposide aqueous dilutions exhibit irregular and unpredictable precipitation, even at low concentrations around 0.1 mg/mL.

The teniposide formulation contains a surfactant which causes extraction of DEHP plasticizer from PVC bags of solutions and PVC administration sets. Consequently, glass or polyethylene containers and non-DEHP plasticized administration sets are recommended. PVC containers and administration sets should be avoided.

Compatibility Table

Solutions	Compatible	Incompatible	Variable
Dextrose 5%	●	...	...
Ringer's injection, lactated	●	...	...
Sodium chloride 0.9%	●	...	...

Drugs	Compatible	Incompatible	Variable
Acyclovir sodium	●	...	...
Allopurinol sodium	●	...	...
Amifostine........................	●	...	...
Amikacin sulfate	●	...	...
Aminophylline	●	...	...
Amphotericin B	●	...	...
Ampicillin sodium	●	...	...
Ampicillin sod.–sulbactam sod.	●	...	...
Aztreonam	●	...	...
Bleomycin sulfate	●	...	...
Bumetanide	●	...	...
Buprenorphine HCl	●	...	...
Butorphanol tartrate	●	...	...
Calcium gluconate	●	...	...
Carboplatin......................	●	...	...
Carmustine	●	...	...
Cefazolin sodium	●	...	...
Cefotaxime sodium................	●	...	...
Cefotetan disodium	●	...	...
Cefoxitin sodium	●	...	...
Ceftazidime......................	●	...	...
Ceftizoxime sodium	●	...	...
Ceftriaxone sodium	●	...	...
Cefuroxime sodium	●	...	...
Chlorpromazine HCl	●	...	...
Cimetidine HCl	●	...	...
Ciprofloxacin	●	...	...
Cisplatin	●	...	...
Cladribine.......................	●	...	...
Clindamycin phosphate	●	...	...
Cyclophosphamide	●	...	...
Cytarabine.......................	●	...	...
Dacarbazine.....................	●	...	...
Dactinomycin....................	●	...	...
Daunorubicin HCl	●	...	...
Dexamethasone sodium phosphate ...	●	...	...
Diphenhydramine HCl	●	...	...
Doxorubicin HCl	●	...	...
Doxycycline hyclate	●	...	...
Droperidol	●	...	...

Drugs	Compatible	Incompatible	Variable
Enalaprilat	●	...	...
Etoposide	●	...	...
Etoposide phosphate	●	...	...
Famotidine	●	...	...
Floxuridine	●	...	...
Fluconazole	●	...	...
Fludarabine phosphate	●	...	...
Fluorouracil	●	...	...
Furosemide	●	...	...
Gallium nitrate	●	...	...
Ganciclovir sodium	●	...	...
Gemcitabine HCl	●	...	...
Gentamicin sulfate	●	...	...
Granisetron HCl	●	...	...
Haloperidol lactate	●	...	...
Heparin sodium	...	●	...
Hydrocortisone sodium phosphate	●	...	...
Hydrocortisone sodium succinate	●	...	...
Hydromorphone HCl	●	...	...
Hydroxyzine HCl	●	...	...
Idarubicin HCl	...	●	...
Ifosfamide	●	...	...
Imipenem–cilastatin sodium	●	...	...
Leucovorin calcium	●	...	...
Lorazepam	●	...	...
Mannitol	●	...	...
Mechlorethamine HCl	●	...	...
Melphalan HCl	●	...	...
Meperidine HCl	●	...	...
Mesna	●	...	...
Methotrexate sodium	●	...	...
Methylprednisolone sod. succ.	●	...	...
Metoclopramide HCl	●	...	...
Metronidazole	●	...	...
Mitomycin	●	...	...
Mitoxantrone HCl	●	...	...
Morphine sulfate	●	...	...
Nalbuphine HCl	●	...	...
Ondansetron HCl	●	...	...
Piperacillin sodium	●	...	...

Drugs	Compatible	Incompatible	Variable
Potassium chloride	●	...	...
Prochlorperazine edisylate	●	...	...
Promethazine HCl	●	...	...
Ranitidine HCl	●	...	...
Sargramostim	●	...	...
Sodium bicarbonate	●	...	...
Streptozocin	●	...	...
Thiotepa	●	...	...
Ticarcillin disod.–clavulanate pot.	●	...	...
Tobramycin sulfate	●	...	...
Trimethoprim–sulfamethoxazole	●	...	...
Vancomycin HCl	●	...	...
Vinblastine sulfate	●	...	...
Vincristine sulfate	●	...	...
Vinorelbine tartrate	●	...	...
Zidovudine	●	...	...

Theophylline

Handbook on Injectable Drugs pp. 1534–1537.

Description: A xanthine derivative used as a bronchodilator.

Products: Available in concentrations ranging from 0.4 to 4 mg/mL in dextrose 5% packaged in various container sizes. *pH:* From 3.5 to 6.5.

Administration: Administer by continuous or intermittent IV infusion. Slow administration, not exceeding 20 mg/min, has been recommended. Loading doses are usually given over 20 to 30 minutes.

Stability: Store intact containers at room temperature protected from freezing and excessive heat. No decrease in theophylline content was found after autoclaving for 20 minutes at 120 °C.

Compatibility Table

Drugs	Compatible	Incompatible	Variable
Acyclovir sodium	●	…	…
Ampicillin sodium	●	…	…
Ampicillin sod.–sulbactam sod.	●	…	…
Ascorbic acid injection	…	●	…
Aztreonam	●	…	…
Bivalirudin	●	…	…
Cefazolin sodium	●	…	…
Cefepime HCl	●	…	…
Cefotetan disodium	●	…	…
Ceftazidime	●	…	…
Ceftriaxone sodium	…	…	●
Chlorpromazine HCl	●	…	…
Cimetidine HCl	…	…	●
Cisatracurium besylate	●	…	…
Clindamycin phosphate	●	…	…
Dexamethasone sodium phosphate	●	…	…
Dexmedetomidine HCl	●	…	…
Diltiazem HCl	●	…	…
Dobutamine HCl	●	…	…
Dopamine HCl	●	…	…
Doxycycline hyclate	●	…	…
Erythromycin lactobionate	●	…	…
Famotidine	●	…	…
Fenoldopam mesylate	●	…	…
Fluconazole	●	…	…

Drugs	Compatible	Incompatible	Variable
Furosemide	●	...	...
Gentamicin sulfate	●	...	...
Haloperidol lactate	●	...	...
Heparin sodium	●	...	...
Hetastarch in sodium chloride 0.9%	...	●	...
Hextend	●	...	...
Hydrocortisone sodium succinate	●	...	...
Lansoprazole	...	●	...
Lidocaine HCl	●	...	...
Linezolid	●	...	...
Methyldopate HCl	●	...	...
Methylprednisolone sod. succ.	●	...	...
Metronidazole	●	...	...
Midazolam HCl	●	...	...
Milrinone lactate	●	...	...
Nafcillin sodium	●	...	...
Nitroglycerin	●	...	...
Oxaliplatin	●	...	...
Papaverine HCl	●	...	...
Penicillin G potassium	●	...	...
Phenytoin sodium	...	●	...
Piperacillin sodium	●	...	...
Potassium chloride	●	...	...
Ranitidine HCl	●	...	...
Remifentanil HCl	●	...	...
Sodium nitroprusside	●	...	...
Ticarcillin disod.–clavulanate pot.	●	...	...
Tobramycin sulfate	●	...	...
Vancomycin HCl	●	...	...
Verapamil HCl	●	...	...

Thiopental Sodium

Handbook on Injectable Drugs pp. 1541–1548.

Description: A short-acting barbiturate anesthetic.

Products: **Pentothal Sodium;** Available in sizes from 250 mg to 5 g. *pH:* A 2.5% solution in water has a pH of 10 to 11.

Preparation: Reconstitute only with sterile water for injection, sodium chloride 0.9%, or dextrose 5% in the 2 to 5% thiopental sodium concentration range. Reconstitute with dextrose 5%, sodium chloride 0.9%, or Normosol R, pH 7.4 for the 0.2 to 0.4% thiopental sodium concentration range.

Administration: Administer by slow IV infusion only. For intermittent IV administration in sterile water for injection, dextrose 5%, or sodium chloride 0.9%, usual concentrations are 2 to 2.5% but may range up to 5%. By continuous IV drip, concentrations of 0.2 to 0.4% in dextrose 5%, sodium chloride 0.9%, or Normosol R, pH 7.4 are used. Sterile water for injection should not be used for these low concentrations because of the danger of hemolysis from the hypotonic solutions. Extravasation and intra-arterial administration of the highly alkaline solutions should be avoided.

Stability: Store intact containers at room temperature. Reconstituted solutions are stable for three days at room temperature and seven days under refrigeration. Extensive sorption of thiopental to plastic infusion solution bags and administration sets has been found, particularly at lower pH values.

Compatibility Table

Solutions	Compatible	Incompatible	Variable
Dextrose 5%	●	...	...
Dextrose 5% in Ringer's injection, lactated	...	●	...
Dextrose 5% in sodium chloride 0.2 & 0.45%	●	...	...

Solutions	Compatible	Incompatible	Variable
Dextrose 5% in sodium chloride 0.9%	...	...	●
Normosol R, pH 7.4	●	...	...
Other Normosol solutions	...	●	...
Ringer's injection	...	●	...
Ringer's injection, lactated	...	●	...
Sodium chloride 0.9%	●	...	...

Drugs	Compatible	Incompatible	Variable
Alfentanil HCl	...	●	...
Amikacin sulfate	...	●	...
Aminophylline	●	...	...
Ascorbic acid injection	...	●	...
Atracurium besylate	...	●	...
Atropine sulfate	...	●	...
Bivalirudin	●	...	...
Chloramphenicol sodium succinate	●	...	...
Chlorpromazine HCl	...	●	...
Cimetidine HCl	...	●	...
Cisatracurium besylate	...	...	●
Clindamycin phosphate	...	●	...
Diltiazem HCl	...	●	...
Dimenhydrinate	...	●	...
Diphenhydramine HCl	...	●	...
Dobutamine HCl	...	●	...
Dopamine HCl	...	●	...
Doxapram HCl	...	●	...
Droperidol	...	●	...
Ephedrine sulfate	...	...	●
Epinephrine HCl	...	●	...
Fenoldopam mesylate	...	●	...
Fentanyl citrate	...	...	●
Furosemide	...	●	...
Glycopyrrolate	...	●	...
Heparin sodium	●	...	...
Hextend	●	...	...
Hyaluronidase	●	...	...
Hydrocortisone sodium succinate	●	...	...
Hydromorphone HCl	...	●	...
Insulin, regular	...	●	...
Isoproterenol HCl	...	●	...
Labetalol HCl	...	●	...
Lidocaine HCl	...	●	...

Drugs	Compatible	Incompatible	Variable
Lorazepam	...	...	●
Meperidine HCl	...	●	...
Midazolam HCl	...	●	...
Milrinone lactate	●	...	...
Mivacurium chloride	●	...	...
Morphine sulfate	...	...	●
Neostigmine methylsulfate	●	...	...
Nicardipine HCl	...	●	...
Nitroglycerin	●	...	...
Norepinephrine bitartrate	...	●	...
Oxytocin	●	...	...
Pancuronium bromide	...	●	...
Pantoprazole sodium	...	●	...
Penicillin G potassium	...	●	...
Pentazocine lactate	...	●	...
Pentobarbital sodium	●	...	...
Phenobarbital sodium	●	...	...
Phenylephrine HCl	...	●	...
Potassium chloride	●	...	...
Prochlorperazine edisylate	...	●	...
Promethazine HCl	...	●	...
Propofol	●	...	...
Ranitidine HCl	●	...	...
Remifentanil HCl	●	...	...
Scopolamine HBr	●	...	...
Sodium bicarbonate	...	...	●
Succinylcholine chloride	...	●	...
Sufentanil citrate	...	●	...
Thiamine HCl	...	●	...
Tubocurarine chloride	...	...	●
Vecuronium bromide	...	●	...

Ticarcillin Disodium–Clavulanate Potassium

Handbook on Injectable Drugs pp. 1557–1561.

Description: A combination of a semisynthetic penicillin and an inhibitor of penicillin inactivation.

Products: Timentin; Vials containing ticarcillin 3 g as the disodium salt with clavulanic acid 100 mg as the potassium salt (3.1-g vials and piggyback bottles). *pH:* From 5.5 to 7.5.

Preparation: Reconstitute the vials with 13 mL of sterile water for injection or sodium chloride 0.9% and shake well to yield a ticarcillin solution of 200 mg/mL with 6.7 mg/mL of clavulanic acid. For IV infusion, dilute to 10 to 100 mg/mL of ticarcillin in a compatible diluent.

Reconstitute the piggyback bottles with 50 to 100 mL of sodium chloride 0.9%, dextrose 5%, or lactated Ringer's injection.

Administration: Administer by intermittent IV infusion over 30 minutes.

Stability: Store the white to pale yellow powder at 24 °C or less. Higher temperatures cause degradation of clavulanate potassium, leading to darkening.

Concentrated solutions are colorless to pale yellow and are stable for six hours at 21 to 24 °C or 72 hours when refrigerated.

Compatibility Table

Solutions	Compatible	Incompatible	Variable
Dextrose 5%*	●	...	...
Ringer's injection, lactated*	●	...	...
Sodium chloride 0.9%*	●	...	...
Sterile water for injection*	●	...	...

*Diluted to a ticarcillin concentration of 10 to 100 mg/mL.

Drugs	Compatible	Incompatible	Variable
Allopurinol sodium	●	...	...
Amifostine	●	...	...
Aminoglycosides	...	●	...
Amphotericin B cholesteryl sulfate complex	...	●	...

Drugs	Compatible	Incompatible	Variable
Azithromycin	...	●	...
Aztreonam	●	...	...
Bivalirudin	●	...	...
Cefepime HCl	●	...	...
Ciprofloxacin	...	...	●
Cisatracurium besylate	...	...	●
Cyclophosphamide	●	...	...
Dexmedetomidine HCl	●	...	...
Diltiazem HCl	●	...	...
Docetaxel	●	...	...
Doxorubicin HCl liposome injection	●	...	...
Drotrecogin alfa (activated)	...	●	...
Etoposide phosphate	●	...	...
Famotidine	●	...	...
Fenoldopam mesylate	●	...	...
Filgrastim	●	...	...
Fluconazole	●	...	...
Fludarabine phosphate	●	...	...
Foscarnet sodium	●	...	...
Gallium nitrate	●	...	...
Gemcitabine HCl	●	...	...
Granisetron HCl	●	...	...
Heparin sodium	●	...	...
Hextend	●	...	...
Insulin, regular	●	...	...
Lansoprazole	...	●	...
Melphalan HCl	●	...	...
Meperidine HCl	●	...	...
Milrinone lactate	●	...	...
Morphine sulfate	●	...	...
Ondansetron HCl	●	...	...
Pantoprazole sodium	●	...	...
Pemetrexed disodium	●	...	...
Propofol	●	...	...
Remifentanil HCl	●	...	...
Sargramostim	●	...	...
Sodium bicarbonate	...	●	...
Teniposide	●	...	...
Theophylline	●	...	...
Thiotepa	●	...	...
Topotecan HCl	...	...	●
Vancomycin HCl	...	...	●
Vinorelbine tartrate	●	...	...

Ticarcillin Disodium–Clavulanate Potassium

Tobramycin Sulfate

Handbook on Injectable Drugs pp. 1564–1576.

Description: An aminoglycoside antibiotic.

Products: **Nebcin;** 40 mg/mL in 2- and 30-mL vials and 1.5- and 2-mL disposable syringes; also 10 mg/mL (pediatric) in 2-mL vials. It is also available premixed in sodium chloride 0.9% in 0.8-mg/mL (80 mg), 1.2-mg/mL (60 mg), and 1.6-mg/mL (80 mg) concentrations. *pH:* From 3 to 6.5.

Preparation: For IV infusion to adults, dilute the dose in 50 to 100 mL of compatible infusion solution. For children, the volume should be proportionately less.

Administration: Administer by IM injection or IV infusion over 20 to 60 minutes.

Stability: Store intact containers at room temperature protected from heat and freezing. The drug is very stable in solution and may be autoclaved without loss of potency. No sorption to plastic IV bags, sets, filters, or syringes has been noted.

Compatibility Table

Solutions	Compatible	Incompatible	Variable
Dextrose 5 & 10%	●	...	...
Dextrose 5% in Polysal	...	●	...
Dextrose 5% in sodium chloride 0.9%	●	...	...
Isolyte E, M, & P in dextrose 5%	...	●	...
Ringer's injection	●	...	...
Ringer's injection, lactated	●	...	...
Sodium chloride 0.9%	●	...	...

Drugs	Compatible	Incompatible	Variable
Acyclovir sodium	●	...	...
Aldesleukin	●	...	...
Allopurinol sodium	...	●	...
Amifostine	●	...	...
Amiodarone HCl	●	...	...

Drugs	Compatible	Incompatible	Variable
Amphotericin B cholesteryl sulfate complex	...	•	...
Azithromycin	...	•	...
Aztreonam	•	...	...
Bivalirudin	•	...	...
Bleomycin sulfate	•	...	...
Calcium gluconate	•	...	...
Cefamandole nafate	...	•	...
Cefepime HCl	...	...	•
Cefotaxime sodium	...	•	...
Cefotetan disodium	...	•	...
Cefoxitin sodium	•	...	...
Ceftazidime	•	...	...
Ciprofloxacin	•	...	...
Cisatracurium besylate	•	...	...
Clindamycin phosphate	...	...	•
Cyclophosphamide	•	...	...
Dexmedetomidine HCl	•	...	...
Diltiazem HCl	•	...	...
Dimenhydrinate	•	...	...
Docetaxel	•	...	...
Doxapram HCl	•	...	...
Doxorubicin HCl liposome injection	•	...	...
Drotrecogin alfa (activated)	...	•	...
Enalaprilat	•	...	...
Esmolol HCl	•	...	...
Etoposide phosphate	•	...	...
Fenoldopam mesylate	•	...	...
Filgrastim	•	...	...
Fluconazole	•	...	...
Fludarabine phosphate	•	...	...
Foscarnet sodium	•	...	...
Furosemide	•	...	...
Gemcitabine HCl	•	...	...
Granisetron HCl	•	...	...
Heparin sodium	...	•	...
Hetastarch in sodium chloride 0.9%	...	•	...
Hextend	•	...	...

Drugs	Compatible	Incompatible	Variable
Hydromorphone HCl	●	...	...
Indomethacin sodium trihydrate	...	●	...
Insulin, regular	●	...	...
Labetalol HCl	●	...	...
Lansoprazole	...	●	...
Linezolid	●	...	...
Magnesium sulfate	...	...	●
Melphalan HCl	●	...	...
Meperidine HCl	●	...	...
Metronidazole	●	...	...
Midazolam HCl	●	...	...
Milrinone lactate	●	...	...
Morphine sulfate	●	...	...
Nicardipine HCl	●	...	...
Pantoprazole sodium	...	●	...
Pemetrexed disodium	...	●	...
Piperacillin sodium	...	●	...
Propofol	...	●	...
Ranitidine HCl	●	...	...
Remifentanil HCl	●	...	...
Sargramostim	...	●	...
Tacrolimus	●	...	...
Teniposide	●	...	...
Theophylline	●	...	...
Verapamil HCl	●	...	...
Vinorelbine tartrate	●	...	...
Zidovudine	●	...	...

Trimethoprim-Sulfamethoxazole

Handbook on Injectable Drugs pp. 1585–1592.

Description: A fixed combination of two synthetic folate-antagonist anti-infectives.

Products: Bactrim, Septra; Trimethoprim 16 mg/mL with sulfamethoxazole 80 mg/mL in 5-, 10-, and 20-mL vials as a concentrate that must be diluted for use. *pH:* Approximately 10.

Preparation: For IV infusion, each 5 mL of drug should be diluted in 100 to 125 mL (or 75 mL if fluid is restricted) of dextrose 5%.

Administration: Administer only by IV infusion over 60 to 90 minutes.

Stability: Store vials at room temperature. Do not refrigerate. The solubility of trimethoprim in aqueous solutions is partially dependent on solution pH; its solubility is lower at alkaline pH.

No sorption to plastic IV bags, sets, or syringes has been noted.

Compatibility Table

Solutions	Compatible	Incompatible	Variable
NOTE: Precipitation from infusion solutions occurs in varying time periods depending on solution pH and drug concentration. Caution and close inspection are warranted for all admixtures.			
Dextrose 5%	...	...	●
Dextrose 5% in sodium chloride 0.45%	...	...	●
Ringer's injection, lactated	...	...	●
Sodium chloride 0.45 & 0.9%	...	...	●

Drugs			
Acyclovir sodium	●	...	...
Aldesleukin	●	...	...
Allopurinol sodium	●	...	...
Amifostine	●	...	...
Amphotericin B cholesteryl sulfate complex	●	...	...

Drugs	Compatible	Incompatible	Variable
Atracurium besylate	●	...	...
Aztreonam	●	...	...
Bivalirudin	●	...	...
Cefepime HCl	●	...	...
Cisatracurium besylate	...	...	●
Cyclophosphamide	●	...	...
Dexmedetomidine HCl	●	...	...
Diltiazem HCl	●	...	...
Dimenhydrinate	●	...	...
Docetaxel	●	...	...
Doxorubicin HCl liposome injection	●	...	...
Enalaprilat	●	...	...
Esmolol HCl	●	...	...
Etoposide phosphate	●	...	...
Fenoldopam mesylate	●	...	...
Filgrastim	●	...	...
Fluconazole	...	●	...
Fludarabine phosphate	●	...	...
Foscarnet sodium	...	...	●
Gallium nitrate	●	...	...
Gemcitabine HCl	●	...	...
Granisetron HCl	●	...	...
Heparin sodium	●	...	...
Hextend	●	...	...
Hydromorphone HCl	●	...	...
Labetalol HCl	●	...	...
Lansoprazole	●	...	...
Linezolid	...	●	...
Lorazepam	●	...	...
Magnesium sulfate	●	...	...
Melphalan HCl	●	...	...
Meperidine HCl	●	...	...
Midazolam HCl	...	●	...
Morphine sulfate	●	...	...
Nicardipine HCl	●	...	...
Pancuronium bromide	●	...	...
Pantoprazole sodium	...	●	...
Pemetrexed disodium	●	...	...
Piperacillin sod.–tazobactam sod.	●	...	...

Drugs	Compatible	Incompatible	Variable
Remifentanil HCl	●	...	...
Sargramostim	●	...	...
Tacrolimus	●	...	...
Teniposide	●	...	...
Thiotepa	●	...	...
Vecuronium bromide	●	...	...
Verapamil HCl	...	●	...
Vinorelbine tartrate	...	●	...
Zidovudine	●	...	...

Trimethoprim–Sulfamethoxazole

Vancomycin Hydrochloride

Handbook on Injectable Drugs pp. 1595–1609.

Description: A glycopeptide antibiotic active against many gram-positive organisms.

Products: **Vancocin Hydrochloride;** 500-mg and 1-g vials as the base and 500-mg and 1-g frozen premixed solutions. *pH:* From 2.5 to 4.5 when reconstituted.

Preparation: Reconstitute the 500-mg vial with 10 mL and the 1-g vial with 20 mL of sterile water for injection to yield a 50-mg/mL solution. For intermittent infusion, add the dose to 100 to 200 mL of dextrose 5% or sodium chloride 0.9%.

Administration: Administer by continuous or intermittent IV infusion over at least one hour. Do not give IM and avoid extravasation during IV administration because of extreme irritation and possible necrosis. Thrombophlebitis may be minimized by using dilute solutions of 2.5 to 5 mg/mL and rotating injection sites.

Stability: Store intact containers at controlled room temperature. Reconstituted solutions are stable for 14 days under refrigeration and room temperature. Little loss occurs when frozen at –20 °C for up to 12 weeks. Thawed premixed solutions are stable for 72 hours at room temperature and 30 days refrigerated. No sorption to plastic IV bags, syringes, or filters has been noted.

Compatibility Table

Solutions	Compatible	Incompatible	Variable
Dextrose 5 & 10%	●	...	...
Dextrose 5% in Ringer's injection, lactated	●	...	...
Dextrose 5% in sodium chloride 0.9%	●	...	...
Ringer's injection, lactated	●	...	...
Sodium chloride 0.9%	●	...	...

Drugs	Compatible	Incompatible	Variable
Acyclovir sodium	●	...	...
Albumin	...	●	...
Aldesleukin	●	...	...
Allopurinol sodium	●	...	...
Amifostine	●	...	...
Amikacin sulfate	●	...	...
Aminophylline	...	...	●
Amiodarone HCl	●	...	...
Amobarbital sodium	...	●	...
Amphotericin B cholesteryl sulfate complex	...	●	...
Ampicillin sodium	...	...	●
Ampicillin sod.–sulbactam sod.	...	...	●
Atracurium besylate	●	...	...
Aztreonam	...	...	●
Bivalirudin	...	●	...
Caffeine citrate	●	...	...
Calcium gluconate	●	...	...
Cefazolin sodium	...	...	●
Cefepime HCl	...	...	●
Cefotaxime sodium	...	...	●
Cefotetan disodium	...	...	●
Cefoxitin sodium	...	...	●
Ceftazidime	...	...	●
Ceftizoxime sodium	...	...	●
Ceftriaxone sodium	...	...	●
Cefuroxime sodium	...	...	●
Chloramphenicol sodium succinate	...	●	...
Chlorothiazide sodium	...	●	...
Cimetidine HCl	●	...	...
Cisatracurium besylate	●	...	...
Corticotropin	●	...	...
Cyclophosphamide	●	...	...
Dexamethasone sodium phosphate ...	...	●	...
Dexmedetomidine HCl	●	...	...
Diltiazem HCl	●	...	...
Dimenhydrinate	...	...	●
Docetaxel	●	...	...
Doxapram HCl	●	...	...
Doxorubicin HCl liposome injection	●	...	...

Drugs	Compatible	Incompatible	Variable
Drotrecogin alfa (activated)	...	●	...
Enalaprilat	●	...	...
Esmolol HCl	●	...	...
Etoposide phosphate	●	...	...
Famotidine	●	...	...
Fenoldopam mesylate	●	...	...
Filgrastim	●	...	...
Fluconazole	●	...	...
Fludarabine phosphate	●	...	...
Foscarnet sodium	...	...	●
Gallium nitrate	●	...	...
Gemcitabine HCl	●	...	...
Granisetron HCl	●	...	...
Heparin sodium	...	...	●
Hextend	●	...	...
Hydrocortisone sodium succinate	...	...	●
Hydromorphone HCl	●	...	...
Idarubicin HCl	...	●	...
Insulin, regular	●	...	...
Labetalol HCl	●	...	...
Lansoprazole	...	●	...
Levofloxacin	●	...	...
Linezolid	●	...	...
Lorazepam	●	...	...
Magnesium sulfate	●	...	...
Melphalan HCl	●	...	...
Meperidine HCl	●	...	...
Meropenem	●	...	...
Methotrexate sodium	●	...	...
Midazolam HCl	●	...	...
Milrinone lactate	●	...	...
Morphine sulfate	●	...	...
Nafcillin sodium	...	...	●
Nicardipine HCl	●	...	...
Ondansetron HCl	●	...	...
Paclitaxel	●	...	...
Pancuronium bromide	●	...	...
Pantoprazole sodium	●	...	...
Pemetrexed disodium	●	...	...
Penicillin G potassium	...	●	...

Drugs	Compatible	Incompatible	Variable
Pentobarbital sodium	...	●	...
Phenobarbital sodium	...	●	...
Phenytoin sodium	...	●	...
Piperacillin sodium	...	...	●
Piperacillin sod.–tazobactam sod.	...	...	●
Potassium chloride	●	...	...
Propofol	●	...	...
Ranitidine HCl	●	...	...
Remifentanil HCl	●	...	...
Sargramostim	...	...	●
Sodium bicarbonate	...	...	●
Tacrolimus	●	...	...
Teniposide	●	...	...
Theophylline	●	...	...
Thiotepa	●	...	...
Ticarcillin disod.–clavulanate pot.	...	...	●
Vecuronium bromide	●	...	...
Verapamil HCl	●	...	...
Vinorelbine tartrate	●	...	...
Warfarin sodium	...	...	●
Zidovudine	●	...	...

Vancomycin Hydrochloride

Vecuronium Bromide

Handbook on Injectable Drugs pp. 1611–1614.

Description: A synthetic, nondepolarizing, neuromuscular blocking agent.

Products: Norcuron; 10- and 20-mg vials. *pH:* Approximately 4.

Preparation: Reconstitute the 10- and 20-mg vials with 10 and 20 mL, respectively, of the accompanying bacteriostatic water for injection or sterile water for injection to yield a 1-mg/mL solution. The bacteriostatic water for injection is not for use in newborns. For IV infusion, add to a compatible diluent to yield a 0.1 to 0.2-mg/mL solution.

Administration: Administer by rapid IV injection or IV infusion using an infusion control device after dilution to a concentration of 0.1 to 0.2 mg/mL.

Stability: Store intact containers at room temperature protected from light. When reconstituted with bacteriostatic water for injection, the drug is stable for up to five days at room temperature or under refrigeration. When reconstituted with sterile water for injection, the drug should be used within 24 hours.

Vecuronium bromide is unstable with alkaline drugs.

Compatibility Table

Solutions	Compatible	Incompatible	Variable
Dextrose 5%	●	...	...
Dextrose 5% in sodium chloride 0.9%	●	...	...
Ringer's injection, lactated	●	...	...
Sodium chloride 0.9%	●	...	...

Drugs	Compatible	Incompatible	Variable
Aminophylline	●	...	...
Amiodarone HCl	●	...	...
Amphotericin B cholesteryl sulfate complex	...	●	...
Cefazolin sodium	●	...	...

Drugs	Compatible	Incompatible	Variable
Cefuroxime sodium	●	...	...
Cimetidine HCl	●	...	...
Ciprofloxacin	●	...	...
Diazepam	...	●	...
Diltiazem HCl	●	...	...
Dobutamine HCl	●	...	...
Dopamine HCl	●	...	...
Epinephrine HCl	●	...	...
Esmolol HCl	●	...	...
Etomidate	...	●	...
Fenoldopam mesylate	●	...	...
Fentanyl citrate	●	...	...
Fluconazole	●	...	...
Furosemide	...	●	...
Gentamicin sulfate	●	...	...
Heparin sodium	●	...	...
Hextend	●	...	...
Hydrocortisone sodium succinate	●	...	...
Hydromorphone HCl	●	...	...
Isoproterenol HCl	●	...	...
Labetalol HCl	●	...	...
Linezolid	●	...	...
Lorazepam	●	...	...
Midazolam HCl	●	...	...
Milrinone lactate	●	...	...
Morphine sulfate	●	...	...
Nicardipine HCl	●	...	...
Nitroglycerin	●	...	...
Norepinephrine bitartrate	●	...	...
Pantoprazole sodium	...	●	...
Propofol	●	...	...
Ranitidine HCl	●	...	...
Sodium nitroprusside	●	...	...
Thiopental sodium	...	●	...
Trimethoprim–sulfamethoxazole	●	...	...
Vancomycin HCl	●	...	...

Verapamil Hydrochloride

Handbook on Injectable Drugs pp. 1614–1620.

Description: An antiarrhythmic drug which acts as a slow-channel inhibitor of calcium ions.

Products: **Isoptin**; 2.5-mg/mL in 2- and 4-mL sizes. *pH:* From 4 to 6.5.

Administration: Administer slowly IV. Direct IV injection should be performed over at least two to three minutes. IV infusion has also been performed.

Stability: Store at room temperature and protect from light and freezing. It is physically compatible over a pH range of 3 to 6 but may precipitate at pH greater than 6. No sorption to glass, PVC, or polyolefin containers has been noted.

Compatibility Table

Solutions	Compatible	Incompatible	Variable
Dextrose 5%	●	...	...
Dextrose 5% in Ringer's injection	●	...	...
Dextrose 5% in Ringer's injection, lactated	●	...	...
Ringer's injection	●	...	...
Ringer's injection, lactated	●	...	...
Sodium chloride 0.45 & 0.9%	●	...	...

Drugs	Compatible	Incompatible	Variable
Albumin	...	●	...
Amikacin sulfate	●	...	...
Aminophylline	...	...	●
Amiodarone HCl	●	...	...
Amphotericin B	...	●	...
Amphotericin B cholesteryl sulfate complex	...	●	...
Ampicillin sodium	...	...	●
Argatroban	●	...	...
Ascorbic acid injection	●	...	...

Drugs	Compatible	Incompatible	Variable
Atropine sulfate	●	...	...
Bivalirudin	●	...	...
Calcium chloride	●	...	...
Calcium gluconate	●	...	...
Cefamandole nafate	●	...	...
Cefazolin sodium	●	...	...
Cefotaxime sodium	●	...	...
Cefoxitin sodium	●	...	...
Chloramphenicol sodium succinate	●	...	...
Cimetidine HCl	●	...	...
Ciprofloxacin	●	...	...
Clindamycin phosphate	●	...	...
Dexamethasone sodium phosphate	●	...	...
Dexmedetomidine HCl	●	...	...
Diazepam	●	...	...
Digoxin	●	...	...
Dimenhydrinate	●	...	...
Dobutamine HCl	...	...	●
Dopamine HCl	●	...	...
Epinephrine HCl	●	...	...
Erythromycin lactobionate	●	...	...
Famotidine	●	...	...
Fenoldopam mesylate	●	...	...
Furosemide	...	...	●
Gentamicin sulfate	●	...	...
Heparin sodium	●	...	...
Hextend	●	...	...
Hydralazine HCl	...	...	●
Hydrocortisone sodium phosphate	●	...	...
Hydrocortisone sodium succinate	●	...	...
Hydromorphone HCl	●	...	...
Insulin, regular	●	...	...
Isoproterenol HCl	●	...	...
Lansoprazole	...	●	...
Lidocaine HCl	●	...	...
Linezolid	●	...	...
Magnesium sulfate	●	...	...
Mannitol	●	...	...
Meperidine HCl	●	...	...

Drugs	Compatible	Incompatible	Variable
Methyldopate HCl	●	...	...
Methylprednisolone sod. succ.	●	...	...
Metoclopramide HCl	●	...	...
Milrinone lactate	●	...	...
Morphine sulfate	●	...	...
Multivitamins	●	...	...
Nafcillin sodium	...	...	●
Naloxone HCl......................	●	...	...
Nitroglycerin	●	...	...
Norepinephrine bitartrate	●	...	...
Oxacillin sodium	...	...	●
Oxaliplatin	●	...	...
Oxytocin	●	...	...
Pancuronium bromide	●	...	...
Pantoprazole sodium	...	●	...
Penicillin G potassium	●	...	...
Penicillin G sodium	●	...	...
Pentobarbital sodium	●	...	...
Phenobarbital sodium	●	...	...
Phenytoin sodium	●	...	...
Piperacillin sodium	●	...	...
Potassium chloride	●	...	...
Potassium phosphates	●	...	...
Procainamide HCl	●	...	...
Propofol	...	●	...
Propranolol HCl	●	...	...
Protamine sulfate	●	...	...
Quinidine gluconate	●	...	...
Sodium bicarbonate................	...	...	●
Sodium nitroprusside	●	...	...
Theophylline	●	...	...
Tobramycin sulfate	●	...	...
Trimethoprim–sulfamethoxazole	...	●	...
Vancomycin HCl	●	...	...
Vasopressin	●	...	...

Vinorelbine Tartrate

Handbook on Injectable Drugs pp. 1634–1641.

Description: A semisynthetic vinca alkaloid antineoplastic agent.

Products: **Navelbine;** 10 mg/mL in 1- and 5-mL single-use vials.
pH: Approximately 3.5.

Preparation: The product must be diluted for use. The product may be diluted to 1.5 to 3 mg/mL for injection by syringe or 0.5 to 2 mg/mL for administration from a minibag into the side port of a free-flowing infusion solution.

Administration: Administer IV from a syringe or minibag over six to 10 minutes into the side port of a free-flowing infusion solution. After administration, flush with 75 to 125 mL of solution. Avoid extravasation because of possible tissue irritation, necrosis, and thrombophlebitis.

Individual doses should be labeled with this statement:
Warning: Navelbine for intravenous use only.
Fatal if given intrathecally.

Stability: Intact vials of the colorless to pale yellow clear solution should be stored under refrigeration and protected from light and freezing. Intact vials are stable for 72 hours at room temperature. Diluted solutions are stable for 24 hours at room and refrigerator temperatures. No vinorelbine loss due to sorption to PVC plastic has been found.

Compatibility Table

Solutions	Compatible	Incompatible	Variable
Dextrose 5%	●	...	...
Dextrose 5% in sodium chloride 0.45%	●	...	...
Ringer's injection	●	...	...
Ringer's injection, lactated	●	...	...
Sodium chloride 0.45 & 0.9%	●	...	...

Drugs	Compatible	Incompatible	Variable
Acyclovir sodium	...	●	...
Allopurinol sodium	...	●	...
Amikacin sulfate	●	...	...
Aminophylline	...	●	...
Amphotericin B	...	●	...
Amphotericin B cholesteryl sulfate complex	...	●	...
Ampicillin sodium	...	●	...
Aztreonam	●	...	...
Bleomycin sulfate	●	...	...
Bumetanide	●	...	...
Buprenorphine HCl	●	...	...
Butorphanol tartrate	●	...	...
Calcium gluconate	●	...	...
Carboplatin	●	...	...
Carmustine	●	...	...
Cefazolin sodium	...	●	...
Cefotaxime sodium	●	...	...
Cefotetan disodium	...	●	...
Ceftazidime	●	...	...
Ceftizoxime sodium	●	...	...
Ceftriaxone sodium	...	●	...
Cefuroxime sodium	...	●	...
Chlorpromazine HCl	●	...	...
Cimetidine HCl	●	...	...
Ciprofloxacin	●	...	...
Cisplatin	●	...	...
Clindamycin phosphate	●	...	...
Cyclophosphamide	●	...	...
Cytarabine	●	...	...
Dacarbazine	●	...	...
Dactinomycin	●	...	...
Daunorubicin HCl	●	...	...
Dexamethasone sodium phosphate ...	●	...	...
Diphenhydramine HCl	●	...	...
Doxorubicin HCl	●	...	...
Doxorubicin HCl liposome injection	●	...	...
Doxycycline hyclate	●	...	...
Droperidol	●	...	...

Drugs	Compatible	Incompatible	Variable
Enalaprilat	●	…	…
Etoposide	●	…	…
Famotidine	●	…	…
Filgrastim	●	…	…
Floxuridine	●	…	…
Fluconazole	●	…	…
Fludarabine phosphate	●	…	…
Fluorouracil	…	●	…
Furosemide	…	●	…
Gallium nitrate	●	…	…
Ganciclovir sodium	…	●	…
Gemcitabine HCl	●	…	…
Gentamicin sulfate	●	…	…
Haloperidol lactate	●	…	…
Heparin sodium	…	…	●
Hydrocortisone sodium phosphate	●	…	…
Hydrocortisone sodium succinate	●	…	…
Hydromorphone HCl	●	…	…
Hydroxyzine HCl	●	…	…
Idarubicin HCl	●	…	…
Ifosfamide	●	…	…
Imipenem–cilastatin sodium	●	…	…
Lansoprazole	…	●	…
Lorazepam	●	…	…
Mannitol	●	…	…
Mechlorethamine HCl	●	…	…
Melphalan HCl	●	…	…
Meperidine HCl	●	…	…
Mesna	●	…	…
Methotrexate sodium	●	…	…
Methylprednisolone sod. succ.	…	●	…
Metoclopramide HCl	●	…	…
Metronidazole	●	…	…
Minocycline HCl	●	…	…
Mitomycin	…	●	…
Mitoxantrone HCl	●	…	…
Morphine sulfate	●	…	…
Nalbuphine HCl	●	…	…
Ondansetron HCl	●	…	…
Oxaliplatin	●	…	…

Drugs	Compatible	Incompatible	Variable
Piperacillin sodium	...	●	...
Potassium chloride	●	...	...
Prochlorperazine edisylate	●	...	...
Promethazine HCl	●	...	...
Ranitidine HCl	●	...	...
Sodium bicarbonate	...	●	...
Streptozocin	●	...	...
Teniposide	●	...	...
Thiotepa	...	●	...
Ticarcillin disod.–clavulanate pot.	●	...	...
Tobramycin sulfate	●	...	...
Trimethoprim–sulfamethoxazole	...	●	...
Vancomycin HCl	●	...	...
Vinblastine sulfate	●	...	...
Vincristine sulfate	●	...	...
Zidovudine	●	...	...

Zidovudine

Handbook on Injectable Drugs pp. 1647–1652.

Description: A synthetic nucleoside antiviral agent.

Products: Retrovir; 10 mg/mL in 20-mL single-use vials. *pH:* Approximately 5.5.

Preparation: Dilute in dextrose 5% to a concentration no greater than 4 mg/mL.

Administration: Administer by IV infusion at a constant rate over one hour or as a continuous IV infusion. Avoid IM injection, IV bolus, and rapid IV infusion.

Stability: Intact vials of zidovudine should be stored at controlled room temperature and protected from light.

Compatibility Table

Solutions	Compatible	Incompatible	Variable
Dextrose 5%	●	…	…
Sodium chloride 0.9%	●	…	…

Drugs	Compatible	Incompatible	Variable
Acyclovir sodium	●	…	…
Allopurinol sodium	●	…	…
Amifostine	●	…	…
Amikacin sulfate	●	…	…
Amphotericin B	●	…	…
Amphotericin B cholesteryl sulfate complex	●	…	…
Aztreonam	●	…	…
Cefepime HCl	●	…	…
Ceftazidime	●	…	…
Ceftriaxone sodium	●	…	…
Cimetidine HCl	●	…	…
Cisatracurium besylate	●	…	…
Clindamycin phosphate	●	…	…
Dexamethasone sodium phosphate	●	…	…
Dobutamine HCl	●	…	…
Docetaxel	●	…	…
Dopamine HCl	●	…	…
Doxorubicin HCl liposome injection	●	…	…
Erythromycin lactobionate	●	…	…

Drugs	Compatible	Incompatible	Variable
Etoposide phosphate	●	...	...
Filgrastim	●	...	...
Fluconazole	●	...	...
Fludarabine phosphate	●	...	...
Gemcitabine HCl	●	...	...
Gentamicin sulfate	●	...	...
Granisetron HCl	●	...	...
Heparin sodium	●	...	...
Imipenem–cilastatin sodium	●	...	...
Lansoprazole	...	●	...
Linezolid	●	...	...
Lorazepam	●	...	...
Melphalan HCl	●	...	...
Meropenem	...	...	●
Metoclopramide HCl	●	...	...
Morphine sulfate	●	...	...
Nafcillin sodium	●	...	...
Ondansetron HCl	●	...	...
Oxacillin sodium	●	...	...
Oxytocin	●	...	...
Paclitaxel	●	...	...
Pantoprazole sodium	●	...	...
Pemetrexed disodium	●	...	...
Pentamidine isethionate	●	...	...
Phenylephrine HCl	●	...	...
Piperacillin sodium	●	...	...
Piperacillin sod.–tazobactam sod.	●	...	...
Potassium chloride	●	...	...
Ranitidine HCl	●	...	...
Remifentanil HCl	●	...	...
Sargramostim	●	...	...
Teniposide	●	...	...
Thiotepa	●	...	...
Tobramycin sulfate	●	...	...
Trimethoprim–sulfamethoxazole	●	...	...
Trimetrexate glucuronate	●	...	...
Vancomycin HCl	●	...	...
Vinorelbine tartrate	●	...	...

Index